CITY COLLEGE LIBRARY
1825 MAY ST.
BROWNSVILLE, TEXAS 78520

W9-ASR-464

Perinatal medicine
review and comments

VOLUME TWO

Perinatal medicine
review and comments

Edited by

FREDERICK C. BATTAGLIA, M.D.

Professor and Chairman, Department of Pediatrics,
University of Colorado Medical Center,
Denver, Colorado

DWAIN D. HAGERMAN, M.D.

Professor, Department of Biochemistry and
Department of Obstetrics and Gynecology,
University of Colorado Medical Center,
Denver, Colorado

GIACOMO MESCHIA, M.D.

Professor, Department of Physiology,
University of Colorado Medical Center,
Denver, Colorado

E. J. QUILLIGAN, M.D.

Professor and Chairman, Department of Obstetrics
and Gynecology, University of Southern
California School of Medicine,
Los Angeles, California

with 118 *illustrations*

The C. V. Mosby Company

Saint Louis 1978

CITY COLLEGE LIBRARY
1825 MAY ST.
BROWNSVILLE, TEXAS 78520

VOLUME TWO

Copyright © 1978 by The C. V. Mosby Company

All rights reserved. No part of this book may be reproduced
in any manner without written permission of the publisher.

Volume one copyrighted 1976

Printed in the United States of America

Distributed in Great Britain by Henry Kimpton, London

The C. V. Mosby Company
11830 Westline Industrial Drive, St. Louis, Missouri 63141

Library of Congress Cataloging in Publication Data (Revised)

Main entry under title:

Perinatal medicine.

   Includes bibliographical references and index.
    1. Fetus—Physiology—Abstracts. 2. Fetus—
Diseases—Abstracts. 3. Infants (Newborn)—Physi-
ology—Abstracts. 4. Infants (Newborn)—Dis-
eases—Abstracts. 5. Pregnancy, Complications
of—Abstracts. I. Battaglia, Frederick C.
II. Meschia, Giacomo. III. Quilligan, Edward J.
[DNLM: 1. Fetal diseases—Collected works.
2. Infant, Newborn, Diseases—Collected works.
3. Fetus—Collected works. 4. Infant, Newborn—
Collected works. WQ210 P4422]
RG600.P416   618.3′2   76-4845
ISBN 0-8016-0513-X

CB/CB/B 9 8 7 6 5 4 3 2 1

Preface

Volume two of *Perinatal Medicine: Review and Comments* covers the literature for 1975 and 1976. In the preface to the first volume we stated that it was aimed at residents and postdoctoral fellows in subspecialty training, as well as those physicians interested in keeping current with the scientific basis of perinatal medicine. With these objectives in mind, we have continued to review the literature, searching primarily for those scientific developments which point the way to significant contributions in clinical medicine or provide new insights into perinatal biology. An attempt has been made to provide a conceptual basis and a critical evaluation for the developments presented in the literature. However, no attempt has been made to review clinical management in obstetrics or pediatrics, since many current publications provide extensive reviews of these areas. A stronger scientific basis for perinatal medicine is being established each year, and our intent is to bring significant developments to the attention of obstetricians and pediatricians.

Frederick C. Battaglia
Dwain D. Hagerman
Giacomo Meschia
E. J. Quilligan

Contents

8 *Immunology,* 134

9 *Parturition,* 139

Perinatal medicine
review and comments

CHAPTER 1

Fetal and neonatal metabolism

Amino acid transport

■ Guidotti, G. G., Gazzola, G. C., Borghetti, A. F., and Franchi-Gazzola, R.: Adaptive regulation of amino acid transport across the cell membrane in avian and mammalian tissues, Biochim. Biophys. Acta **406:**264-279, 1975.

An adaptive transport mechanism for certain amino acids is described. Apparently, this mechanism is controlled by alterations of transport activity by means of amino acid substrates of the transport system. The amino acids may regulate the synthesis of one or more proteins involved in the transport process. A variety of tissues were examined for the presence of this transport mechanism. Only the transport system that acted on α-aminoisobutyric acid (AIB), proline, glycine, alanine, and serine (the A amino transport system) is responsive to regulation. In chick embryo corneal fibroblast, for example, the transport of sensitive substrates is increased 119% to 366% by a 2-hour exposure to the amino acid before measuring transport kinetics. The sensitive A transport system is found in many mesenchymal cells, including fibroblasts, chondroblasts, osteoblasts, and myoblasts, and in the epithelial cells from embryonal crystalline lens. Adaptive control of transport in other cells, such as macrophages and thymic lymphocytes, is restricted to a smaller number of amino acids (α-aminoisobutyrate, proline, and glycine). It is of special interest that the sensitive A transport system is present in cells from the immature rat uterus. The adaptive regulation mechanism is absent from erythrocytes and adult epithelial tissues.

■ Enders, R. H., Judd, R. M., Donohue, T. M., and Smith, C. H.: Placental amino acid uptake. III. Transport systems for neutral amino acids, Am. J. Physiol. **230:**706-710, 1976.

This study characterizes the amino acid transport systems in human placental tissue in vitro. Using competitive inhibition techniques to characterize the specificity of the principal placental amino acid transport system, the investigators were able to demonstrate three transport systems with somewhat overlapping specificity. These correspond to the A, L, and ASC systems of Christensen and associates. The A system includes α-aminoisobutyric acid, glycine, proline, N-methylalanine, serine, threonine, and glutamine; the L sysetm includes isoleucine, valine, phenylalanine, BCH, alanine, serine, threonine, and glutamine; and the ASC system includes alanine, serine, threonine, and glutamine. The study further demonstrated that the facilitation phenomenon for amino acid transport following preincubation in amino acid–free solutions was confined to the A system. Fig. 1-1 from the article demonstrates that alanine, α-aminoisobutyric acid, and glycine responded to preincubation with an increased intracellular/extracellular concentration ratio in amino acid–free solutions, compared with control tissues not subject to a preincubation phase.

■ Gusseck, D. J., Yuen, P., and Longo, L. D.: Amino acid transport in placental slices: mechanism of increased accumulation by prolonged incubation, Biochim. Biophys. Acta **401:**278-284, 1975.

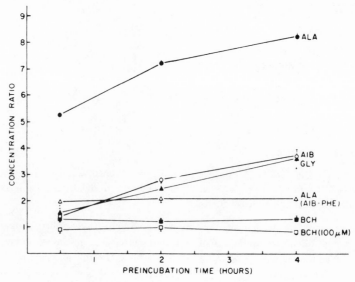

FIG. 1-1

Effects of preincubation on uptake of various amino acid substrates. Placental tissue was preincubated in a 250 ml Erlenmeyer flask containing a balanced salts-glucose medium. Tissue was transferred at three time intervals to 50 ml Erlenmeyer flasks for incubation with an amino acid substrate. *Abscissa,* length of preincubation period before incubation with substrate. *Ordinate,* concentration ratio attained in 8-minute incubation period. Lines are labeled with substrate used. Alanine uptake was measured uninhibited and in the presence of AIB-phenylalanine as inhibitors. Except when indicated, substrate concentrations were 10 μmolar. Only the NMA-inhibitable system responds to a preincubation period. (From Enders, R. H., Judd, R. M., Donohue, T. M., and Smith, C. H.: Placental amino acid uptake. III. Transport systems for neutral amino acids, Am. J. Physiol. **230:**706-710, 1976.)

This study presents additional data on the facilitation of amino acid transport into placental tissue in vitro when the placental tissue is preincubated in an amino acid–free solution. It confirmed the observation of Smith et al. (Placental amino acid uptake: tissue preparation, kinetics, and preincubation effect, Am. J. Physiol. **224:**558-564, 1973) that the facilitation of amino acid transport by preincubation in an amino acid–free medium is associated with an increased V_{max} and a decreased K_m. The increase in V_{max} with preincubation suggests synthesis of an increased number of carrier proteins. Fig. 1-2 demonstrates that incubation with inhibitors of protein synthesis blocks the facilitation phenomenon, thus supporting the hypothesis that the facilitation phenomenon is associated with the synthesis of an increased number of carrier proteins.

COMMENT: The three articles by Guidotti et al., Gusseck et al., and Enders et al. confirm the fact that a very different rate of amino acid transport into some tissues in vitro can be obtained by the conditions under which each tissue is preincubated. When placental tissue is incubated in amino acid–free solutions, a much higher rate of transport is obtained. The facilitation, or "adaptive," phenomenon has been demonstrated in a wide variety of embryonic and fetal tissues and serves to emphasize that in vitro conditions under which tissues are studied may alter markedly the determinations of transport capacity for those tissues. This has particular significance in studies with fetal and embryonic tissues, since the concen-

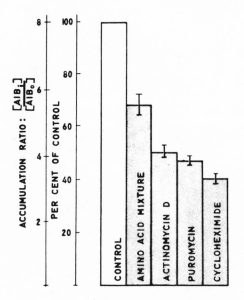

FIG. 1-2
Influence of inhibitors of protein synthesis and an amino acid mixture on the AIB accumulation
ratios after 1 hour. Placental slices were preincubated for 2 hours in the presence of
cycloheximide (0.1 mmolar), puromycin (0.1 mmolar), actinomycin D (1 mmolar), an
amino acid mixture (0.1 mmolar in each of the nineteen common amino acids, excluding
asparagine and glutamine), or no inhibitor. At the end of the preincubation period, the slices
were blotted and transferred to a flask containing 0.1 mmol α-aminoiso(^{14}C)butyrate
for a 1-hour incubation at 37° C. Each value represents the average of 6 measurements on
each of three placentas ± SEM. (From Gusseck, D. J., Yuen, P., and Longo, L. D.: Amino
acid transport in placental slices: mechanism of increased accumulation by prolonged
incubation, Biochim. Biophys. Acta **401:**278-284, 1975.)

trations of a variety of solutes in both fetal and embryonic extracellular fluids are very different from those found in postnatal life. For example, studies in vitro comparing liver tissue
from fetuses with liver tissue from adults and in which the incubation medium contains
solutes in concentrations perhaps more appropriate to adult rather than fetal interstitial
fluid may not be giving us information that can be easily extrapolated to in vivo conditions. The study of Guidotti et al. is more comprehensive than the other two studies in
searching for a common denominator among those developing tissues which exhibit this phenomenon.

Gluconeogenesis in the newborn period

■ Arinze, I. J.: On the development of phosphoenolpyruvate carboxykinase and gluconeogenesis in guinea pig liver, Biochem. Biophys. Res. Commun. **65:**184-189, 1975.

The activity of phosphoenolpyruvate carboxykinase (PEPCK) was measured in fetal
guinea pig liver. The fetal liver tissue was obtained from pregnant guinea pigs 2 to 5 days
prior to delivery. The fetuses were removed by cesarean section and the livers removed from
the animals and perfused in vitro with a nonrecirculating system. The study demonstrated
that PEPCK activity in the cytosol fraction of fetal liver tissue is virtually zero prior to
delivery and increases rapidly in the immediate neonatal period.

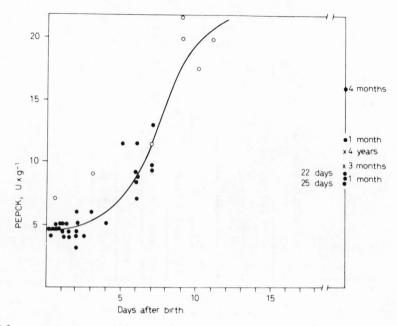

FIG. 1-3

Development of PEPCK activity as a function of age after birth. ●, Premature; ○, full term; and ×, biopsies. (From Marsac, C., Saundubray, J. M., Moncion, A., and Leroux, J. P.: Development of gluconeogenic enzymes in the liver of human newborns, Biol. Neonate 28: 317-325, 1976; S. Karger AG, Basel.)

■ Robinson, B. H.: Development of gluconeogenic enzymes in the newborn guinea pig, Biol. Neonate **29:**48-55, 1976.

This study measured some gluconeogenic enzymes in liver tissue of newborn guinea pigs delivered vaginally at term. Several of the enzymes including glucose-6-phosphatase and fructose-1,6-diphosphatase did not change significantly in the immediate postnatal period (the first 72 hours of postnatal life). Both pyruvate carboxylase in the mitochondria and PEPCK in the cytosol increased significantly in the first 24 hours of life. The study showed that there was rapid depletion of liver glycogen in guinea pigs even though the animals did not become hypoglycemic after birth. The rapid fall in liver glycogen in the immediate postnatal period is similar to that seen with many other mammalian species.

■ Marsac, C., Saundubray, J. M., Moncion, A., and Leroux, J. P.: Development of gluconeogenic enzymes in the liver of human newborns, Biol. Neonate **28:**317-325, 1976.

The activity of three enzymes—fructose diphosphatase, pyruvate carboxylase, and PEPCK were determined on liver tissue obtained in infants of a variety of postnatal ages. Forty-one samples were obtained after death in infants and children and four tissue samples were obtained from living children by needle biopsy of the liver carried out for diagnostic purposes. All three enzymes showed an increase in activity expressed per gram of wet weight of tissue. Fig. 1-3 from their report shows the rather striking increase in PEPCK activity per unit of wet weight of tissue in the first 2 weeks of life.

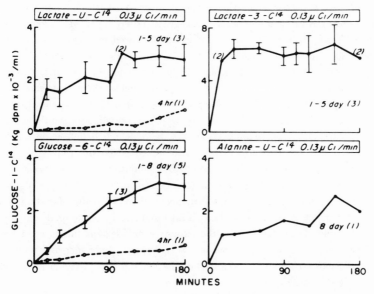

FIG. 1-4

Incorporation of ^{14}C substrates into l-^{14}C-glucose (mean ± SEM). Number of pups in each group is indicated by the number in parentheses after the age range. (From Adam, P. A. J., Glazer, G., and Rogoff, F.: Glucose production in the newborn dog. I. Effects of glucagon in vivo, Pediatr. Res. 9:816-820, 1975.)

■ Adam, P. A. J., Glazer, G., and Rogoff, F.: Glucose production in the newborn dog. I. Effects of glucagon in vivo, Pediatr. Res. 9:816-820, 1975.

This study attempts to determine a glucose production rate and glucose turnover rate by the simultaneous infusion of 1-^{14}C-glucose and 2-^{3}H-glucose into newborn puppies. Glucose production rate in the absence of glucagon averaged 55 μmol/min/kg, or approximately 5.5 mg/kg/min. The glucose production rate was increased 81 μmol/min/kg during a glucagon infusion. The glucose production rate estimated with 1-^{14}C-glucose was consistently less than that estimated with ^{3}H tracer, averaging 88% in the control period and 77% of the ^{3}H estimate during glucagon infusion. Additional evidence for gluconeogenesis other than the discrepancy between [14]C- and ^{3}H-glucose was obtained by the infusion of ^{14}C-labeled lactate and alanine. There was significant incorporation of radioactivity into 1-^{14}C-glucose with the infusion of ^{14}C-lactate and alanine. These data are presented in Fig. 1-4 and demonstrate that both ^{14}C-lactate and ^{14}C-alanine were incorporated in significant quantities into 1-^{14}C-glucose. The rate did not differ between 1 and 8 days postnatal age; however, there did seem to be significantly lower incorporation of these substrates into glucose when the puppies were studied 4 hours after birth.

■ Girard, J. R., Guillet, I., Marty, J., and Marliss, E. B.: Plasma amino acid levels and development of hepatic gluconeogenesis in the newborn rat, Am. J. Physiol. 229:466-473, 1975.

Numerous studies have demonstrated no evidence of gluconeogenesis in fetal rat liver in contrast to studies in many other mammalian species, in which gluconeogenesis and gluconeogenic pathways can be demonstrated in fetal liver. This study compares the postnatal changes in some substrates, including gluconeogenic amino acids, in newborn rats that are fasted for 16 hours versus a similar group that are allowed to suckle. In addition, labeled gluconeogenic substrates—including ^{14}C-labeled lactate, alanine, serine, and glutamine—were injected intraperitoneally into both groups of animals and the conversion to ^{14}C-glucose studied. In contrast to newborn animals permitted to suckle, those that were fasted for 16 hours showed a fall in concentration of most of the amino acids. Two conspicuous exceptions to this were lysine and taurine, both of which increased significantly. In all animals the hepatic accumulation of ^{14}C-aminoisobutyric acid, which had been injected intraperitoneally, showed a progressive rise after birth. Gluconeogenesis from labeled precursors (lactate, alanine, serine, and glutamine) could be demonstrated in all animals both fasted and suckled. In the fasted animals the in vivo conversion of labeled precursors increased during the first 6 hours after birth and then declined by 16 hours of fasting. In contrast, the in vitro conversion increased with time in all instances. Fasted animals developed a profound hypoglycemia. From these data, the authors conclude that the entry of amino acids into liver and the potential for gluconeogenesis in newborn liver increases with time. They suggest that the most probable explanation for the marked hypoglycemia in the fasted newborn rat is an inadequate supply of gluconeogenic substrates.

COMMENT: **The first three reports by Arinze, Robinson, and Marsac et al. describe changes in enzyme activity in liver tissue of newborn guinea pigs and newborn infants. It is always difficult to interpret changes in enzyme activity as reflecting changes in various metabolic pathways, providing ultimately for fuel and growth needs to the various organs of the newborn infants. In vitro enzyme activity measurements determine the maximal capability of various metabolic pathways. They do not define the degree to which pathways are used under in vivo conditions. In cerebral metabolism, for example, it has been found that an increased uptake of keto acids by the brain can be demonstrated considerably before changes in the various enzyme activities related to keto-acid utilization can be shown. In considering the capability for gluconeogenesis, ultimately one needs direct measurements of the quantity of new glucose produced from other carbon sources over a given period of time; such measurements should relate glucose production to the fuel and growth requirements of the organisms to decide whether significant gluconeogenesis is occurring at a particular stage in development.**

The changes described by Arinze parallel those found in fetal rat liver tissue. However, in contrast to the rat, liver tissue from guinea pig fetuses had a high activity of PEPCK in the mitochondrial fraction; in fact, the activity was comparable to that found in adult guinea pig tissue. Furthermore, as shown in Fig. 1-5, when the fetal livers were perfused with pyruvate, lactate, or glycerol, a net production of glucose from these substrates could be demonstrated. This study, coupled with those of Jones and Ashton (The development of some enzymes of gluconeogenesis in the liver and kidney of the foetal guinea pig [abst.], Biochem. J. 130:23p-24p, 1972), clearly demonstrates that the guinea pig fetus has a capacity for gluconeogenesis prior to birth.

Robinson's study confirms Arinze's observations and clearly demonstrates the difference in enzyme activity changes after birth between one enzyme located in two different places in the cell; that is, PEPCK in the mitochondria was found to be at a high level immediately after birth and did not change significantly during the first 3 days of life. In contrast, PEPCK activity in the cytoplasm was very low at the time of birth and increased markedly

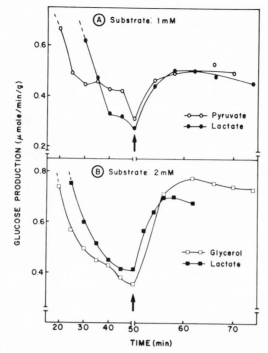

FIG. 1-5

Gluconeogenesis by isolated perfused livers from fetal guinea pigs. Livers were perfused in a nonrecirculating fashion with Krebs-Ringer bicarbonate buffer, pH 7.4, at 30° to 32° C. After a 50-minute washout to reduce the level of endogenous glucose release, the substrates were introduced into the perfusion system at the points indicated by the arrows and maintained at, **A,** 1 mmolar and, **B,** 2 mmolar. Each point in **A** represents results from three experiments. The glycerol and lactate curves in **B** were from five and four experiments, respectively. (From Arinze, I. J.: On the development of phosphoenolpyruvate carboxykinase and gluconeogenesis in guinea pig liver, Biochem. Biophys. Res. Commun. 65:184-189, 1975.)

during the first 24 hours of life. These changes are illustrated in Fig. 1-6 taken from Robinson's report. The author points out that the physiologic role of PEPCK in regulating the rate of postnatal gluconeogenesis is still not established. The study does show clearly that a rapid postnatal increase in cytosol PEPCK activity can occur in animals without any overt hypoglycemia.

In the Marsac et al. study all the material obtained in the immediate newborn period was obtained from postmortem tissue. The needle biopsies of the liver were carried out in older children. Furthermore, although the authors refer to the extensive work in rats describing a sharp postnatal increase in PEPCK activity, it might have been more appropriate to refer to the studies of Robinson in guinea pig liver. In that species and in man approximately one half of the PEPCK activity is in the mitochondria and half in the cytosol fraction.

In the study by Adam et al., glucose turnover rates in newborn dogs were estimated with 1-^{14}C-glucose and 2-^{3}H-glucose. They found, as has every other group of investigators, that the estimate of glucose turnover rate was higher when 2-^{3}H-glucose was used for the determination than those made with 1-^{14}C-glucose. This discrepancy between the turnover

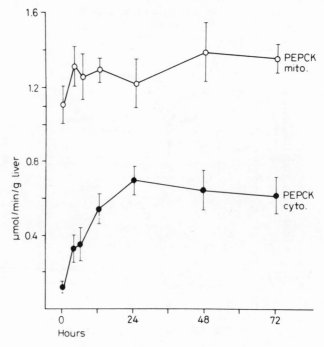

FIG. 1-6
Levels of cytosolic (●—●) and mitochondrial (O—O) PEPCK in liver of newborn guinea
pigs in the first 3 days of life. Values are the means ± SEM of determination on six or eight
animals. (From Robinson, B. H.: Development of gluconeogenic enzymes in the newborn
guinea pig, Biol. Neonate **29:**48-55, 1976; S. Karger AG, Basel.)

rates estimated with glucose labeled in positions 1 and 2 has been found in adult as well as
growing organisms. One cannot ascribe this discrepancy directly to gluconeogenesis, but the
higher rate with the 2-^{3}H-glucose does reflect significant recycling. More direct evidence
was provided by their infusions of ^{14}C-lactate and alanine, and those studies certainly do
demonstrate gluconeogenesis occurring in the newborn dog. However, the rates of glucose
production cannot be calculated from the data provided. There is no information regarding
the total carbon requirements of the newborn dog both for new tissue accretion and for carbon dioxide production. It would seem that such studies in gluconeogenesis could be placed
in better perspective if the quantity of new carbon produced as glucose was evaluated
against a background requirement of total carbon needs of the organism. The study by Girard
et al. points to the fact that inflow concentrations of substrates to the liver of the newborn
rat may be crucial in determining the rate of gluconeogenesis rather than changes in enzyme
activity or in amino acid transport across the liver. In this regard the importance of inflow
concentration of substrates in determining the rate of gluconeogenesis is similar to the
correlation observed in cerebral metabolism between arterial keto acid concentrations and
cerebral utilization rates.

Glycogen synthesis in fetal life

■ Sparks, J. W., Lynch, A., Chez, R. A., and Glinsmann W. H.: Glycogen regulation in
  isolated perfused near-term monkey liver, Pediatr. Res. **10:**51-56, 1976.

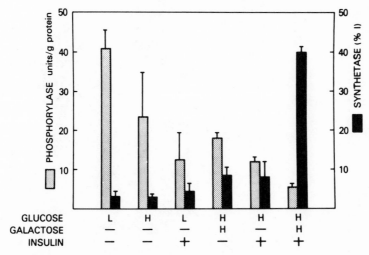

FIG. 1-7

Glycogen synthetase and phosphorylase activities with various combinations of glucose, galactose, and insulin in the perfusate. Values shown are means ± SEM of synthetase and phosphorylase activity after 30 minutes of perfusion under conditions shown. For comparison, animals are grouped by presence (+) or absence (−) of insulin, at 10^{-7} mol, and by glucose and galactose concentration. High concentrations, *H,* are between 275 and 400 mg/dl; lower concentrations, *L,* are between 100 and 250 mg/dl. (From Sparks, J. W., Lynch, A., Chez, R. A., and Glinsmann, W. H.: Glycogen regulation in isolated perfused near-term monkey liver, Pediatr. Res. **10:**51-56, 1976.)

Fetal rhesus monkeys with gestational ages between 144 and 152 days (term is approximately 164 days) were used in these studies. The umbilical vein of the fetal monkey was cannulated for inflow perfusion of the fetal liver and the inferior vena cava cannulated for collection of the perfusate and recirculation. The technique of liver perfusion was that described for perfusion of the adult rat liver (Buschiazzo et al.: Effects of glucose on glycogen synthetase, phosphorylase and glycogen deposition in the perfused rat liver, Proc. Natl. Acad. Sci. USA **65:**383-387, 1970). The perfusate varied in concentrations of glucose, galactose, and insulin in different experiments. Serial measurements were made of glucose and galactose concentration in the perfusate and of phosphorylase and glycogen synthetase activities in the liver at the conclusion of the perfusion. Fig. 1-7 from the report of Buschiazzo et al. demonstrates that phosphorylase activity was much higher when the perfusate contained a low glucose concentration and no galactose or insulin. Thus mobilization of liver glycogen was accelerated with these perfusate conditions. In contrast, glycogen synthetase activity, expressed as a percentage of synthetase in the form independent of glucose-6-phosphate, increased markedly when galactose and insulin were added to the perfusate in the presence of extremely high glucose concentration. Glycogen synthetase activity was not increased even in the presence of very high glucose concentrations when galactose and insulin were absent from the perfusate. The net uptake of carbon by the liver occurred only in the presence of galactose in the perfusate. This is illustrated in Fig. 1-8 taken from their report.

■ Randall, G. C. B., and L'Ecuyer, C.: Tissue glycogen and blood glucose and fructose levels in the pig fetus during the second half of gestation, Biol. Neonate **28:**74-82, 1976.

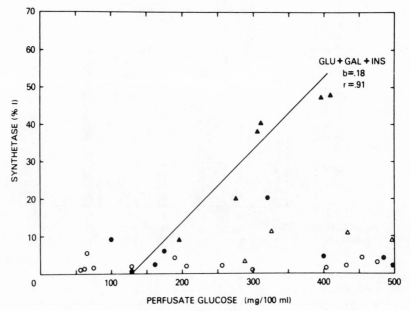

FIG. 1-8
Synthetase activities as a function of perfusate glucose concentration. Each point is the activity observed after 30 minutes of perfusion with glucose as shown. Circles represent perfusions with glucose added to perfusate with (●) and without (○) added insulin. Triangles represent perfusions with both glucose, *GLU,* and galactose, *GAL,* added to perfusate with (▲) and without (△) added insulin, *INS*. Regression line for combination of glucose, galactose, and insulin added to perfusate was calculated by the least squares method. (From Sparks, J. W., Lynch, A., Chez, R. A., and Glinsmann, W. H.: Glycogen regulation in isolated perfused near-term monkey liver, Pediatr. Res. **10**:51-56, 1976.)

This study presents the glucose and fructose concentrations in amniotic fluid, umbilical venous and arterial blood, and uterine arterial blood in fetuses of from 60 to 112 days' gestational age. In addition, tissue samples were taken at the time of acute severe infection from the cardiac ventricles, liver, muscles, lateral aspect of the thigh, lung, kidney, and placental tissue. All specimens were frozen immediately in liquid nitrogen. The samples were used for the measurement of tissue concentrations of glycogen. Fig. 1-9 taken from this report presents the changes in fetal tissue glycogen concentrations in the various studies over this period of gestation. Liver and muscle glycogen concentrations increased sharply during the latter half of gestation. Cardiac muscle glycogen was virtually unchanged throughout the latter half of pregnancy, and lung glycogen concentrations began to fall in the latter part of pregnancy. The authors could find no significant arteriovenous difference for fructose concentration across the umbilical circulation, confirming an observation made earlier for the sheep fetus studied chronically (Tsoulos et al.: Comparison of glucose, fructose, and oxygen uptakes by fetuses of fed and starved ewes, Am. J. Physiol. **221**:234-237, 1971). Amniotic fluid glucose and fructose concentrations were lower than those in the umbilical circulation—again, similar to findings for the lamb fetus. There was a significant arteriovenous difference for glucose concentration across the umbilical circulation throughout the gestational ages studied. The coefficient of extraction for glucose across the umbilical circulation was approximately 10%, a figure very close to that found for the lamb fetus in chronic studies. Fetal glucose

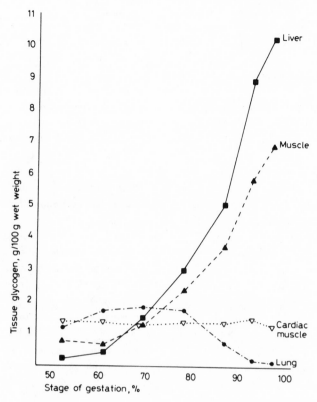

FIG. 1-9

Changes in fetal tissue glycogen levels with fetal age. (From Randall, G. C. B., and L'Ecuyer, C.: Tissue glycogen and blood glucose and fructose levels in the pig fetus during the second half of gestation, Biol. Neonate **28**:74-82, 1976; S. Karger AG, Basel.)

concentrations were approximately half the maternal concentrations at all gestational ages studied.

COMMENT: These two articles present important information concerning glycogen metabolism during fetal life. The findings by Sparks et al. suggest a key role of galactose in initiating glycogen synthesis in fetal monkey liver. The study demonstrated that under the conditions of the in vitro perfusion, glucose was not used as a carbon source for glycogen synthesis in the absence of galactose and insulin. In this respect the results are different from those of studies with perfused adult rat liver. Fetal monkey liver was similar to adult rat liver in regard to the stimuli that prompted glucose release; that is, glucose release in the liver was stimulated in both fetal monkey liver and adult rat liver by glucagon, cyclic AMP, or hypoglycemia. This had been previously demonstrated by the same investigators involved in the study of Sparks et al. (Glinsmann et al.: Glucose regulation by isolated near-term fetal monkey liver, Pediatr. Res. **9**:600-604, 1975). Fetal monkey liver is different from adult rat liver in that the regulation of glycogen synthesis in the former is dependent on the presence of galactose as well as glucose concentration. This is an important observation with considerable significance in the neonatal period, when the infant is feeding on a high-lactose diet. Undoubtedly, the study of Sparks et al. will stimulate further clinical research evaluating plasma clearance of galactose versus that of other carbohydrates in newborn infants. It is not clear how this dependence of liver on galactose uptake would explain the high glycogen deposition, which occurs in late fetal life in all mammals studied. Although one might expect galactose concentration to be elevated in the pregnant animal as lactogenesis increases in the mammary gland, one would not expect galactose concentrations in fetal blood to be comparable to the very high portal venous concentrations occurring postnatally with a high lactose diet. These data do suggest, however, that glycogen deposition in the fetal liver (and perhaps in fetal skeletal muscle; see Randall et al. review) may be dependent on other carbon sources than glucose from the circulation.

The pattern of change in tissue glycogen concentrations within the different tissues was elegantly presented in the study by Randall et al. The striking finding that cardiac muscle glycogen is relatively constant throughout the latter half of pregnancy is difficult to reconcile with the hypothesis proposed in the past: that very high cardiac glycogen concentration in late fetal life helps explain the resistance to hypoxia found after birth. The fall in lung glycogen in late gestation may reflect the effect of increased adrenocorticosteroid concentrations on mobilization of lung glycogen. The striking parallelism in the time during gestation when skeletal muscle and liver glycogen concentrations are changing rapidly suggests that perhaps the same substrates are involved in glycogen synthesis. In two mammals, both characterized by high fetal fructose concentrations, it has now been shown that no significant umbilical uptake of fructose can be demonstrated, suggesting that under normal conditions exogenous or placental fructose is not a major source of carbon for the developing fetus.

Amino acid infusions in newborn infants

■ Williams, P. R., Fiser, R. H., Jr., Sperling, M. A., and Oh, W.: Effects of oral alanine feeding on blood glucose, plasma glucagon and insulin concentrations in small-for-gestational-age infants, N. Engl. J. Med. 292:612-614, 1975.

The effect of an infusion of alanine on alanine, glucose, insulin, and glucagon concentrations was studied in 21 SGA and 26 AGA infants. They varied in gestational age from 34 to 42 weeks. Following an increase in plasma alanine concentrations, plasma glucagon concentrations were elevated in both SGA and AGA infants. Blood glucose and insulin concentrations were elevated in AGA infants alone.

■ Falorni, A., Massi-Benedetti, F., Gallo, S., and Romizi, S.: Levels of glucose in blood and insulin in plasma and glucagon response to arginine infusion in low birth weight infants, Pediatr. Res. 9:55-60, 1975.

This study is similar to that of Williams et al. In this case an arginine infusion rather than an alanine infusion was used as a stimulus to test a response of the infant's pancreas in AGA infants, SGA infants, and SGA hypoglycemic infants. As with the alanine infusions, an infusion of arginine raised the glucagon level significantly in all three groups of infants. In contrast to the alanine infusions in which insulin concentrations were not altered in SGA infants, the infusion of arginine increased plasma insulin concentration significantly in both AGA and SGA infants. The net effect of the increase in glucagon and insulin concentrations in the SGA hypoglycemic infant was a significant reduction in blood sugar, with glucose concentration falling from 42.4 to 32.4 mg/dl over a 60-minute infusion.

COMMENT: These two studies compared the effect of an infusion of an amino acid on insulin, glucose, and glucagon concentrations in the plasma of newborn infants, including AGA and SGA infants. It is clear that SGA infants differed from AGA infants in both studies in one respect: an amino acid infusion sufficient to trigger an increase in plasma glucagon concentrations did not produce a significant increase in glucose concentration in SGA infants, although it did in AGA infants. Studies of this kind cannot be regarded as definitive in clarifying the reasons why an increase in plasma gluconeogenic amino acids might not lead to an increase in blood glucose concentration. Alanine and arginine are two of several amino acids that have been used as test solutes to stimulate the release of glucagon or insulin from the pancreas. However, in studies in both children and adults there has been no attempt to obtain any form of dose-response relationship between the various amino acids on the one hand and the increase in hormonal concentrations on the other. These studies do suggest that one of the main problems responsible for hypoglycemia in SGA infants may be an inadequate hepatic response to apparently adequate stimuli, not an abnormality in pancreatic secretion. Beyond that, it is difficult to see how infusions of amino acids at this time can provide much clarification of the mechanisms responsible for neonatal hypoglycemia so characteristic of many mammals, including man.

Environmental changes and metabolism

■ Kervran, A., Gilbert, M., Girard, J. R., Assan R., and Jost, A.: Effect of environmental temperature on glucose-induced insulin response in the newborn rat, Diabetes 25:1026-1030, 1976.

This study compares the insulin release from the pancreas of newborn rats at two different environmental temperatures. The stimulus for insulin release was a bolus intraperitoneal injection of a 30% glucose solution, providing between 5 and 30 mg of glucose per animal. The two environmental temperatures compared were 37° C in a relative humidity of 70% (a thermal neutral environment for the newborn rat) and room temperature, 23° to 25° C.

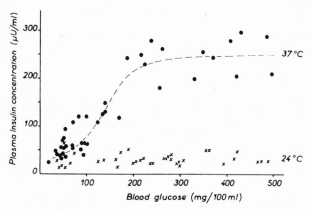

FIG. 1-10
Effect of environmental temperature on plasma insulin response to a 1-hour intraperitoneal glucose load in 1-hour-old newborn rats. (From Kervran, A., Gilbert, M., Girard, J. R., Assan, R., and Jost, A.: Effect of environmental temperature on glucose-induced insulin response in the newborn rat, Diabetes 25:1026-1030, 1976.)

It is clear from Fig. 1-10 taken from their report that the animals maintained in a cold environment developed no insulin response to the hyperglycemia, whereas those maintained in a thermal neutral zone developed a brisk insulin response. The study demonstrated that insulin responsiveness could be reintroduced even in a cold environment if the newborn rats received an alpha-adrenergic blockade produced by the subcutaneous injection of phentolamine, 20 mg/kg of body weight, 10 minutes prior to the bolus glucose injection. These findings suggest that increased sympathetic activity induced by cold stress is at least in part responsible for the insulin unresponsiveness.

■   Stave, U., and Armstrong, M. D.: Free amino acids in newborn and adult rabbit liver after prolonged hypoxia, Biol. Neonate 28:247-352, 1976.

This report presents interesting data on the changes in free amino acid concentration within liver tissue after 12 and 24 hours' exposure to hypoxia. Fig. 1-11 taken from this report demonstrates the fact that there was a different response in adult liver tissue compared with newborn liver tissue. The adult liver tissue showed an increase in amino acid levels that were significant in a few instances at both 12 and 24 hours of hypoxia. Tissue from newborn animals first showed a decrease in some of the amino acids and then a rather striking increase in the concentration or lysine, histidine, alanine, and glutamine.

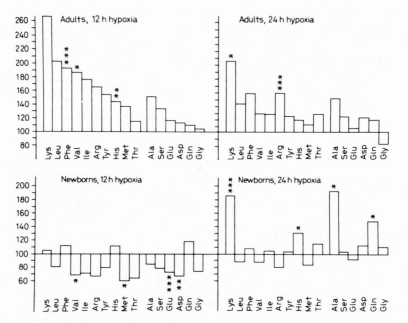

FIG. 1-11

Changes in liver free amino acids after hypoxia. *Abscissa,* levels of free amino acids as percentage of those in control animals, which were not subjected to hypoxia. Values for glutamine are actually glutamine plus asparagine, and for valine are valine plus cystine.
*, p < .05; **, p < .01; and ***, p < .005. (From Stave, U., and Armstrong, M. D.: Free amino acids in newborn and adult rabbit liver after prolonged hypoxia, Biol. Neonate **28:** 347-352, 1976; S. Karger AG, Basel.)

COMMENT: These two studies present the impact of environmental changes on various aspects of metabolism. The first report by Kervran et al. demonstrates how maintaining animals in a cold environment blocks the demonstration of any pancreatic response with insulin release to hyperglycemia in the newborn rat. The dramatic effect of environmental temperature on insulin release in response to hyperglycemia may help explain some of the conflicting data in the literature regarding the response of the fetal pancreas to infusions of glucose into the fetal circulation. Earlier work from some centers had been unable to demonstrate any increase in plasma insulin concentrations in the fetal circulation after hyperglycemia induced by intravenous injections of glucose. More recent studies have been able to define not only that there is invariably an insulin response but also the kinetics of this response. This variability in the literature might be introduced in some measure by alterations in tempreature when the glucose infusions were of large volume and at room temperature.

The second report begins to investigate changes in amino acid metabolism induced by hypoxia. It is not clear why the authors chose to concentrate solely on liver tissue, nor is it clear why there was no attempt to compare changes in different lobes of the liver, particularly in the newborn animals, since there may be differences in the perfusion of each lobe and thus differences in the level of tissue hypoxia, especially in the immediate neonatal period. The comparison of the changes in plasma amino acids at the time these tissue amino acid concentrations were occurring would also be helpful.

Developmental changes with taurine concentration

■ Sturman, J. A., and Gaull, G. E.: Taurine in the brain and liver of the developing human and monkey, J. Neurochem. 25:831-835, 1975.

Data are presented for the taurine concentrations in brain and liver tissue from human fetuses and adults and from fetal, newborn, and adult rhesus monkeys. The taurine

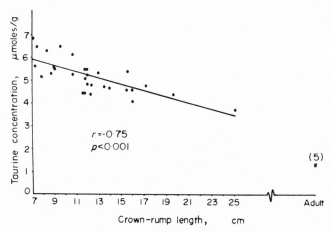

FIG. 1-12
Concentration of taurine in human fetal occipital lobe as a function of crown-rump length. The line of best fit was determined by computer using the method of least squares. The value for adult occipital lobe represents the mean ± SEM of the number of separate samples indicated. (From Sturman, J. A., and Gaull, G. E.: Taurine in the brain and liver of the developing human and monkey, J. Neurochem. 25:831-835, 1975.)

concentration in fetal brain tissue was found to be much higher (four or five times higher) in the fetuses of both humans and monkeys than in adult monkey brain. The concentration in fetal brain tissue decreased linearly with increasing crown-rump length in man. This is shown in Fig. 1-12 taken from their report. In the monkey the concentration of taurine in the brain tissue decreased during postnatal life, reaching adult values by 8 or 9 months after birth. In contrast, the concentrations of taurine in liver tissue from fetuses of humans and monkeys was only twofold that of adult liver tissue and decreased rapidly after birth, reaching adult concentrations within a few days. Fig. 1-13 presents comparative data from several studies, including the present one, for taurine concentrations in brain tissue related to weaning time. It is clear that several mammalian species widely different in dietary intake, gestation length, and size at birth experience similar postnatal changes in taurine concentration. The authors suggest that the changes in taurine concentration may be associated with brain development per se, in addition to any functional role this compound may have in brain tissue.

COMMENT: The changes during development in the concentration of taurine, which is widely distributed in the body, reminds one of the changes in inositol concentration, a cyclohexitol also found in very high concentration in the water-soluble extracts of fetal brain tissue (Battaglia et al.: The free myo-inositol concentration of adult and fetal tissues of several species, Q. J. Exp. Physiol. 46:188-193, 1961). As with inositol, we find a rela-

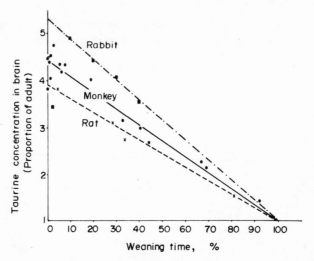

FIG. 1-13
Concentrations of taurine in brain of infant monkeys (●), rabbits (■), and rats (×) plotted as proportion of the concentration of taurine in the brain of the appropriate adult as a function of weaning time for each species. The line of best fit for each set of data was determined by computer using the method of least squares. Data for rabbits from Chanda and Himwich (Taurine levels in developing rabbit brain and other organs, Dev. Psychobiol. 3:191-196, 1970) and data for rats from Agrawal et al. (Subcellular distribution of taurine and cysteinesulphinate decarboxylase in developing rat brain, Biochem. J. 122:759-763, 1971). (From Sturman, J. A., and Gaull, G. E.: Taurine in the brain and liver of the developing human and monkey, J. Neurochem. 25:831-835, 1975.)

tively small molecule present in extremely high concentrations within the brain during fetal and immediate postnatal life. The significance of these changes in taurine concentration, and for that matter in free inositol concentration, are not clear at this time.

Fetal cardiac metabolism

■ Wildenthal, K., Allen, D. O., Karlsson, J., Wakeland, J. R., and Clark, C. M., Jr.: Responsiveness to glucagon in fetal hearts: species variability and apparent disparities between changes in beating, adenylate cyclase activation, and cyclic AMP concentration, J. Clin. Invest. 57:551-558, 1976.

Two species were compared for their cardiac response to glucagon. Isolated fetal hearts of mice and rats from 13 to 22 days' gestational age were studied under identical in vitro conditions. Changes in atrial rate, ventricular contractility, and adenylate cyclase activity were measured after exposure to varying concentrations of glucagon. Fig. 1-14 illustrates the response to glucagon at various fetal ages in mice. A developmental sequence is clearly demonstrated in the response of atrial rate to 10^{-5} μmol glucagon concentration. Ventricular inotropic responsiveness also appeared after 17 to 19 days' gestational age in fetal hearts of mice. In contrast, there were no changes in atrial rate or strength of contraction in the hearts of fetal rats at any gestational age.

At any concentration tested, glucagon failed to increase adenylate cyclase activity in homogenates of myocardial tissue from fetal mice. In contrast, liver obtained from fetal

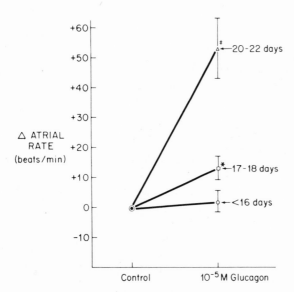

FIG. 1-14
Atrial rate response to glucagon in fetal mouse hearts. Each point represents the mean of sixteen hearts, and the vertical bars represent ± SEM. *, p < .05 compared to control (Student's *t* test for paired observations); ‡, p < .01. (From Wildenthal, K., Allen, D. O., Karlsson, J., Wakeland, J. R., and Clark, C. M., Jr.: Responsiveness to glucagon in fetal hearts: species variability and apparent disparities between changes in beating, adenylate cyclase activation, and cyclic AMP concentration, J. Clin. Invest. 57:551-558, 1976.)

CITY COLLEGE LIBRARY
1825 MAY ST.
BROWNSVILLE, TEXAS 78520

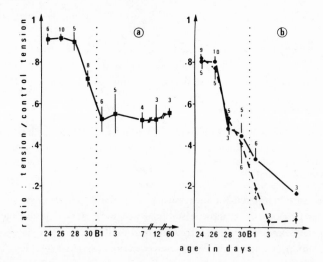

FIG. 1-15
Effect of substrate deprivation on the isometric tension during perinatal period. **a,** In normoxia, the plot shows the ratio: tension developed after 30 minutes without glucose/tension with 11 mmolar glucose. **b,** In hypoxia, comparison of the action of hypoxia (5 minutes) in the presence (solid line) and in the absence (dotted line) of glucose. Each plot is expressed as the ratio of hypoxic to prehypoxic tension. The prehypoxic tension was measured after 30 minutes of equilibration either in 11 mmolar (solid line) glucose or in 0 mmolar (dotted line) glucose. (From Hoerter, J.: Changes in the sensitivity to hypoxia and glucose deprivation in the isolated perfused rabbit heart during perinatal development, Pflügers Arch. **363**:1-6, 1976.)

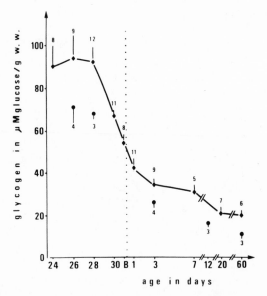

FIG. 1-16
Perinatal evolution of the myocardial glycogen content. Continuous line and rhombus, immediately frozen hearts; isolated circles, hearts paced at 90 minutes and perfused during 1 hour in 11 mmolar glucose. (From Hoerter, J.: Changes in the sensitivity to hypoxia and glucose deprivation in the isolated perfused rabbit heart during perinatal development, Pflügers Arch. **363**:1-6, 1976.)

mice showed a concentration-dependent increase in adenylate cyclase activity with varying glucagon concentrations. Glycogen content was reduced in hearts of fetal mice exposed to glucagon but not in those of fetal rats. Thus interspecies differences could be demonstrated in the effect of glucagon on both cardiac rate and metabolism. In addition, the maturational changes in response to glucagon were well demonstrated in fetal mice.

■ Hoerter, J.: Changes in the sensitivity to hypoxia and glucose deprivation in the isolated perfused rabbit heart during perinatal development, Pflügers Arch. **363:**1-6, 1976.

This study presents data on the contractile forces that develop in perfused fetal rabbit hearts obtained at different stages of gestation and during the immediate neonatal period. The effect of hypoxia and changes in glucose concentration on measurements of isometric tension and intracellular action potentials was determined. Fig. 1-15 presents the data for fetuses of 26 days postconception. For these young fetuses, neither hypoxia nor hypoglycemia altered the intracellular action potentials compared with control values under normoxia and in the presence of glucose. In contrast, for term fetal hearts studied under hypoxic conditions there was a marked difference in tension ratios in the presence or absence of

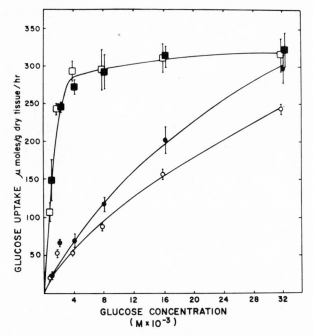

FIG. 1-17
Effect of initial glucose concentration in incubation medium on glucose uptake by chick embryo hearts. Five-day-old hearts with (■—■) or without (□—□) insulin; 9-day-old hearts with (●—●) or without (○—○) insulin. Hearts incubated 1 hour at 37.5° C in Krebs-Henseleit medium, pH 7.4 in an atmosphere of 95% oxygen and 5% carbon dioxide. Osmolarity of the medium was 0.306. Insulin concentration, 0.01 U/ml. Each point represents means of five experiments ± SEM (8). (From Foá, P. P., Melli, M., Berger, C. K., Billinger, D., and Guidotti, G. G.: Action of insulin on chick embryo heart, Fed. Proc. 24:1046-1050, 1965.)

glucose. The changes in myocardial glycogen concentrations during late fetal and early neonatal life in the rabbit myocardium are presented in Fig. 1-16.

COMMENT: The differences in metabolism of individual organs such as the heart at different developmental stages are just beginning to be described. Perhaps the two organs that have been best studied include the brain and the heart. In 1965 Foà et al. (Action of insulin on chick embryo heart, Fed. Proc. 24:1046-1050) demonstrated that in chick embryo hearts insulin stimulated the incorporation of radioactivity from ^{14}C-labeled acetate or glucose into lipids several days before an insulin effect on glucose uptake in the hearts could be demonstrated. Fig. 1-17 taken from their report shows the absence of any insulin effect on glucose uptake by the myocardium in the 5-day-old hearts versus a demonstrable effect later in development.

Table 1-1 presents data on the glucose/oxygen quotients and the lactate/oxygen quotients for the myocardium of puppies and adult dogs. These values are calculations from the data on coronary arteriovenous differences presented by Breuer et al. (Developmental changes of myocardial metabolism. I. Peculiarities of cardiac carbohydrate metabolism in the early postnatal period in dogs, Biol. Neonate 11:367-377, 1967). These authors clearly demonstrated that in the early postnatal period—that is, in puppies 7 to 12 days of age— glucose could account for all the metabolic requirements of the heart. The glucose/oxygen quotient expressed stoichiometrically across the coronary circulation was 1.1. This changed during development so that in puppies from 13 to 21 days the glucose/oxygen quotient fell to 0.9 and the lactate/oxygen quotient, which was negative at 7 to 12 days, became positive (0.14). Thus in puppies at 13 to 21 days, carbohydrate in the form of glucose plus lactate could account for all the oxygen consumption. In sharp contrast, glucose plus lactate combined still accounted for no more than 30% of the oxygen consumption in adult dog hearts. These data received confirmation in a subsequent report by the same investigators (Breuer et al., Developmental changes of myocardial metabolism. II. Myocardial metabolism of fatty acids in the early postnatal period in dogs, Biol. Neonate 12:54-64, 1968). In that report the investigators showed that they could not demonstrate any uptake of free fatty acids in puppies from 7 to 12 days of age; in fact, they showed a small but significant arteriovenous difference of free fatty acids at that age. In contrast, free fatty acids represented the bulk of the fuel taken up by the adult heart, a finding in agreement with studies in many other mammalian species showing free fatty acids as the major fuel for the myocardium when it is normally oxygenated and perfused.

TABLE 1-1
Myocardial metabolism in puppies*

Age in days	Coronary arteriovenous differences (mmol/L)			Glucose/ oxygen quotients	Lactate/ oxygen quotients
	Glucose	Lactate	O_2		
7-12	0.63	−0.30	3.44	1.10	−0.26
13-21	0.57	0.18	3.79	0.90	0.14
Adult	0.13	0.56	6.92	0.11	0.24

*Calculated from data of Breuer, E., Barta, E., Pappová, E., and Zlatoš, L.: Developmental changes of mycardial metabolism. I. Peculiarities of cardiac carbohydrate metabolism in the early postnatal period in dogs, Biol. Neonate 11:367-377, 1967; S. Karger AG, Basel.

The importance of glucose as the major fuel for the heart in early development has considerable clinical significance when considered against a background of several reports in the pediatric literature documenting heart failure in newborn infants in the presence of severe hypoglycemia. When one considers the increased brain/body weight ratio of a newborn infant and the fact that the brain is also dependent on glucose as its major substrate, it becomes clear that hypoglycemia, possibly coupled with poor organ perfusion in the immediate newborn period, might produce severe dysfunction of both the brain and the heart at a critical time in postnatal development. The hypothesis that the newborn heart is dependent on glucose metabolism and thus might be prone to cardiac failure secondary to hypoglycemia received additional strength from the report by Gennser (Influence of hypoxia and glucose on contractility of papillary muscles from adult and neonatal rabbits, Biol. Neonate 21:90-106, 1972). Gennser showed that although many of the properties of the newborn and adult heart (that is, maximum active force in the presence or absence of hypoxia and in the presence or absence of glucose) were similar, there was one striking difference between neonatal and adult heart. Fig. 1-18, taken from their report, demonstrates that in the absence of glucose the neonatal heart that is made hypoxic (open circles) shows no increase in the maximum active force with an increase in frequency of

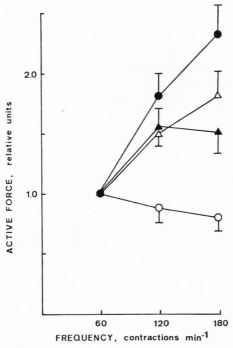

FIG. 1-18

Relation between contraction frequency and maximum active force of adult (solid symbols) and neonatal (open symbols) rabbit papillary muscles during perfusion with 3.3 mmolar glucose with 95% nitrogen (circles), and 33 mmolar glucose with 95% nitrogen (triangles) (n = 8 in all muscle groups). Force at 60 contractions $\cdot$ min^{-1} = 1.0. (From Gennser, G.: Influence of hypoxia and glucose on contractility of papillary muscles from adult and neonatal rabbits, Biol. Neonate 21:90-106, 1972; S. Karger AG, Basel.)

contractions. This is strikingly different from the adult heart and is almost totally corrected by a tenfold increase in glucose concentration in the presence of hypoxia (open triangles).

The study by Wildenthal et al. illustrates nicely the maturational sequence that occurs in the heart's response to glucagon. Studies that aim at defining differences in fetal metabolism among species are fraught with difficulties of interpretation. Some of the difficulties stem from the fact that one is attempting to compare fetuses which may vary greatly in their growth rate, length of gestation, degree of maturity at birth, and relative size with respect to the mother. Another difficulty stems from the fact that the surgical techniques and/or the in vitro conditions used during any given study may define an artificial state which has little relevance to normal conditions in vivo. It is difficult to design experiments in which these variables are carefully controlled; however, the study by Wildenthal et al. appears to overcome most of these difficulties in documenting a difference in the response of fetal mice and fetal rats to glucagon.

Amino acid catabolism in the fetus and newborn

■ Lemons, J. A., Adcock, E. W., III, Jones, M. D., Jr., Naughton, M. A., Meschia, G., and Battaglia, F. C.: Umbilical uptake of amino acids in the unstressed fetal lamb, J. Clin. Invest. 58:1428-1434, 1976.

This study presents the whole blood amino acid concentrations across the umbilical circulation and in maternal arterial blood. In addition, oxygen contents were determined in blood for the umbilical arterial and venous samples. The latter measurements were made

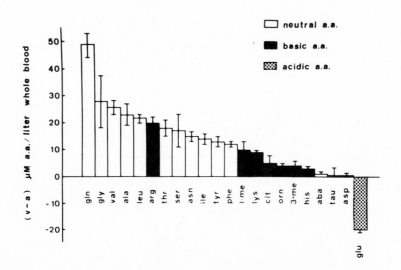

FIG. 1-19
The mean umbilical arteriovenous concentration differences ± SEM for each amino acid are depicted in the order of decreasing value. The acidic amino acids (taurine, aspartate, glutamate) show either no net flux or a negative (arteriovenous) difference, whereas the neutral amino acids demonstrate a large positive uptake by the fetus from the placenta.
(From Lemons, J. A., Adcock, E. W., III, Jones, M. D., Jr., Naughton, M. A., Meschia, G., and Battaglia, F. C.: Umbilical uptake of amino acids in the unstressed fetal lamb, J. Clin. Invest. 58:1428-1434, 1976.)

to reflect changes in umbilical blood flow and thus attempt to relate fetal oxygen consumption to amino acid uptake across the umbilical circulation. Seventy-three sets of samples from the umbilical artery and vein and the maternal artery were analyzed in fetal lambs studied from 118 to 146 days' gestational age. Special precautions were taken to ensure an accurate estimation of glutamine concentration in the whole blood analysis. In addition, modification was introduced (Lemons et al.: Removal of glutathione interference in blood amino acid analysis, Biochem. Med. **15**:282-288, 1976) to oxidize completely the high concentrations of glutathione present in sheep blood and thus keep glutathione from interfering with the analysis of alanine and glycine. Fig. 1-19 taken from their reviewed report summarizes the arteriovenous differences in micromoles per liter of whole blood for the individual amino acids. With the exception of glutamate, which was transferred from the umbilical circulation to the placenta, the amino acids appeared in increased concentration in the umbilical venous blood. For sixteen of the twenty-two amino acids, there was a significant mean umbilical arteriovenous difference ($p < .005$). Neutral amino acids and the basic amino acid arginine account for approximately 94% of the total amino acid flux into the umbilical circulations. Acidic amino acids were unique in that there were no significant arteriovenous differences for aspartate and taurine in either direction and a significant venous arteriovenous difference for glutamate into the placenta. From the arteriovenous differences in oxygen content, an estimate of umbilical blood flow was calculated from the equation $F = 30.5 + 222/(A - V)$ oxygen. The net nitrogen flux into the umbilical circulation represented by the amino acids was 1.52 gm of nitrogen per kilogram of fetal body weight per day. The net uptake of carbon from amino acids was 3.94 gm of carbon per kilogram of fetal body weight per day.

TABLE 1-2

Effect of age and nutritional status on specific activity of liver glycogen*†

	Substrate	
	^{14}C-alanine, dpm/mg glycogen	^{14}C-leucine, dpm/mg glycogen
Group	dpm/μmol alanine‡	dpm/μmol leucine‡
3-day-old		
Fed	1.08 ± 0.14	0.37 ± 0.025
Starved 4 hr	0.98 ± 0.33	0.53 ± 0.022
19-day-old		
Fed	0.15 ± 0.03§	0.003 ± 0.001
Starved 15 hr	6.41 ± 3.62	0.032 ± 0.015
3-month-old		
Fed	0.00 ± 0.00§‖	0 ± 0¶
Starved 48 hr	0.25 ± 0.17	0 ± 0
−CHO#	0.28 ± 0.22	0 ± 0

*From White, P. K., and Miller, S. A.: Utilization of dietary amino acids for energy production in neonatal rat liver, Pediatr. Res. **10**:158-164, 1976.
†Mean ± SEM ($n = 3$).
‡Specific activity of amino acid in hepatic free amino acid pools.
§Different from 3-day fed value, $p < .005$.
‖Different from 19-day fed value, $p < .01$.
¶Different from 19-day fed value, $p < .02$.
#Animals fed high-fat, low-carbohydrate diet.

■ White, P. K., and Miller, S. A.: Utilization of dietary amino acids for energy production in neonatal rat liver, Pediatr. Res. 10:158-164, 1976.

This study presents data on the incorporation of ^{14}C-leucine or ^{14}C-alanine into carbon dioxide and liver glycogen in rats. The studies were carried out in rats at 3 days, 19 days, and 3 months of age. The amino acids were fed to the animals orally. In addition, the activity of hepatic PEPCK was measured. In each age group the animals were studied both in a fed state and a starved state. In all three groups, liver glycogen concentration fell with starvation. Table 1-2 presents the data on the incorporation of orally administered ^{14}C-alanine or ^{14}C-leucine to the fed and starved animals in the three age groups. In the 3-day-old, incorporation of labeled amino acids into glycogen was much higher in the fed state than in the older animals and did not increase significantly with starvation. In the 19-day-old and 3-month-old animals, incorporation of the labeled amino acids was extremely low when they were in the fed state and increased markedly with starvation. In fed animals the percentage of radioactivity represented by expired ^{14}CO$_2$ decreased with age for both amino acids. Urinary nitrogen concentration increased significantly between 3 and 19 days of age. Starvation did not alter urinary nitrogen concentration in the 3-day-old or in the adult rats but decreased urinary nitrogen concentration in the 19-day-old animals.

COMMENT: The reviewed study by Lemons et al. demonstrates that amino acid transfer across the placenta provides nitrogen to the fetus in amounts considerably greater than those required for new tissue growth. The bulk of the amino acid nitrogen is provided by the neutral amino acids. Previously Gresham et al. (Production and excretion of urea by the fetal lamb, Pediatrics 50:372-379, 1972) had measured the urea production rate of the fetal lamb and found it to be equal to 0.54 ml/kg/min. This corresponded to approximately 25% of the oxygen consumption accounted for by the catabolism of amino acids. White and Miller's study also shows in rapidly growing newborn rats that approximately 25% of their total caloric requirements was met by catabolism of amino acids. Thus two rapidly growing organisms, the fetal lamb and the newborn rat, derive an appreciable proportion of their total caloric requirements from catabolism of amino acids. White and Miller arrived at their figure based upon the fact that their own studies had shown that 54% of dietary protein and 59% of dietary fat were not incorporated into body mass (Dymsza et al.: Influence of artificial diet on weight gain and body composition of the neonatal rat, J. Nutr. 84:100-106, 1964). The following equations taken from their report illustrate that approximately 0.9 cal were derived from protein per 24 hours from a total of 3.6 cal/24 hr.

$$\frac{1.5 \text{ gm protein}}{7 \text{ days}} \times \frac{4 \text{ cal}}{\text{gm protein}} = \frac{6 \text{ cal}}{7 \text{ days}} = 0.9 \text{ cal/24 hr from protein}$$

$$\frac{2.1 \text{ gm fat}}{7 \text{ days}} \times \frac{9 \text{ cal}}{\text{gm fat}} = \frac{18.9 \text{ cal}}{7 \text{ days}} = 2.7 \text{ cal/24 hr from fat}$$

White and Miller's study demonstrates that the newborn rat has a high rate of gluconeogenesis from amino acids even in the fed-state. Because of its high basal rate, there is little further increase in the incorporation of amino acids into liver glycogen with starvation. However, the 19-day-old and 3-month-old rats with a lower basal rate of gluconeogenesis do respond dramatically to starvation by an increase in gluconeogenesis. White and Miller measured the urinary nitrogen concentration in the newborn rats and confirmed that it increases markedly from a low value of 4.7 ml of nitrogen/ml of urine in the newborn up to 13.4 ml of nitrogen/ml of urine in the 3-month-old rats. Previously Hoy had shown

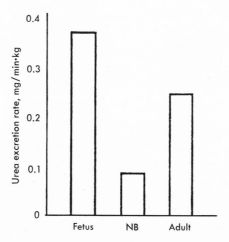

FIG. 1-20
The urea excretion rates for newborn infants *(NB)* and adults represent urinary excretion rates, that for the fetus represents the estimate of transplacental urea excretion. The data for the figure were obtained from the following studies: for the fetus, from Gresham et al. (Maternal-fetal urea concentration difference in man: metabolic significance, J. Pediatr. **79:** 809-811, 1971); for the adult, from McCance and Widdowson (Metabolism and renal function in the first two days of life, Cold Spring Harbor Symp. Quant. Biol. **19:**161-166, 1954); and for the newborn infant from the present study. (From Jones, M. D., Jr., Gresham, E. L., and Battaglia, F. C.: Urinary flow rates and urea excretion rates in newborn infants, Biol. Neonate **21:**321-329, 1972; S. Karger AG, Basel.)

an increasing urinary flow rate with increasing age (Diuresis in newborn rat given intravenous water or salt solution, Proc. Soc. Exp. Biol. Med. 122:358-361, 1966). The low urinary nitrogen excretion in newborns is not confined to rats but has been reported for newborn infants as well. Barlow and McCance (The nitrogen partition in newborn infants' urine, Arch. Dis. Child. 23:225-230, 1948), for instance, reported a urea excretion rate of between 0.27 and 0.05 ml/kg/min in a group of normal term infants during the first 1 to 6 postnatal days. Jones et al. (Urinary flow rates and urea excretion rates in newborn infants, Biol. Neonate 21:321-329, 1972) similarly found a low rate of urea excretion in newborn infants compared with fetuses and adults. Fig. 1-20 taken from their report summarizes those observations. The basis for the low urinary nitrogen excretion in newborn infants is unclear at this time.

Glucose homeostasis in pregnancy

■ Gillmer, M. D. G., Beard, R. W., Brooke, F. M., and Oakley, N. W.: Carbohydrate metabolism in pregnancy. I. Diurnal plasma glucose profile in normal and diabetic women, Br. Med. J. 3:399-402, 1975.

The aim of this study was to investigate diurnal variability of plasma glucose in normal and diabetic pregnant women. Of the fifty patients studied, thirteen were insulin-dependent diabetic women who had all been receiving insulin treatment before pregnancy for 6 to 26 years, thirteen were classified as "chemical diabetics," and twenty-four were normal controls. Patients were assigned to either a normal or a chemical diabetic group, depending on the result of a glucose tolerance test performed in the last trimester. The response to this test was assessed in terms of area under the 3-hour glucose curve. The insulin-dependent diabetic women were studied between 32 and 36 weeks, after at least 2 weeks in the hospital, when optimal diabetic control had been achieved with careful dietary carbohydrate management and twice-daily injections of soluble and isophane insulin. Results in normal patients are shown in Fig. 1-21. Mean plasma glucose remained below 5.6 mmol (100 mg/dl) except

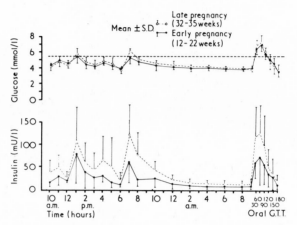

FIG. 1-21

Plasma glucose and insulin concentrations during diurnal profile and oral glucose tolerance tests in nine normal women studied in early and late pregnancy. Conversion: SI to traditional units—1 mmol/L = 18 mg/dl. (From Gillmer, M. D. G., Beard, R. W., Brooke, F. M., and Oakley, N. W.: Carbohydrate metabolism in pregnancy. I. Diurnal plasma glucose profile in normal and diabetic women, Br. Med. J. **3:**399-402, 1975.)

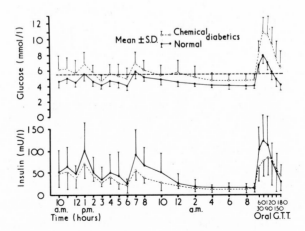

FIG. 1-22

Plasma glucose and insulin concentrations during diurnal profile and oral glucose tolerance tests in twenty-four normal and thirteen chemical diabetic women studied during last trimester of pregnancy. (From Gillmer, M. D. G., Beard, R. W., Brooke, F. M., and Oakley, N. W.: Carbohydrate metabolism in pregnancy. I. Diurnal plasma glucose profile in normal and diabetic women, Br. Med. J. **3:**399-402, 1975.)

during the hour after a meal. The diurnal plasma glucose range was greater in late than in early pregnancy. In late pregnancy, plasma insulin concentrations were increased throughout the day, particularly after meals. Also, in late pregnancy the insulin/glucose ratio was almost twice that observed in early pregnancy. Fig. 1-22 shows a comparison of chemical diabetics with normal patients. The pattern of diurnal variation was similar for the two groups, but there were higher glucose and lower insulin concentrations in the diabetic group. Mean glucose values and diurnal fluctuations were greater in the insulin-requiring diabetics than in the normal group (Fig. 1-23). In addition, there was a strong tendency to hypoglycemia during the night.

■ Gillmer, M. D. G., Beard, R. W., Brooke, F. M., and Oakley, N. W.: Carbohydrate metabolism in pregnancy. II. Relation between maternal glucose tolerance and glucose metabolism in the newborn, Br. Med. J. 3:402-404, 1975.

The infants of thirty-one women whose carbohydrate metabolism had been documented during the last trimester of pregnancy were studied. Twenty-one of the women were classified as normal and ten as chemical diabetics on the basis of a glucose tolerance test. At birth the infants were transferred to an incubator and feedings withheld for 2 hours after delivery. At that time, capillary blood was obtained for glucose and insulin measurements. There was an inverse relationship between the neonatal plasma glucose concentration determined 2 hours after delivery and the total area under the curve obtained from a 3-hour glucose tolerance test performed on the mother approximately 4 weeks before birth. The mean insulin/glucose ratio of infants born to chemically diabetic women was significantly higher than that of those born to normal women.

COMMENT: These two articles provide quantitative evidence of the impairment of maternal glucose homeostasis in insulin-dependent diabetics and in patients with abnormal glucose tolerance tests. In addition, they show that such an impairment has a demonstrable effect on the ability of the newborn to regulate its own plasma glucose. Much remains to be learned about the chain of events that connects maternal, fetal, and neonatal glucose metabolism, but the following explanation is suggested by clinical and experimental studies. In late fetal life, as in neonatal and adult life, hyperglycemia stimulates hypersecretion of

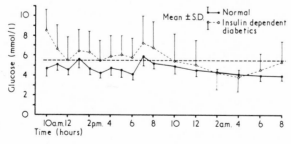

FIG. 1-23
Diurnal glucose concentrations in thirteen insulin-dependent diabetics and nine women with normal glucose tolerance studied between 32 and 35 weeks of pregnancy. (From Gillmer, M. D. G., Beard, R. W., Brooke, F. M., and Oakley, N. W.: Carbohydrate metabolism in pregnancy. I. Diurnal plasma glucose profile in normal and diabetic women, Br. Med. J. 3: 399-402, 1975.)

insulin. However, it is a unique characteristic of the fetus that hypersecretion of insulin by the fetal pancreas cannot bring plasma glucose back to normal because placental transfer of glucose will maintain a high level of glucose in the fetus as long as the mother is hyperglycemic. In other words, glucose and insulin in the fetus are *not* linked by a regulatory negative feedback loop as they are in extrauterine life. If the maternal and fetal hyperglycemia persist, the pattern of fetal hypersecretion of insulin becomes established, perhaps because of hypertrophy of the beta cells. The fetus then becomes unable to rapidly reduce its secretion of insulin when glucose becomes scarce, for example, in the period of fasting that follows birth. A temporary shortage of glucose may also occur in utero, as shown in Fig. 1-23, despite attempts to attain an optimal control of the diabetes. In this case the fetus is likely to develop an inappropriately high insulin/glucose ratio. It is conceivable that failure to control this ratio causes serious metabolic disturbances in the fetus, but there is no experimental basis for this conjecture.

Lactate metabolism in the fetus

- Burd, L. I., Jones, M. D., Jr., Simmons, M. A., Makowski, E. L., Meschia, G., and Battaglia, F. C.: Placental production and foetal utilisation of lactate and pyruvate, Nature (Lond.) 254:710-711, 1975.

This study presents data on the lactate and pyruvate concentrations in the umbilical arterial and venous blood as well as the uterine arterial and venous blood in pregnant sheep from 67 days' gestational age to term (term is approximately 145 days). Blood samples were obtained from the four vessels supplying and draining the placenta in chronic unstressed animal preparations. The blood samples were used for both lactate and pyruvate concentrations as well as the determination of oxygen contents. A significant arteriovenous difference of lactate was found across both the umbilical and uterine circulations. Lactate/oxygen quotients were calculated as given in the following equation:

$$\text{Lactate/oxygen quotient} = 3(\text{v-a lactate/v-a oxygen})$$

The lactate/oxygen quotient across the umbilical circulation was 0.25 (95% confidence limits calculated by Fieller's theorem was 0.16 to 0.32). No significant arteriovenous differences for pyruvate concentration across the umbilical circulation was found. There was a small arteriovenous difference of 0.01 mmolar across the uterine circulation for pyruvate.

COMMENT: The demonstration that placental tissue in a variety of mammals is characterized by a high rate of production of lactate under aerobic conditions has now been extended by Burd et al. to sheep and to a demonstration of placental lactate production under in vivo conditions. Beginning with an initial report in 1925 of lactate production by the rat placenta (Murphy et al.: Comparative studies on metabolism of normal and malignant cells, J. Gen. Physiol. 8:115-130, 1925), lactate production by the placenta was next demonstrated for human placental tissue incubated in vitro (Loeser: Atmung und Gärung der überlebenden Placenta des Menschen sowie deren Beeinflussung durch Hormone nebst dem Milschsäurestoffwechsel der lebenden Placenta im trächtigen Tiere, Arch. Gynaekol. 148:118-148, 1932). This was later confirmed in studies by Villee (The metabolism of human placenta in vitro, J. Biol. Chem. 205:113-123, 1953). However, the study by Burd et al. demonstrates that lactate production is a characteristic of placental tissue in vivo and that the lactate produced by that organ is delivered into both the uterine and umbilical circulations, since the venous concentration of lactate is higher in both the umbilical and uterine veins. Furthermore, since the lactate/oxygen quotients were equal to 0.25, their study demonstrates that lactate utilization by the fetus represents a significant percentage of the total carbon needs of the fetus despite a high arterial lactate concentration.

Fetal and neonatal cerebral metabolism

■ Dahlquist, G., and Persson, B.: The rate of cerebral utilization of glucose, ketone bodies, and oxygen: a comparative in vivo study of infant and adult rats, Pediatr. Res. **10**:910-917, 1976.

In this study cerebral blood flow was measured using [141]Ce-labeled microspheres and the arteriovenous differences of acetoacetate, beta-hydroxybutyrate, glucose, lactate, and oxygen were determined. In addition, the DNA content of the brain was measured. These measurements were carried out in both the 20-day-old infant rats and 3-month-old adult rats. Fig. 1-24 summarizes the results. There were no differences between the adult and infant rats in terms of the solutes used to meet metabolic requirements with the animals in the fed state. However, during starvation of 48 or 72 hours' duration, infant rats met their substrate requirements with a higher percentage of ketoacid utilization than that of adult rats. In infant rats the utilization of acetoacetate and beta-hydroxybutyrate was related to the arterial plasma concentration of these compounds. In infant rats the glucose plus ketone body/oxygen quotients were significantly greater than 1, whereas in the adult rats the glucose plus ketone body "oxygen quotient" was equal to 1 in both the fed and starved groups. Thus in infant rats, carbon from glucose and ketone bodies was used for purposes other than carbon dioxide production.

■ Jones, M. D., Jr., Burd, L. I., Makowski, E. L., Meschia, G., and Battaglia, F. C.: Cerebral metabolism in sheep: a comparative study of the adult, the lamb, and the fetus, Am. J. Physiol. **229**:235-239, 1975.

The uptake of a variety of solutes across the cerebral circulation in adult, newborn, and fetal sheep was measured under chronic unstressed conditions. Samples were obtained from

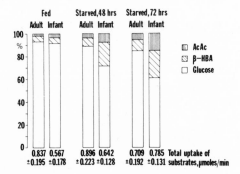

FIG. 1-24
Cerebral uptake of acetoacetate (AcAc) D-β-hydroxybutyrate (β-HBA), and glucose in adult and infant (20-day-old) rats fed or starved for 48 to 72 hours. The values are expressed as a percentage of total substrate uptake in micromoles per minute. (From Dahlquist, G., and Persson, B.: The rate of cerebral utilization of glucose, ketone bodies, and oxygen: a comparative in vivo study of infant and adult rats, Pediatr. Res. **10**:910-917, 1976.)

TABLE 1-3

Summary of arterial (A) concentrations (mmolar) and cerebral arteriovenous differences (A-V) in nonpregnant ewes, lambs, and fetuses*

	Adults	Lambs	Fetuses
A_{O_2} content	6.228 ± .137 (40)	5.832 ± .217 (41)	4.219 ± .131 (51)
$(A-V)_{O_2}$ content	3.300 ± .063 (40)	2.543 ± .091 (41)	1.373 ± .041 (51)
$A_{glucose}$	2.807 ± .070 (40)	5.389 ± .112 (42)	0.994 ± .036 (50)
$(A-V)_{glucose}$	0.566 ± 0.10 (40)	0.419 ± .017 (42)	0.223 ± .008 (50)
$A_{lactate}$	0.668 ± .024 (19)	1.471 ± .116 (38)‡	1.598 ± .058 (40)‡
$(A-V)_{lactate}$	−0.031 ± .015 (18)†	−0.021 ± .013 (35)	0.010 ± .014 (40)
$A_{pyruvate}$	0.153 ± .010 (14)	0.137 ± .029 (3)	0.307 ± .037 (40)‡
$(A-V)_{pyruvate}$	−0.013 ± .002 (14)†	−0.053 ± .032 (3)	−0.020 ± .010 (40)†
$A_{\beta\text{-hydroxybutyrate}}$	0.289 ± .024 (23)	0.195 ± .019 (25)	0.070 ± .005 (11)
$(A-V)_{\beta\text{-hydroxybutyrate}}$	0.001 ± .007 (23)	0.003 ± .003 (25)	0.002 ± .001 (11)
$A_{acetoacetate}$	0.039 ± .007 (22)	0.049 ± .003 (25)	0.037 ± .004 (11)
$(A-V)_{acetoacetate}$	−0.003 ± .001 (22)†	−0.001 ± .001 (25)	−0.007 ± .001 (11)†
$\dfrac{6 \times (A-V)_{glucose}}{(A-V)_{O_2 \text{ content}}}$	0.98 < 1.03 < 1.08§	0.92 < 0.99 < 1.06§	0.92 < 0.98 < 1.03§
$\dfrac{A_{lactate}}{A_{pyruvate}}$	3.59 < 4.37 < 5.37§		5.14 < 5.21 < 6.97§

*From Jones, M. D., Jr., Burd, L. I., Makowski, E. L., Meschia, G., and Battaglia, F. C.: Cerebral metabolism in sheep: a comparative study of the adult, the lamb, and the fetus, Am. J. Physiol. **229:**235-239, 1975.

Values are mean ± 1 SE. All units, except ratios, are mmolar. Numbers of determinations are given in parentheses.

†Less than 0 (p < .05).
‡Higher than adult (p < .05).
§Mean and 95% confidence limits.

arterial blood above the ductus and from sagittal sinus blood beginning 1 to 2 days after surgery and continuing for periods up to 2 weeks. Whole blood arteriovenous differences were measured for glucose, lactate, pyruvate, acetoacetate, and beta-hydroxybutyrate, and these were compared to the arteriovenous differences of oxygen content. The results are summarized in Table 1-3 taken from their report. The data demonstrate that the glucose/oxygen quotient for all three age groups was approximately equal to 1. There was no significant production of lactate by the fetal brain. Since keto acid concentrations in the arterial blood were very low in all three age groups, it is not surprising that there was no significant uptake of keto acids across the cerebral circulation. The lactate/pyruvate ratios in adult and fetal blood were not significantly different.

■ Settergren, G., Lindblad, B. S., and Persson, B.: Cerebral blood flow and exchange of oxygen, glucose, ketone bodies, lactate, pyruvate, and amino acids in infants, Acta Paediatr. Scand. **65:**343-353, 1976.

This study reports on cerebral blood flow measurements and venous arterial differences for oxygen, glucose, lactate, pyruvate, and keto acids in a group of children varying in age. The children were divided into two age groups: one group ranging from 11 days postnatal

TABLE 1-4

Arterial concentration, cerebral arteriovenous difference and cerebral exchange of oxygen, glucose, lactate, pyruvate, acetoacetate, and D-β-hydroxybutyrate in nine infants*

	Arterial concentration (mmols/L)	Cerebral av-difference (mmols/L)	Cerebral exchange (μmols/100 gm brain tissue × min⁻¹)
Oxygen	6.17 ± 0.35	+1.62 ± 0.18	+104.4 ± 8.0†
Glucose	7.02 ± 0.66	+0.38 ± 0.07	+ 27.2 ± 6.2†
Lactate	1.05 ± 0.16	−0.04 ± 0.01	− 2.4 ± 0.8‡
Pyruvate	0.085 ± 0.000	−0.01 ± 0.00	− 0.8 ± 0.2
Acetoacetate	0.250 ± 0.081	+0.021 ± 0.007	+ 0.9 ± 0.3†
D-β-hydroxybu-tyrate	0.833 ± 0.185	+0.032 ± 0.003	+ 2.3 ± 0.6†

*From Settergren, G., Lindblad, B. S., and Persson, B.: Cerebral blood flow and exchange of oxygen, glucose, ketone bodies, lactate, pyruvate, and amino acids in infants, Acta Paediatr. Scand. **65:**343-353, 1976.

Values are given as mean ± SE.

†+ indicates uptake.
‡− indicates release.

age to 12 months postnatal age with a mean age of 5 months, and a second group ranging in age from 10 to 15 years with a mean age of 12 years and 1 month. Cerebral blood flow was measured by a modification of the nitrous oxide technique. Blood samples were obtained by means of catheterization of the radial artery and jugular vein for plasma amino acid determinations. A cerebral uptake that was statistically significant could be documented only for two of the dibasic amino acids—histidine and arginine. For all other amino acids no significant arteriovenous differences in either direction were obtained. Table 1-4 from this report describes the significant findings for the cerebral arteriovenous differences and cerebral uptake; that is, arteriovenous difference multiplied by cerebral blood flow for the compounds listed. Table 1-4 points out the fact that glucose uptake alone could more than account for the oxygen uptake with the glucose/oxygen quotient of 1.41. The combined uptake of acetoacetate and β-hydroxybutyrate was equivalent to approximately 13% of the oxygen consumption, or approximately one tenth of the glucose uptake.

■ DeVivo, D. C., Leckie, M. P., and Agrawal, H. C.: D-beta-Hydroxybutyrate: a major precursor of amino acids in developing rat brain, J. Neurochem. **25:**161-170, 1975.

This study compares incorporation of ¹⁴C-labeled glucose and beta-hydroxybutyrate (β-OHB) into amino acids of newborn rats. The experimental design consisted of a subcutaneous injection of either 3-¹⁴C-β-OHB or 2-¹⁴C-glucose. Following the subcutaneous injection, blood samples and brain tissue samples were obtained for analysis. Fig. 1-25 taken from this report illustrates the fact that specific activity of two amino acids, glutamate and asparate, increased markedly when 3-¹⁴C-β-OHB was used as the precursor compared to 2-¹⁴C-glucose. Alanine presented a striking contrast in that the specific activity increased solely with the injection of 2-¹⁴C-glucose. Figs. 1-26 and 1-27 taken from the report compare the incorporation of ¹⁴C from either glucose or β-hydroxybutyrate in two different age groups of suckling rats: 6-day-old (Fig. 1-26) and 15-day-old (Fig. 1-27). At both age

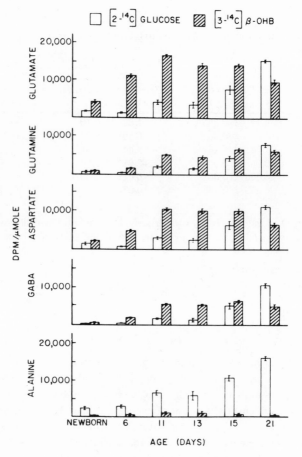

FIG. 1-25

The specific activities of brain amino acids 20 minutes after the subcutaneous injection of 2-14C-glucose or 3-14C-β-hydroxybutyrate. Suckling rats at 12 hours and at 6, 11, 13, 15, and 21 days of age were injected with 0.1 μCi/gm of body weight and decapitated 20 minutes later. Brain acid-soluble extracts were fractionated by column chromatography. The amino acids eluted from the column containing AG50-W resin were converted into DNP-derivatives and separated on silica gel chromagram sheets for determination of their specific activities. (From DeVivo, D. C., Leckie, M. P., and Agrawal, H. C.: D-β-Hydroxybutyrate: a major precursor of amino acids in developing rat brain, J. Neurochem. 25:161-170, 1975.)

groups it is clear that there was far more incorporation of radioactivity into amino acids from β-hydroxybutyrate than from glucose. In fact, in the 15-day-old animals virtually all the radioactivity in the acid-soluble fraction was represented by the radioactivity in the amino acid compartment. However, far more glucose was incorporated into the amino acids in the 15-day-old animals.

COMMENT: The studies by Dahlquist et al. and Jones et al. compare cerebral metabolism in newborn versus adult animals in both rats and sheep. No significant differences in the metabolic profile of substances used by the brain was found for newborn animals compared

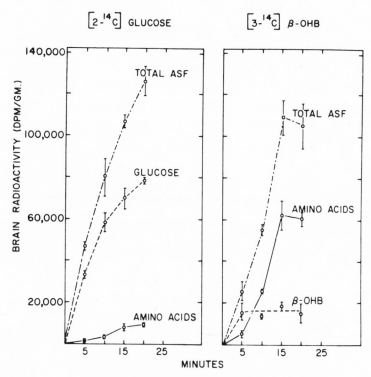

FIG. 1-26

The distribution of the brain acid-soluble radioactivity at various time points after the subcutaneous injection of 2-¹⁴C-β-hydroxybutyrate into 6-day-old suckling rats. After the injection of the (¹⁴C) precursor, animals were decapitated at 5, 10, 15, and 20 minutes. Neutralized acid-soluble fractions (ASF) were prepared as outlined under experimental procedures and then separated into glucose, organic acid, and amino acid fractions. The radioactivity in these fractions is expressed as dpm/gm of wet weight. (From DeVivo, D. C., Leckie, M. P., and Agrawal, H. C.: D-β-Hydroxybutyrate: a major precursor of amino acids in developing rat brain, J. Neurochem. **25:**161-170, 1975.)

with adult animals until some change such as fasting was introduced. There was no evidence of significant anaerobic metabolism by the fetal brain, although a high rate of lactate production by fetal brain tissue in vitro had been reported previously. These in vivo studies did not confirm the in vitro observations. When one considers that oxygen consumption by the fetus is high and is not increased by oxygen administration and that the lactate/pyruvate ratio is within normal adult limits, there is then no reason to suppose that any fetal organ including the brain must rely on anaerobic metabolism to meet its energy needs under normal circumstances.

The study by Settergren et al. confirms in human newborn infants the observations of Dahlquist et al. in newborn rats. In both studies a significant uptake of both glucose and keto acids was found. In Settergren's study the glucose/oxygen quotient alone was greater than 1, and the combined glucose plus keto acid/oxygen quotient was approximately 1.5. Thus in two different newborn species a much greater carbon uptake by the brain in the form of glucose plus keto acids was demonstrated compared with that required for carbon dioxide production. The newborn sheep differed in this respect in that no significant keto

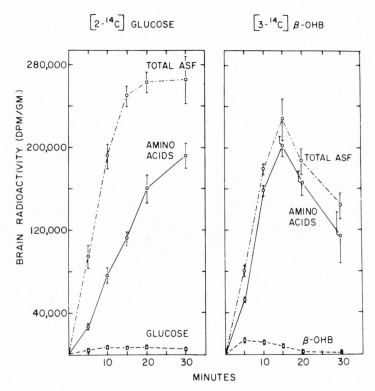

FIG. 1-27

The distribution of the brain acid-soluble radioactivity at various time points after the subcutaneous injection of 2-¹⁴C-glucose or 3-¹⁴C-β-hydroxybutyrate into 15-day-old suckling rats. After the injection of the (¹⁴C) precursor, animals were decapitated at 5, 10, 15, 20, and 30 minutes. Brain tissues were extracted and analyzed as outlined in the legend of Fig. 1-26. (From DeVivo, D. C., Leckie, M. P., and Agrawal, H. C.: D-β-Hydroxybutyrate: a major precursor of amino acids in developing rat brain, J. Neurochem. 25:161-170, 1975.)

acid uptake could be demonstrated. This may be a reflection of the extremely low arterial keto acid concentrations in the sheep and raises the question of what other sources may be supplying additional carbon to the brain in sheep. The study by DeVivo et al. suggests how some of the carbon derived from keto acids may be used by the brain. It appears that β-hydroxybutyrate is being used for the synthesis of glutamate, asparate, and γ-amino-isobutyric acid (GABA) by brain tissue in the newborn. It is possible that in those species in which a high cerebral uptake of keto acids cannot be demonstrated in the newborn period, the uptake of glutamate and aspartate by the brain may be increased. The role of keto acids in the synthesis of cerebral lipids should also be studied. Part of the difficulty with the tracer studies such as those used in the report by DeVivo et al. is that one is not in a position to quantitate the amounts of carbon represented in the various forms of amino acids derived from keto acids. It will be important to describe the carbon balance for the brain at a stage of rapid growth, lipid deposition, and protein synthesis and to see to what extent a common pattern emerges in the principal carbon sources used by the growing brain to meet its fuel and growth requirements.

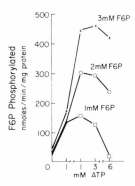

FIG. 1-28

Effect of increasing levels of fructose-6-phosphate, *F6P,* on the inhibitory effect of high levels of ATP in an extract of skeletal muscle from a 100-day fetal rhesus monkey. Incubation time, 4 minutes; 0.6 to 0.7 mg protein/ml incubation medium. The incubation medium was 80 mmol *N*-tris(hydroxymethyl)methyl-2-aminomethanesulfonic acid, 80 mmol KCl, 2 mmol NAD, 0.2 mmol $MgCl_2$, 1 mmol fructose-6-PO$_4$, ATP added as indicated ($MgCl_2$ maintained at equimolar concentrations), 200 mg/100 ml bovine serum albumin, and pH 7.0, at 37° C. Endogenous levels of ATP in the medium were 0.02 mmol or less and P$_i$ was 0.2 to 0.3 mmol with an incubation time of 10 minutes. (From Beatty, C. H., Young, M. K., and Bocek, R. M.: Control of glycolysis in skeletal muscle from fetal rhesus monkeys, Pediatr. Res. **10:** 149-153, 1976.)

Metabolites and fetal tissues

■ Beatty, C. H., Young, M. K., and Bocek, R. M.: Control of glycolysis in skeletal muscle from fetal rhesus monkeys, Pediatr. Res. **10:**149-153, 1976.

Skeletal muscle was obtained from both adult and fetal rhesus monkeys of 90 to 155 days gestational age. The level of metabolic intermediates and cofactors of the glycolytic pathway in the tissues were measured and mass-action ratios calculated for the various reactions. Their data suggests that pyruvate kinase, hexokinase, and phosphofructokinase (PFK) were rate-limiting for glycolysis in fetal skeletal muscle as early as approximately 50% through gestation. There was a striking effect of ATP concentration on PFK activity in both fetal and adult muscle. The data for the effect of ATP on PFK activity at various fructose-6-phosphate concentrations is presented in Fig. 1-28 taken from their report. The amount of fructose-6-phosphate phosphorylated milligrams of protein was two or three times greater in fetal than in adult muscle. This study demonstrated that citrate at concentrations up to 1.2 mmolar decreased PFK activity markedly even in tissue obtained from 100-day gestation fetuses.

■ Herrera, E., and Freinkel, N.: Metabolites in the liver, brain and placenta of fed or fasted mothers and fetal rats, Horm. Metab. Res. **7:**247-249, 1975.

The concentrations of acetyl-CoA and citrate were determined in the liver of both the pregnant rats and their fetuses and in the fetal brain and placenta. The pregnant rats were divided into two groups: one group fed ad libitum and the others deprived of food for 48 hours prior to study. Acetyl-CoA and citrate were chosen for study because previous work had shown that the concentrations of both these compounds in liver tissue were markedly altered by starvation. These studies confirmed previous work that citrate concentration in maternal liver fell and acetyl-CoA concentration in maternal liver increased with fasting. In contrast, there were no changes in either compound in fetal liver. The citrate concentration in the placenta and fetal brain increased. These changes are compatible with an increased rat of fatty acid oxidation in placental and fetal brain in response to maternal starvation.

COMMENT: The observations of Beatty et al. demonstrate that at least one key feature of the glucose fatty acid cycle proposed by Randle et al. (The glucose fatty-acid cycle, Lancet 1:785, 1963) occurs in fetal as well as adult tissue: an increased concentration of citrate in muscle tissue would decrease glucose uptake and utilization. Therefore this report demonstrates that citrate inhibition of PFK activity is a general property of skeletal muscle in both fetuses and adults, a tissue mass considerably larger than cardiac and diaphragm muscle, tissues in which this phenomenon had previously been demonstrated. In summary, the concentrations of substrates and cofactors in tissues and their effect on PFK activity were shown to be similar in fetal and adult muscle tissue.

Whether the observations reported by Beatty et al. are relevant to the citrate concentration changes in placenta and fetal brain described by Herrera and Freinkel is unclear at this time. Herrera and Freinkel's study certainly points out differences in the response of maternal and fetal liver to fasting. Their interpretation that the increase in citrate concentrations reflects perhaps an increased rate of fatty acid oxidation in the placenta and brain is an interesting speculation, particularly since no one at this time has demonstrated significant fatty acid oxidation by fetal brain in direct measurements across the cerebral circulation.

CHAPTER 2

Nutrition

Nutritional factors affecting reproductive performance

- Riopelle, A. J., and Hale, P. A.: Nutritional and environmental factors affecting gestation length in rhesus monkeys, Am. J. Clin. Nutr. 28:1170-1176, 1975.

This study reports data on the length of gestation in forty-seven live-born infant rhesus monkeys. The data were obtained in rhesus monkeys who had first been acclimated to a semisynthetic diet providing approximately 4 gm of protein per kilogram of body weight daily. The animals were divided into three groups: those receiving a diet providing 4, 2, and 1 gm/kg/24 hr. At the end of the study, gestation length was analyzed against the independent variables of infant sex, maternal weight at the time of conception, dietary intake, and ambient temperature. It was found that the higher the protein intake in the diet, the shorter the length of gestation. The gestation length was shortened approximately 8½ days in the animals receiving a diet of 4 gm/kg/24 hr. The length of gestation was consistently shorter for female infants at any maternal dietary protein intake. In addition, there was a correlation between ambient temperature and the length of gestation. Gestation length was significantly longer when conceptions occurred in the summer (an approximate increase of 1 day in the length of gestation for every 2° C rise in average ambient temperature at the time of conception). There was no statistically significant correlation between maternal conception weight and gestation length. Thus the study demonstrated an effect of the pregnant monkeys' diet, the infants' sex, and the season of pregnancy on the length of gestation.

- Shevah, Y., Black, W. J. M., Carr, W. R., and Land, R. B.: The effects of nutrition on the reproductive performance of Finn x Dorset ewes. I. Plasma progesterone and LH concentrations during late pregnancy, J. Reprod. Fertil. 45:283-288, 1975.

This study compared progesterone and luteinizing hormone (LH) concentrations with free fatty acid concentrations in the plasma of forty-eight pregnant ewes. The ewes were divided into two groups of twenty-four based on caloric intake and were studied at 120 and 134 days of gestation. The division of animals into two groups was made on day 100 when caloric intake in the two groups was altered as follows. In group I at the higher plane of nutrition, the ewes were provided with a pelleted diet consisting of 33 Kcal/kg of live weight of the ewe, plus 365 Kcal/kg of anticipated total lamb birth weights. An approximation of 3.5, 6.5, and 8.2 kg of total fetal weight was used respectively for singleton, twin, and triplet pregnancies. Thus the animals carrying more fetuses were provided with more calories from 100 days to term. In Group II at the lower level of nutrition, the ewes were provided with half the diet allowed those in Group I. At day 100 before these caloric adjustments of diet were introduced, the concentration of plasma progesterone was significantly correlated with litter size; but there was no correlation of plasma progesterone concentration with litter size on days 120 and 134 when ewes were fed according to litter size. The lower caloric intake in the group of ewes fed fewer calories resulted in a significant increase in plasma progesterone concentration regardless of litter size. In contrast, leuteinizing hormone concentrations showed no major changes during pregnancy and were not altered by the level of nutrition or by litter size. Thus it would appear that maternal nutrition is the determining factor in the correlation of plasma progesterone concentrations with litter size. There was a highly significant correlation between progesterone and free fatty acid concentrations at all stages of gestation. This correlation was found at all nutritional levels. It is possible, therefore, that the impact of maternal nutrition on plasma progesterone concentrations may be mediated through changes in free fatty acid concentration. At any rate, changes in maternal plasma progesterone concentration do provide an indication of the nutritional state of the pregnant sheep.

COMMENT: These two studies provide further information regarding the subtle effects of nutrition on reproduction. Both studies, directly or indirectly, point out how nutritional factors in pregnancy might alter the overall function of the endocrine system and thus affect growth rate and gestation length. In the report by Riopelle and Hale the animals fed a high-protein diet had significantly shorter gestation lengths. The effect of a high-protein diet on gestation length may in part be mediated by the mechanism reported in the study by Shevah et al. in which it was shown that plasma progesterone concentrations were increased in pregnant ewes fed lower total calories, regardless of litter size. If there is a relationship between the normal fall in progesterone concentration in late pregnancy and the onset of parturition, it would be a satisfying teleologic explanation for the impact of nutrition on progesterone concentrations: one would be lengthening gestation and providing more time at a slower growth rate to achieve the same approximate fetal mass at the time of birth. It is interesting in the Riopelle report that gestation lengths were shorter in female infants than in male infants, considering the well-established sexual dimorphism found in most mammals at birth with males being larger than females (Bruce and Norman: Influence of sexual dimorphism on foetal and placental weights in the rat, Nature [Lond.] 257:62-63, 1975).

The study of Shevah et al. elegantly confirms that the alterations in progesterone concentration related to litter size simply reflect a discrepancy between the total caloric intake of the pregnant ewe and the total amount of fetal tissue to be produced; that is, when they adjusted caloric intake at two different planes but provided additional calories based on litter size, then progesterone concentration became independent of litter size and reflected simply the plane of nutrition. The correlation found between progesterone concentrations and maternal free fatty acid concentration provides at least one mechanism by which alterations in the mother's nutritional state might have a direct bearing on fetal metabolism and fetal tissue composition.

Mineral and vitamin deficiencies

■ Shaw, J. C. L.: Evidence for defective skeletal mineralization in low-birthweight infants: the absorption of calcium and fat, Pediatrics 57:16-25, 1976.

Calcium balance studies were conducted in eleven preterm and two full-term small-for-gestational age (SGA) infants. The studies were done during the first 2 months of life. The infants were compared in terms of the percentage of calcium absorbed and retained and the percentage of fat absorbed using four different milk formulas: whole cow's milk, half-skim cow's milk, a modified cow's milk formula, and breast milk. The study showed that all infants absorbed less calcium than would have been required at a comparable postconceptual age in utero. The infants fed breast milk had an absolute dietary deficiency of calcium, and those fed other milk had a deficiency in calcium accretion reflecting inadequate absorption.

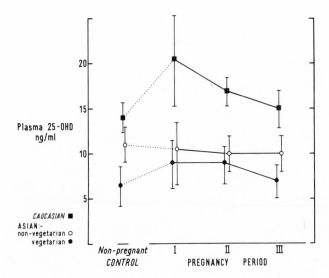

FIG. 2-1
Plasma 25-OHD levels in controls and three groups of patients during their pregnancies.
(From Dent, C. E., and Gupta, M. M.: Plasma 25-hydroxyvitamin-D levels during pregnancy
in Caucasians and in vegetarian and non-vegetarian Asians, Lancet **2:**1057-1060, 1975.)

The retention of calcium in preterm infants averaged 38%, 27%, and 17% for cow's milk,
SMA., and breast milk, respectively. There was no apparent relationship between the percentage of fat absorption on the various milk diets and the percentage of dietary calcium
absorbed.

■ Dent, C. E., and Gupta, M. M.: Plasma 25-hydroxyvitamin-D levels during pregnancy in
   Caucasians and in vegetarian and non-vegetarian Asians, Lancet **2:**1057-1060, 1975.

This study reports data on plasma 25-hydroxyvitamin D (25-OHD) levels and on calcium phosphorus and alkaline phosphorus levels during pregnancy in pregnant women. The
pregnant women included both Causasians and Asians. In the latter group were included
both vegetarians and those taking a nonvegetarian diet. Fig. 2-1 taken from their report
presents the data on 25-OHD levels. It is clear that in all periods of pregnancy the Asian
women, particularly those taking a vegetarian diet, had significantly lower 25-OHD levels
than did Caucasian women. However, there was no demonstrable fall in 25-OHD levels
throughout pregnancy. A relationship between maternal 25-OHD levels and the infant's birth
weight was demonstrated. 25-OHD levels in the umbilical cord blood were approximately
80% to 90% of the maternal levels.

■ Williams, M. L., Shott, R. J., O'Neal, P. L., and Oski, F. A.: Role of dietary iron and fat
   on vitamin E deficiency anemia of infancy, N. Engl. J. Med. **292:**887-890, 1975.

This study presents data on hemoglobin concentrations, reticulocyte counts, vitamin E
concentrations, and susceptibility to hydrogen peroxide hemolysis for newborn infants fed
four different formulas. The composition of the formulas is presented in Table 2-1. They
varied in two important respects: first, in the presence or absence of iron supplementation,
and second, in the percentage of the total fatty acids in the formula represented by polyunsaturated linoleic acid. The infants fed formula B, which contained both a high percent-

TABLE 2-1
Composition of formulas*†

| | Fatty acids (%) | | | | |
Formula	c16:0	c18:1	c18:2	Iron (mg/l)	E:PUFA‡
A	10.4	18.7	32.4	0	1.3
B	10.4	18.7	32.4	12.0	1.3
C	12.4	39.8	12.8	0	1.3
D	12.4	39.8	12.8	13.3	1.3

*From Williams, M. L., Shott, R. J., O'Neal, P. L., and Oshi, F. A.: Role of dietary iron and fat on vitamin E deficiency anemia of infancy, reprinted by permission of The New England Journal of Medicine 292:887-890, 1975.
†Formula A, Similac (Ross Laboratories, Columbus, Ohio); formula B, Similac with iron (Ross Laboratories); formula C, SMA (prepared specifically without iron, not commercially available, Wyeth Laboratories, Radnor, Pa.); Formula D, SMA (Wyeth Laboratories). All formulas had fat content of 3.5 gm/100 dl and vitamin E content of 10 IU/liter.
‡Ratio of vitamin E to amount of polyunsaturated fatty acids.

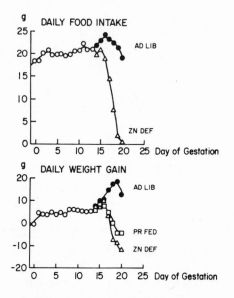

FIG. 2-2
Daily food intake and weight gain of the three groups of rats. The zinc-deficient group of dams was placed on the zinc-deficient regimen on the morning of day 14 of gestation. There were 26 dams in the zinc-deficient group, 25 in the pair-fed group, and 27 in the ad libitum–fed group. Weight gains were significantly depressed (p < .01) by day 18 for both zinc-deficient (4.3 ± 1.6 [SEM] gm) and pair-fed dams (5.0 ± 1.7 gm) in comparison with the ad libitum–fed controls (15.2 ± 0.9 gm) and by day 19 (p < .01) for zinc-deficient (−7.4 ± 1.1) compared with pair-fed controls (−0.4 ± 1.4 gm). Food intake was significantly depressed (p < .01) on day 15 for the zinc-deficient dams (19.4 ± 0.8 gm) when compared with the ad libitum–fed controls (22.9 ± 1.0 gm). (From McKenzie, J. M., Fosmire, G. J., and Sandstead, H. H.: Zinc deficiency during the latter third of pregnancy: effects on fetal rat brain, liver, and placenta, J. Nutr. 105:1466-1475, 1975.)

age of polyunsaturated fat and iron supplementation, had significantly lower hemoglobin concentrations and higher reticulocyte counts than did the infants fed the other three formulas. Both groups of infants fed formulas with high polyunsaturated fats showed a higher percentage of hemolysis in the hydrogen peroxide hemolysis tests. Thus it would appear that dietary intake, including iron, vitamin E, and the composition of fatty acids, all play a role conjointly in determining the susceptibility of a newborn infant to develop a significant degree of hemolytic anemia.

■ McKenzie, J. M., Fosmire, G. J., and Sandstead, H. H.: Zinc deficiency during the latter third of pregnancy: effects on fetal rat brain, liver, and placenta, J. Nutr. **105:**1466-1475, 1975.

This study investigated the effects of zinc deficiency introduced in the latter third of gestation in rats. The pregnant rats were divided into three groups: (1) a zinc-deficient group, (2) a pair-fed control group, and (3) an ad libitum–fed control group. Zinc deficiency introduces a marked anorexia and thus a reduction in daily food intake. Fig. 2-2 demonstrates the striking change in daily food intake among the ad libitum and zinc-deficient pregnant animals and the reduction in daily weight gain that occurred in both the pair-fed and zinc-deficient animals. Table 2-2 demonstrates that in the zinc-deficient group both the fetal brain and liver were reduced in weight compared with both the pair-fed and ad libitum–fed controls. The effect on the liver was most striking. The changes in the placenta were of a lesser order of magnitude than the changes in other fetal organs. Both the pair-fed control and the zinc-deficient animal were characterized by a lower total caloric intake. The placenta was spared relative to the fetus, giving a somewhat increased placental/fetal weight ratio compared with the ad libitum–fed controls.

TABLE 2-2
Weight of fetuses, fetal brain, fetal liver, and placentas*†

Group		Fetal weight gm	Brain weight		Liver weight		Placental weight	
			gm	Percent of fetal weight	gm	Percent of fetal weight	gm	Percent of fetal weight
Zinc deficient	$\overline{X}$	3.98‡§	0.166‡§	4.2	0.227‡§	5.7	0.455	11.4
	SEM	0.09	0.004		0.009		0.015	
	n	23	21		21		21	
Pair-fed control	$\overline{X}$	4.25‡	0.178‖	4.2	0.260‡	6.1	0.473	11.1
	SEM	0.08	0.003		0.011		0.017	
	n	24	21		21		21	
Ad libitum–fed control	$\overline{X}$	4.96	0.188	3.8	0.346	7.0	0.489	9.8
	SEM	0.06	0.002		0.008		0.017	
	n	27	27		27		27	

*From McKenzie, J. M., Fosmire, G. J., and Sandstead, H. H.: Zinc deficiency during the latter third of pregnancy: effects on fetal rat brain, liver, and placenta, J. Nutr. **105:**1466-1475, 1975.
†Data are means derived from the eight fetuses nearest the median weight for the litter; n indicates the number of liters analyzed.
‡Significantly different from ad libitum control group, p < .01.
§Significantly different from pair-fed control group by Student's *t* test, p < .05.
‖Significantly different from ad libitum–fed control group by Student's *t* test, p < .01.

COMMENT: The report by Shaw illustrates a study design appearing with increasing frequency in the pediatric literature. Essentially, it examines the impact of various modified milk formulas on nutritional balance studies in preterm babies and compares the adequacy of their intake in terms of the accretion that would have occurred had the preterm infants continued with intrauterine development. In this report the focus is on calcium balance and demonstrated the fact that whether modified cow's milk or human breast milk was used, all infants had deficiency in calcium accretion when compared with calcium accretion rates that would have occurred in utero.

The article by Dent and Gupta challenges earlier reports, presented in Chapter 14 of the first volume of *Perinatal Medicine: Review and Comments.* Earlier reports in *Lancet* had suggested a relationship between vitamin D intake in the latter third of pregnancy and calcium deposition, enamel deposition in the deciduous teeth, and incidence of neonatal tetany. The suggestion from those earlier studies was that in a high-risk group of pregnant women for vitamin D deficiency, vitamin D intakes may be marginal. In that group, the degree of exposure to sunlight may alter the amounts of 25-OHD available for placental transfer to the fetus and thus alter calcium metabolism within the fetus. This, in turn, would be reflected by changes in the newborn infant's calcium concentration immediately after birth. Dent and Gupta's report points out that there certainly were lower 25-OHD levels in Asian women than in Caucasian women, but these authors were unable to demonstrate any decrease in vitamin D levels throughout pregnancy. They did confirm earlier studies that showed a relationship between maternal 25-OHD concentrations and cord blood concentrations. Although the data of Dent and Gupta do not provide evidence of a vitamin D deficiency in the fetuses of vegetarian women, one must be cautious in that conclusion. A single determination of vitamin D concentration in umbilical cord blood may be a poor reflection of total vitamin D transfer during the latter third of pregnancy. The changes in enamelization of deciduous teeth and in incidence of tetany in newborn infants may, in fact, be a better reflection of an overall imbalance in calcium metabolism in those fetuses. These changes in enamelization may in part be due to a deficient intake of vitamin D over many days of gestation.

The study by Williams et al. makes evident the complexity of attempting to relate a single dietary factor to changes in red cell metabolism. Their study demonstrated that when the diet contained both a high–polyunsaturated fat intake and an increased amount of iron, there were significantly lower hemoglobin concentrations and higher reticulocyte counts in the infants. In this regard, their study parallels that of Ballabriga and Martinez (also reported in this chapter): alterations in the proportion of polyunsaturated to saturated fats in the diet alter red cell lipid stroma. This altered red cell lipid stroma might then demonstrate an increased susceptibility to vitamin E deficiency and indicate iron supplementation.

The report by McKenzie et al. describing the impact of zinc deficiency on fetal growth is interesting in a number of aspects. To start with, it confirms the striking effect of zinc deficiency on total caloric intake in still another mammalian species. Furthermore, the authors observe that in this instance a reduced caloric intake in pregnant animals was associated with a more marked reduction in fetal body weight than in placental weight, leading to a decreased fetal/placental weight ratio. This is particularly interesting in light of both the Dutch famine studies and the studies in Central America concerning the impact of malnutrition on human pregnancy. A characteristic occurrence accompanying poor nutritional intake by pregnant women is that the reduction in weight is most striking in the mothers, less so in the placenta, and least in the fetus. Zinc deficiency and its concomitant reduction in caloric intake for the pregnant animals is an interesting exception to this general pattern.

Nutrition and pregnancy

■ Stein, H.: Maternal protein depletion and small-for-gestational-age babies, Arch. Dis. Child. **50:**146-148, 1975.

In this study 103 mothers who delivered single low birth weight babies were studied for plasma protein concentration. The infants were given a clinical estimate of gestational age by using the scoring system proposed by Dubowitz et al. (Clinical assessment of gestational age in the newborn infant, J. Pediatr. **77:**1-10, 1970). The pregnant women were selected from a population of underprivileged urban Africans who had been shown to have an exceptionally high incidence of SGA babies (Stein and Ellis: The low birth weight African baby, Arch. Dis. Child. **49:**156-159, 1974). Fig. 2-3 presents the birthweight/gestational age distribution of the infants for mothers whose serum albumin concentrations were below 3 gm/dl and those whose albumin concentrations were 3 gm/dl or higher. The incidence

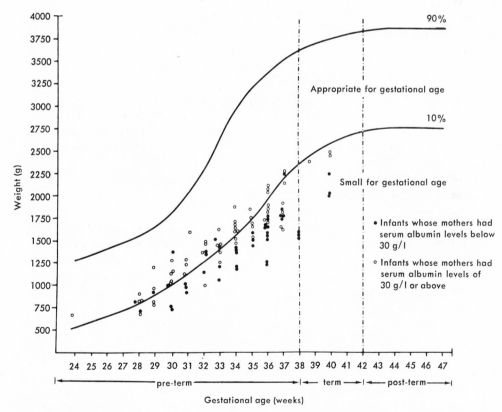

FIG. 2-3
Cases plotted on chart relating birth weights and gestational age of infants to maternal serum albumin levels. (From Stein, H.: Maternal protein depletion and small-for-gestational age babies, Arch. Dis. Child. **50:**146-148, 1975.)

TABLE 2-3

Correlation between maternal factors (independent variables) and each of dependent variables—sample 1 (n = 129)*

	Birth weight	Cranial volume	MOT	MDQ
Maternal height	0.2787§	0.1283	0.1571†	0.1020
Prepregnant weight	0.3793§	0.2563‡	−0.0127	0.0109
Weight gain (N = 125)	0.1815†	0.1260	0.0961	0.0959
Amino acids	0.1477†	0.0735	0.0959	0.0478
Proteins	−0.0162	−0.0731	0.0440	−0.0348
Globulins	−0.0309	−0.1413	−0.0141	−0.0119
Albumin	−0.0014	0.0514	0.0574	−0.0227
Alpha$_1$ globulin	−0.1014	−0.2140‡	−0.2212‡	−0.2387‡
Alpha$_2$ globulin	0.0018	−0.0708	0.0234	0.0491
Beta globulin	0.1002	−0.0361	−0.0514	0.0201
Gamma globulin	−0.0900	−0.1097	0.0876	0.0819

*From Moghissi, K. S., Churchill, J. A., and Kurrie, D.: Relationship of maternal amino acids and proteins to fetal growth and mental development, Am. J. Obstet. Gynecol. **123:**398-410, 1975.
†p < .05.
‡p < .01.
§p < .001.
MOT, motor development; MDQ, mental development.

TABLE 2-4

Contribution (percent variance) of maternal height and weight and significant blood measures (sample 2) to the four infant dependent variables (second set of regression analysis)*

Birth weight	Percent of variance	F value	p
Maternal height	7.6	3.582	NS
Maternal weight (prepregnancy)	8.7	20.122	<0.01
Valine†	3.1	12.555	<0.01
Lysine	4.6	8.136	<0.01
Gamma globulin†	3.3	5.552	<0.05
All together	27.3	9.118	<0.01

*From Moghissi, K. S., Churchill, J. A., and Kurrie, D.: Relationship of maternal amino acids and proteins to fetal growth and mental development, Am. J. Obstet. Gynecol. **123:**398-410, 1975.
†Negative correlation.

of SGAs among those whose albumin concentrations were ≥3 gm/dl was 44% but 76% among those whose albumin concentrations were <3 gm/dl.

■ Moghissi, K. S., Churchill, J. A., and Kurrie, D.: Relationship of maternal amino acids and proteins to fetal growth and mental development, Am. J. Obstet. Gynecol. **123:**398-410, 1975.

This study reports data on plasma concentrations of amino acids and protein at 32 to 34 weeks and 34 to 36 weeks of gestational age in 129 obstetric patients. The maternal weight

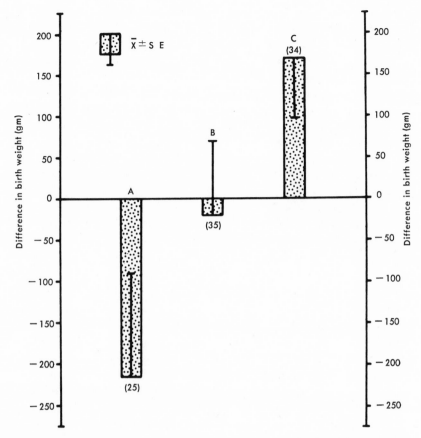

FIG. 2-4
Relationship between differences in caloric supplementation and birth weight for two
consecutive siblings (second birth weight minus first birth weight); n = 94 pairs. Difference
in caloric supplementation during pregnancy: $A = -40,000$ to 0 calories; $B = 100$ to 20,000
cal.; $C = 20,000$ to 120,000 cal. Numbers in parentheses indicate numbers of pairs. Difference
between A and C: $p < .01$. (From Lechtig, A., Habicht, J., Delgado, H., Klein, R. E.,
Yarbrough, C., and Martorell, R.: Effect of food supplementation during pregnancy on
birthweight, Pediatrics **56**:508-520, 1975.)

gain in pregnancy, prepregnancy weight, and nutritional intake were also compared with the
birth weight and length of the newborn infant. Additional measurements made on the infant
included cranial volume and mental and motor development at 8 months of age assessed by
the Bayley scale. Stepwise regression analysis was carried out to determine the correlation, if
any, between each mother's measurements and the infant's body proportions and later mental
and motor development. Table 2-3 demonstrates that maternal size (i.e., maternal height and
prepregnancy weight) was significantly correlated with the infant's birth weight. A rather
striking finding was that only lysine among all the amino acids was shown to have a positive
correlation with infant birth weight independent of maternal prepregnancy weight or maternal height. This is shown in Table 2-4. Cranial volume at birth correlated significantly
with maternal glycine and alpha$_1$ globulin concentrations.

■ Lechtig, A., Habicht, J., Delgado, H., Klein, R. E., Yarbrough, C., and Martorell, R.: Effect of food supplementation during pregnancy on birthweight, Pediatrics 56:508-520, 1975.

The study was conducted in four rural villages of Guatemala. The supplementation included one diet that provided a protein supplement as well as total calories and another that supplied total calories as carbohydrates. Both diets supplemented iron and vitamin intake. Both diets were adequate to achieve an increase in total caloric intake during pregnancy. There was a consistent correlation between the birth weight and the amount of calories supplemented during pregnancy even after the birth weight was corrected for maternal home diet, height, head circumference, parity, gestational age, duration of disease during pregnancy, and socioeconomic status. Fig. 2-4 taken from their report summarizes these results and presents the differences in birth weight versus caloric supplementation for two consecutive siblings. No differences were seen between the two diets used for supplementation; that is, no specific advantage of the diet supplementing calories and protein was found over that supplying calories as carbohydrate alone.

■ Riopelle, A. J., Hill, C. W., and Li, S.: Protein deprivation in primates. V. Fetal mortality and neonatal status of infant monkeys born of deprived mothers, Am. J. Clin. Nutr. 28: 989-993, 1975.

This study presents the outcome of seventy-four pregnancies in forty-five rhesus monkeys who were fed semisynthetic diets offering 1, 2, or 4 gm of protein/kg/24 hr during pregnancies. Dietary intake was arranged to provide approximately the same caloric intake but to vary protein intake. The study demonstrates that the restriction of protein intake did not produce infants with significantly different birth weights or radius lengths, the latter being used as an index of skeletal growth. This is in contrast to previous studies carried out by others in rats. Also, there were no significant differences in fetal survival rates among the three groups, although the lower protein intake was associated with an approximately 40% fetal wastage compared with 20% in the mothers on the 4 gm protein diet. Because of the small numbers of animals involved, these differences were not significant.

TABLE 2-5
Mean skinfold thickness at birth (±1 SD) related to maternal skinfold*

	Maternal triceps skinfold percentiles		
	>*90th (obese)*	*10th-90th (normal)*	<*10th (thin)*
Number of infants	61	179	25
Skinfold thickness (mm)			
Biceps	3.3 ± 0.7†	3.0 ± 0.6‡	2.7 ± 0.5
Triceps	4.4 ± 0.9†	3.9 ± 0.8‡	3.6 ± 0.9
Subcapsular	4.6 ± 1.2†	4.0 ± 1.0	3.6 ± 1.0
Suprailiac	3.7 ± 0.9†	3.3 ± 0.7§	2.8 ± 0.7
Sum of 8 skinfolds	32.2 ± 6.1†	28.6 ± 5.7§	25.4 ± 5.8

*From Whitelaw, A. G. L.: Influence of maternal obesity on subcutaneous fat in the newborn, Br. Med. J. 1:985-986, 1976.
†Significantly greater than skinfolds of babies of normal mothers (p <.001).
Significantly greater than skinfolds of babies of thin mothers:
‡p <.05.
§p <.01.

■ Whitelaw, A. G. L.: Influence of maternal obesity on subcutaneous fat in the newborn, Br. Med. J. 1:985-986, 1976.

Skinfold thickness measurements were made to estimate body fat on 265 full-term new-born infants. The measurements were made bilaterally on the biceps, triceps, and subcapsular and suprailiac sites. The infants were divided into three groups depending on the mother's obesity: (1) 25 in a group in whom the mother's triceps skinfold measurements were less than the 10th percentile, (2) 179 in which they were normal, and (3) 61 in which they were above the 90th percentile. The average birth weights in the three groups were significantly different (p < .01). The mean birth weight in the obese mothers was 3.6 kg; in the normal, 3.4 kg; and in the thin, 3.0 kg. Table 2-5 taken from their report demonstrates that not only was body weight correlated with maternal obesity determined by tricep-skinfold measurements, but also body fat determined by the skinfold caliper measurements was significantly increased in those babies born to mothers with obesity. When mothers in the obese group were subdivided into those who were hypertensive and those who were normotensive, the hypertensive group was shown to deliver infants having lower birth weights and lower skinfold measurements than the normotensive group.

■ Andrew, G., Chan, G., and Schiff, D.: Lipid metabolism in the neonate. I. The effects of Intralipid infusion on plasma triglyceride and free fatty acid concentrations in the neonate, J. Pediatr. 88:273-278, 1976.

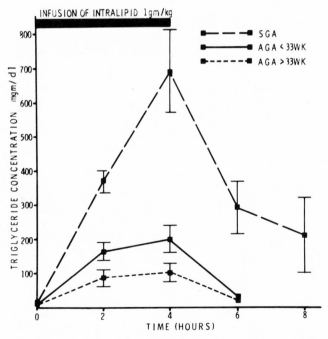

FIG. 2-5
Sequential changes in plasma triglyceride concentration during infusion of Intralipid and the postinfusion period in the three groups of infants (mean ± SEM). (The SEM is not shown where less than 20 mg/dl.) (From Andrew, G., Chan, G., and Schiff, D.: Lipid metabolism in the neonate. I. The effects of Intralipid infusion or plasma triglyceride and free fatty acid concentrations in the neonate, J. Pediatr. 88:273-278, 1976.)

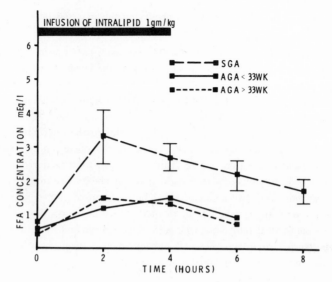

FIG. 2-6

Sequential changes in plasma FFA concentration during the infusion of Intralipid and the postinfusion period in the three groups of infants (mean ± SEM). (The SEM is not shown where less than 0.2 mEq/L.) (From Andrew, G., Chan, G., and Schiff, D.: Lipid metabolism in the neonate. I. The effects of Intralipid infusion on plasma triglyceride and free fatty acid concentrations in the neonate, J. Pediatr. **88:**273-278, 1976.)

This study presents the data on free fatty acid and triglyceride concentrations in the plasma of twenty-seven newborn infants in the first 48 hours of life. The infants were challenged with an Intralipid infusion over a 4-hour period, providing 1 gm/kg of Intralipid. The clearance of triglyceride and free fatty acid from the plasma was much slower in SGA infants than in either group of AGA preterm babies. Within the group consisting of preterm AGA infants, those that were less than 33 weeks' gestation had significantly slower rates of triglyceride clearance than did the more mature preterm infant. There were no differences among the two groups of preterm infants in free fatty acid clearance. Figs. 2-5 and 2-6 taken from their report summarize the data on triglyceride concentrations in the plasma for the three groups of infants during and immediately after the Intralipid infusions.

- Crawford, J. D., and Osler, D. C.: Body composition at menarche: the Frisch-Revelle hypothesis revisited, Pediatrics 56:449-458, 1975.

This study presents an analysis of the relationship between the onset of menarche, figures for height and weight, and derived values for total body water and fat in young girls. The girls included children with a variety of disorders, including unusually tall stature, central idiopathic precocity, precocity associated with hypothyroidism, hypothyroidism without evidence of sexual maturation, obesity, and children with gonadal dysgenesis. The conclusions from this analysis supported the hypothesis proposed by Frisch et al. (Components of weight at menarche and the initiation of the adolescent growth spurt in girls: estimated total water, lean body weight and fat, Hum. Biol. **45:**469-483, 1973) that menarche is highly correlated with the achievement of a characteristic body composition. In most girls this would also mean a correlation with a critical body weight, since body composition and body weight would be intimately related in the absence of disease.

COMMENT: These studies present a variety of effects of maternal nutrition on fetal growth. The report by Stein et al. demonstrates that in a population with an exceptionally high rate of SGA babies (underprivileged urban Africans), a group could be isolated in whom the incidence of SGAs was 76%. This selection could be done simply by a measurement of plasma albumin concentration of the mother. Obviously the albumin concentration represents only one indirect reflection of maternal nutrition status, but it is most impressive that such a simple measurement could isolate a population in whom three fourths of the infants would be SGA. The report by Moghissi et al. presents a more comprehensive study of both maternal plasma protein concentrations and maternal plasma amino acid concentrations in a population whose overall nutritional intake would be far superior to the population studied by Stein et al. The multifactorial analysis of Moghissi et al. demonstrated several interesting correlations. Perhaps the most intriguing was the fact that lysine was singled out among the amino acids, showing a direct correlation in the maternal concentration of this amino acid and the infant's birth weight. This is significant considering the report by Lemons et al. reviewed in Chapter 1. In that report they found that lysine and histidine were crossing the placenta in quantities approximately equal to that required for new tissue deposition. These observations suggest a narrow margin of safety between umbilical uptake of those amino acids and the requirements of fetal growth. The observations of Moghissi et al. certainly need further confirmation. Considering the report by Shevah et al., previously reviewed in this chapter, regarding an effect of nutritional level in pregnancy on progesterone concentrations in sheep, it would have been interesting to couple nutritional intake of the mothers with measurement of progesterone and free fatty acid concentration.

The report by Lechtig et al. from the INCAP* studies in Guatemala extends early observations on nutritional intake and its effect on infant growth. The current report documents that it is a reduction in total caloric intake which reduces infant growth and that this can be corrected by supplementing the diet with additional calories in the form of carbohydrate and does not require specific supplementation with protein. Presumably, when total caloric intake of pregnant women is markedly reduced, the mother uses calories supplied in the form of carbohydrates to meet her own fuel requirements and provides the nitrogen essential for growth to the fetus in the form of amino acids mobilized from her own tissue proteins. In this regard the INCAP studies suggest a similarity to the adaptations made in some other mammals, such as the hibernating bear, which permit the growth of the fetus at a time when there is essentially no nitrogen intake by the mother. Presumably, at that time the mother meets her fuel requirements by the mobilization of fat and again supplies the nitrogen required for the fetus for growth by mobilization of maternal tissue protein. The study by Riopelle et al. in rhesus monkeys also confirms the fact that at a fixed caloric intake, one could vary the protein intake fourfold without demonstrable effect on fetal birth weight.

The report by Whitelaw relates maternal obesity to infant size and body composition. The report demonstrates that maternal obesity correlates with an increase not only in fetal body weight but also in body fat. It confirms elegantly an observation commonly accepted in clinical obstetrical practice. It would be important to know how infant size and body fat composition was altered in a group of obese patients who varied in their weight gain during the pregnancy; that is, what is the impact of reduced caloric intake during pregnancy on

---

*Institute of Nutrition of Central America and Panama.

infant growth when the prepartum weight of the mother reflects her obesity. The study is particularly important considering earlier reports (Brook: Evidence for a sensitive period in adipose-cell replication in man, Lancet 2:624-625, 1972), which related the number of adipose cells in children with obesity and subdivided this group into those who were obese from infancy and those obese after 1 year of age. His report demonstrated that when obesity was present in infancy, the children had an increase in total number of adiposites. Presumably, the same effect of early obesity would apply to those infants born with an increased body fat at birth. The report by Andrew et al. describes the alterations in plasma triglyceride and free fatty acid concentrations introduced in newborn infants by Intralipid infusions. It is clear that there are rather striking differences among newborn infants in their ability to metabolize the complex mixture of lipids provided by Intralipid. Taken against the background of the previous studies described in this chapter, which point out numerous changes introduced in body composition and fat deposition when alterations are made in lipid composition of the diets of newborn infants, as well as the report of Andrew et al., which presents the differences and rates of metabolism, one would have to approach the use of Intralipid in markedly preterm infants with considerable caution. (For related articles on the impact of nutrition on subsequent development, see Chapter 3.)

The study by Crawford and Osler is a continuation of a number of studies initiated by Frisch on an important topic in reproductive biology. This report examines the relationship between body composition, metabolic rate, and onset of menarche in young girls. Because body composition in adolescence can be related to nutrition in the perinatal period, it does provide a link between nutritional state of the fetus and newborn infant and a later impact on reproduction. Crawford and Osler had shown previously that in children who were bedridden, menarche occurred when they reached a body composition similar to that of normal girls at the time of menarche. This meant that in the bedridden girls, menarche was achieved at a much lower total body weight (Osler and Crawford: Examination of the hypothesis of a critical weight at menarche in ambulatory and bedridden mentally retarded girls, Pediatrics 51:675-679, 1973). This study is important in providing further clinical information supporting and strengthening the relationship of the attainment of a critical body composition to the onset of menarche.

■ Davies, D. P., Gray, O. P., Ellwood, P. C., and Abernathy, M.: Cigarette smoking in pregnancy: associations with maternal weight gain and fetal growth, Lancet 1:385-387, 1976.

This study reexamines the effect of smoking during pregnancy on fetal growth. Anthropomorphic measurements were made on the newborn infant, and the changes in body proportions were correlated with the changes in maternal weight gain in pregnancy. Table 2-6 demonstrates that in heavy smokers there was a significant reduction in birth weight. The mean length and head circumferences of the newborn infants were lower in the heavy smokers than in the nonsmokers. It is not clear from the report whether these differences are statistically significant.

COMMENT: When the maternal weight gain is considered, it is clear that a great part of the reduction in infant birth weight can be explained by the fact that the heavy smokers gained less weight in pregnancy. It has previously been demonstrated that maternal weight gain and fetal birth weight were significantly related. Thus, some of the intrauterine growth retardation that occurs with heavy smoking must be ascribed to the reduced weight gain

TABLE 2-6

Means and standard errors of infants' birth weight, length, and head circumference and maternal rate of change of weight by maternal smoking habit*

Variable	Nonsmokers	Light-to-moderate smokers (1-14 cigarettes/24 hr)	Heavy smokers (> 15 cigarettes/24/hr)
Male births			
Birth weight (kg)	3.51 ± 0.026	3.35 ± 0.038	3.27 ± 0.050
Length (cm)	52.5 ± 0.11	51.9 ± 0.17	51.8 ± 0.23
Head circumference (cm)	36.5 ± 0.07	36.3 ± 0.12	36.2 ± 0.13
Maternal weight gain (kg/wk)	0.45 ± 0.024	0.44 ± 0.023	0.32 ± 0.025
Female births·			
Birth weight (kg)	3.38 ± 0.028	3.14 ± 0.050	3.05 ± 0.052
Length (cm)	51.5 ± 0.11	50.8 ± 0.22	50.9 ± 0.25
Head circumference (cm)	35.5 ± 0.07	35.3 ± 0.13	35.1 ± 0.16
Maternal weight gain (kg/wk)	0.45 ± 0.023	0.41 ± 0.035	0.38 ± 0.032

*From Davies, D. P., Gray, O. P., Ellwood, P. C., and Abernathy, M.: Cigarette smoking in pregnancy: associations with maternal weight gain and fetal growth, Lancet 1:385-387, 1976.

of the mother during pregnancy. Chapter 4 discusses the potential effects of smoking on fetal oxygenation.

Dietary intake of lipids and body composition of the infants

■ Crawford, M. A., Hassam, A. G., and Williams, G.: Essential fatty acids and fetal brain growth, Lancet 1:452-453, 1976.

Data are presented on the proportion of longer-chain, polyunsaturated fatty acids, including arachidonic (C20:4,n–6) and docosahexaenoic (C22:6,n–6) acids, in various tissue fluids of pregnant guinea pigs. Pregnant guinea pigs were given ^{14}C-labeled linoleic and linolenic acids orally. The data on the percentage distribution of ^{14}C-labeled phospholipids is presented in Table 2-7. It is clear that most of the radioactivity was still present as the original shorter chain fatty acids in maternal liver, which suggests that chain elongation and desaturation does not occur appreciably in adult liver. However, there was a stepwise increase in the percentage distribution of the isotope within the long-chain polyunsaturated fatty acids, comparing placenta to fetal liver and then to fetal brain tissue. The investigators also examined the phosphoglyceride pattern of fatty acids in human brain tissue; an identical trend was noted. These findings in both the guinea pig and man agree with similar data in rats and imply that in all mammals there is an inability in adult liver to elongate chain length and increase desaturation.

■ Widdowson, E. M., Dauncey, M. J., Gairdner, D. M. T., Jonxis, J. H. P., and Pelikan-Filipkova, M.: Body fat of British and Dutch infants, Br. Med. J. 1:653-655, 1975.

There are remarkable differences in the fatty acid composition of the fat in the milks fed to infants in Britain and the Netherlands. Most British infants who are not breast-fed have received foods based on cow's milk. The most frequently used Dutch food for infants contains maize (corn) oil as a replacement of cow's milk fat. Corn oil has a large percentage of linoleic acid. The fatty acids in the body fat of forty-one British and thirty-seven Dutch infants between birth and 1 year were determined. At birth linoleic acid contributed

TABLE 2-7

Distribution of isotope in fatty acids from total phospholipid of tissues from ginuea pigs dosed orally with either 1-^{14}C-labeled linoleic (18:2,n–6) or linolenic 18:3,n–3) acids with the tissues being sampled 24 hours later*

| | *Percentage distribution of isotope* | | | | | |
| | *n-6 series* | | | *n-3 series* | | |
Tissue	*18:2*	*20:4*	*22:4*	*18:3*	*22:5*	*22:6*
Maternal liver						
Mean ± SEM	86 ± 1.7	1.7 ± 0.2	0.6 ± 0.16	78 ± 1.3	1.05 ± 0.12	0.7 ± 0.09
No. analyzed	8	8	8	6	6	6
Placenta						
Mean ± SEM	72 ± 1.8	10.2 ± 2.3	1.1 ± 0.38	49.2 ± 6.4	6.1 ± 0.62	4.8 ± 0.91
No. analyzed	6	6	6	5	5	5
Fetal liver						
Mean ± SEM	69 ± 4.3	8.3 ± 1.2	3.0 ± 1.0	43.2 ± 2.6	16 ± 1.1	11 ± 0.93
No. analyzed	6	6	6	5	5	5
Fetal brain						
Mean ± SEM	35 ± 1.2	35 ± 3.5	4.0 ± 0.9	12.3 ± 0.6	13 ± 0.67	31 ± 1.42
No. analyzed	5	5	5	6	6	6

*From Crawford, M. A., Hassam, A. G., and Williams, G.: Essential fatty acids and fetal brain growth, Lancet 1: 452-453,1976.

1% to 3% of the total fatty acids of the body fat in infants of both countries. In the subsequent weeks its proportion in the fat of the Dutch infants increased remarkably. (See Fig. 2-7.) This large increase in linoleic acid was accompanied by a fall in the percentage contribution of the saturated acids myristic, palmitic, and stearic. Dutch infants also had a lower concentration of cholesterol in their serum than did British infants. The results show that the triglycerides in the adipose tissue are profoundly influenced by the nature of the fat in the diet.

■ Ballabriga, A., and Martinez, M.: Changes in erythrocyte lipid stroma in the premature infant according to dietary fat composition, Acta Pediatr. Scand. **65:**705-709, 1976.

Eighteen preterm babies of similar gestational age and birth weight were fed milk formulas that provided the same total calories per kilogram per 24 hours. The formulas differed in the percentage of total calories supplied by linoleic acid, formula A supplying 6.1%, formula B 15.9%, and C 0.6%. After 3 weeks on these formulas, the changes in red cell ethanolamine and choline phosphoglycerides were determined. Fig. 2-8 taken from this report demonstrates the fact that in the group fed the low–linoleic acid concentration, changes occurred which were similar to those described in essential fatty acid–deficient rats. There was a marked increase in the concentration of the 20:3,n–6 fatty acid in the red cell stroma. This fatty acid is normally present in trace amounts. It increases with essential fatty acid deficiencies. Despite these changes in the red cell stroma, there was no clinical evidence of essential fatty acid deficiency noted in any of the infants.

■ Räihä, N. C. R., Heinonen, K., Rassin, D. K., and Gaull, G. E.: Milk protein quantity and quality in low-birthweight infants. I. Metabolic responses and effects on growth, Pediatrics **57:**659-674, 1976.

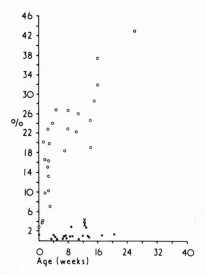

FIG. 2-7

Linoleic acid as percentage of total fatty acids in body fat of British and Dutch infants. British infants fed on cow's milk fat (●), British breast-fed infants (×), and Dutch infants fed on Almiron containing corn oil (○). (From Widdowson, E. M., Dauncey, M. J., Gairdner, D. M. T., Jonxis, J. H. P., and Pelikan-Filipkova, M.: Body fat of British and Dutch infants, Br. Med. J. **1**:653-655, 1975.)

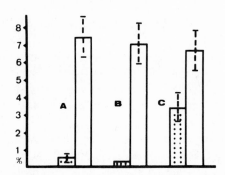

FIG. 2-8

Fatty acid concentrations of 20:3, n–9 to 20:4, n–6 proportion in CPG red cells lipid stroma after 21 days of feeding with the different milk formulas. Blank columns, # 20:4 (n–6); dotted columns, # 20:3 (n–9). (From Ballabriga, A., and Martinez, M.: Changes in erythrocyte lipid stroma in the premature infant according to dietary fat composition, Acta Pediatr. Scand. **65**:705-709, 1976.)

This study compares the four types of formula fed to preterm AGA infants. The groups of infants were subdivided into gestational age categories of 28 to 30 weeks, 31 to 33 weeks, and 34 to 36 weeks. The four formulas differed in two respects. The concentration of protein was either 1.5 or 3 gm/dl and the composition of the protein either 60 parts bovine whey protein to 40 parts bovine casein protein or the same proteins in a proportion of 18 to 82.

The study demonstrated that there was no significant difference among any of the subgroups of infants in terms of their growth rate whether it was measured in crown-rump length, femoral length, head circumference, or weight gain. There were predictable differences in certain biochemical measurements. The infants fed higher protein concentrations showed higher blood urea nitrogens, total serum proteins, serum albumin and globulin concentrations, and urine osmolalities, suggesting that an increasing proportion of total amino acid intake was diverted to amino acid catabolism and the amino acid used as fuels rather than as building blocks for new tissue growth. Ammonia concentrations were increased with all formulas compared with human breast milk or with the formula having a low protein concentration (1.5 gm/dl) and a high proportion of whey to casein proteins (60/40). Metabolic acidosis was associated particularly with the casein-dominant formulas.

■ Mamunes, P., Prince, P. E., Thornton, N. H., Hunt, P. A., and Hitchcock, E. S.: Intellectual deficits after transient tyrosinemia in the term neonate, Pediatrics 57:675-680, 1976.

This study presents follow-up data on the neurologic development of fifteen children who had been born at term and in whom transient neonatal tyrosinemia had been recognized as an outgrowth of newborn screening for phenylketonuria. All the infants were known to have elevated tyrosine concentrations after discharge from the neonatal nursery and all had been receiving an evaporated milk formula providing a high protein content (approximately 5.7 gm/kg/24 hr). None of the infants was receiving supplemental vitamin C until after the diagnosis of severe neonatal tyrosinemia. They were then treated for a 1-month course of a reduced protein intake and vitamin C, 100 mg/24 hr. The mean ± 1 SD for the maximum serum tyrosine concentration was 25.8 ± 9.4 mg/dl. Three psychologic tests were administered to each patient at one time by the same examiner. The three tests were the Peabody Picture Vocabulary Test, the McCarthy Scale of Children's Abilities, and the Illinois Test of Psycholinguistic Ability. Significantly lower scores were obtained on the group of children with transient neonatal tyrosinemia compared with the control group of infants for the McCarthy scale and the Illinois test. These data suggest that transient tyrosinemia may produce specific learning disabilities and indicate the need for further studies regarding appropriate protein intake for newborn infants.

COMMENT: These five reports present additional information regarding the impact of changes of lipid intake on body composition in fetuses and newborn infants. The report by Crawford et al. presents important information regarding the location of synthetic reactions producing compounds essential for normal brain growth. The authors comment that in thirty-two different species of mammals varying widely in food intake there was no difference in the pattern of the long-chain polyunsaturated fatty acid composition in brain tissue, supporting the fact that brain metabolism is rather uniform among mammals. Since the liver of the larger mammals does not seem capable of chain elongation and desaturation, it was an important contribution to document that the synthesis of these long-chain fatty acids presumably takes place in placental tissue in both man and the guinea pig. Perhaps this also occurs in fetal liver, although it is possible that the increasing concentrations of the long-chain fatty acids noted in fetal liver and fetal brain represent accumulation and storage after synthesis in the placenta.

The reports by Widdowson et al. and Ballabriga and Martinez document further changes in tissues of newborn infants fed diets varying in a lipid intake. The report by Widdowson et al. clearly shows that the type of fat stored in the body of an infant is influenced by

the nature of the fat in the diet. Thus, in infants fed a formula containing corn oil as the main source of lipid, linoleic becomes the predominant fatty acid of adipose tissue. It is not known whether this type of fat storage in the first few months of life represents any advantage or disadvantage, although the introduction of corn oil in the diet of Dutch babies was probably due to the current notion that unsaturated fat is preferable. It should be noted that human milk contains relatively small quantities of linoleic acid. Thus careful experimental and clinical observations are needed to decide on a rational basis the pros and cons of diet manipulations in infants. The report of Ballabriga and Martinez documents the changes in red cell lipid stroma that occurred after 3 weeks in preterm babies fed diets varying in linoleic acid concentration. Those receiving the low linoleic acid concentration showed changes in red cell lipid stroma consistent with that found in essential fatty acid deficiency in animals. These studies continue to raise questions concerning the appropriateness of human breast milk as a feeding for markedly preterm infants. In all nurseries there has been a strong impetus to encourage breast milk feeding for the larger and more mature preterm and term infants. This impetus has come from many areas, including an attempt to improve mother-infant contact and the possible advantages of breast milk feeding in avoiding certain infections. (See Chapter 16.) At this stage one can only approach an extension of breast milk feeding to the markedly preterm baby with considerable caution.

Räihä et al. were able to demonstrate that preterm infants grew equally well on milk with large variations in protein concentration from human breast milk up to 3% casein proteins. Whether the biochemical changes they described in the newborn infants—higher urea and ammonia concentrations and a metabolic acidosis associated with the high protein-high casein formulas—have any clinical significance in the preterm is not clear at this time. The need for such studies as that of Räihä et al. is demonstrated in the follow-up studies of Mamunes et al., since they found lower scores in a variety of developmental testing in infants who had transient neonatal tyrosinemia. Such a result should not be construed as reflecting a direct effect of tyrosine concentration on brain development but may, in fact, reflect changes in other amino acids for certain groups of infants fed a high-protein diet, amino acids whose relationship with brain function might be considerably more direct than that of tyrosine.

Technique for feeding low birth weight infants

■ Van Caillie, M., and Powell, G. K.: Nasoduodenal versus nasogastric feeding in the very low birth-weight infant, Pediatrics 56:1065-1072, 1975.

This study reports the results of a comparison between nasoduodenal versus nasogastric feeding for very low birth weight infants. Eleven infants who weighed less than 1300 gm and had gestational ages between 26 and 36 weeks were fed either by nasogastric or nasoduodenal infusions given continuously. The feeding consisted of a modified cow's milk formula (Enfamil, 24 cal/oz). The technique used consisted of placing a relatively stiff plastic catheter (Bardic, Deseret Intracath 1936R) into the nasopharynx and then, with the infant lying on his right side, advancing the tube into the stomach and into the duodenum. The placement of the tube was confirmed by the backflow of bile-stained fluid and was later confirmed radiologically. The infants fed with nasoduodenal tubes tolerated larger volumes (therefore greater calorie intake) per day, with a mean caloric intake of 131 cal/kg/24 hr versus 106 cal/kg/24 hr for those fed with nasogastric tubes. The very low birth weight infants fed by continuous nasoduodenal infusions reached caloric intakes of 120 cal/kg/24 hr within 2 or 3 days after tube placement (approximately half the time required in the nasogastric group).

COMMENT: The report by Van Caillie and Powell examines methods of providing milk feedings to very low birth weight infants. The report is a timely one considering the increase in clinical research aimed directly at describing the most appropriate kind of milk feeding for very immature low birth weight infants. Furthermore, although peripheral alimentation has been used extensively in low birth weight infants, it would seem teleologically much safer to provide nutrition into the gastrointestinal tract, where absorption would lead to delivery of a high concentration of amino acids, fats, and carbohydrates into the portal venous blood rather than into the peripheral venous circulation. The advantage of portal venous infusion essentially is that it allows the liver to continue to function as an effective buffer, altering concentrations of various solutes before they are delivered into the general circulation. Thus, it permits a continuation of the liver's role in buffering change in arterial inflow concentrations to rapidly growing tissues.

In addition, the report by Widdowson et al. reviewed in Chapter 3 points out that feedings placed in the gastrointestinal tract may markedly alter the growth rate of the bowel, and this may represent an extremely important adaptation of the gastrointestinal tract for postnatal survival. In very low birth weight infants, nasoduodenal feedings have been associated with significant complications such as perforations of the small bowel. Duodenal perforations have been reported on several occasions (Shijan et al.: Duodenal perforation: A rare complication of neonatal nasojejunal tube feedings, Pediatrics 55:371-375, 1975; Boros and Reynolds: Duodenal perforation: a complication of neonatal nasojejunal feeding, J. Pediatr. 85:107-108, 1974), as have jejunal perforations (Chen and Wong: Intestinal complications of nasojejunal feeding, J. Pediatr. 85:109-110, 1974) with nasojejunal tubes. Unfortunately, the report of Van Caillie and Powell does not give details regarding the length of time the milk was left at room temperature during the infusion or any data on bacteriology of the milk samples at the point of entry into the infant.

■ Bamford, D. R., and Ingham, P. A.: Sugar absorption by fetal and neonatal rat intestine in vitro, J. Physiol. 248:335-348, 1975.

In this study, tissues were obtained from various areas of the small intestine from fetal, neonatal, and adult rats. The tissues were studied in vitro as everted intestinal rings in terms of their uptake of either ^{14}C-labeled D-galactose or ^{14}C-labeled 3-0-methyl-glucose. The data demonstrate that relatively early in gestation (by the seventeenth day), there is active sugar absorption in the fetal rat intestine, a capacity which persists at that level for approximately the first week of postnatal life. In addition, when various areas of the small intestine were compared in their uptake of ^{14}C-labeled D-galactose, it was found that initially there was a high rate of galactose accumulation in the ileum, but that around the twenty-seventh postnatal day the jejunum became the principal site of galactose accumulation. This coincided with the time at which the absorption of intact protein from the small bowel could no longer be demonstrated.

COMMENT: This study demonstrates one more physiologic characteristic that develops relatively early in gestation and can be interpreted as a preparation of the fetal organ system for the adaptations required for postnatal survival. In this case the ability of the intestine to concentrate sugars begins in late fetal life and would appear to occur before the development of amino acid uptake by the intestine. The continued development and specialization of the small intestine is demonstrated in part by the changing location of the most active site of carbohydrate absorption, which shifts during the first 3 weeks of postnatal life from the ileum to the jejunum. Considering the data that Widdowson et al. (Changes in the organs of pigs in response to feeding for the first 24 hours after birth. II. The digestive tract, Biol. Neonate 28:272-281, 1976) have presented in the pig on the extremely rapid growth of the small intestine immediately after birth, it would be interesting to compare similar changes in the rat in length and weight of different areas of the small intestine and to attempt to relate them to the specific changes described for sugar and amino acid absorption at various points in the gastrointestinal tract.

CHAPTER 3

Growth

Growth of children who were small at birth

■ Beck, G. J., and van den Berg, B. J.: The relationship of the rate of intrauterine growth of low-birth-weight infants to later growth, J. Pediatr. 86:504-511, 1975.

This is part of a longitudinal study of pregnancy, pregnancy outcome, and child health and development. The present report is about 488 single-born infants, surviving the neonatal period, with birth weights from 1501 to 2500 gm, who did not have severe congenital anomalies. The relationship of the rate of intrauterine growth to postnatal growth up to 10 years of age was investigated. Each child was assigned to one of four gestation quartiles that had identical birth weight distribution but differed widely in the lengths of gestation. The mean heights and weights of the children in each of the four quartiles were compared with similar data of a control group who had birth weights above 2500 gm. Height and weight from 1 to 10 years are presented in Fig. 3-1 of the original. The weight curves indicate that the group of infants with short gestation (that is, born prematurely) continue their growth after the first year more rapidly than do those with long gestation (that is, born growth-retarded at term), despite equal birth weights in both groups. The weight of the short gestation group approaches closely the weight of the normal birth weight infants by the age of 2 years and starts diverging from the weight of the long gestation group. It can be seen that at 10 years of age, the children who were growth retarded at birth tend to have a smaller weight than the normal and prematurely born children. The analysis of heights gives analogous results.

■ Clarkson, J. E., Silva, P. A., Buckfield, P. M., and Hardman, J.: The later growth of children who were preterm and small for gestational age, N.Z. Med. J. 81:279-282, 1975.

Weight, height, and head circumference at 4 years of age were compared between 56 preterm, 35 small for gestational age (SGA), and 111 randomly selected normal children. Children who were preterm but were greater than 2500 gm at birth were significantly heavier, taller, and had larger head circumference measurements than the control group. Preterm children who had weighed less than 2500 gm at birth were significantly lighter than the controls. Children who were small for gestational age were significantly shorter and lighter than the control group. The significant differences that are apparent when groups are subdivided according to both gestational age and birth weight emphasize the need to consider both these parameters.

■ Ratten, G. J., Targett, C. S., Drew, J. H., and Beischer, N. A.: The effect of fetal and placental weight at birth on weight during early childhood, Med. J. Aust. 2:735-736, 1975.

This study was on a population of infants born to private patients in Melbourne, Australia. A hundred consecutive infants were selected in four categories according to the position of birth weight or placental weight on percentile charts. The majority of children whose birth weights or placental weights were above the 90th percentile remained oversized

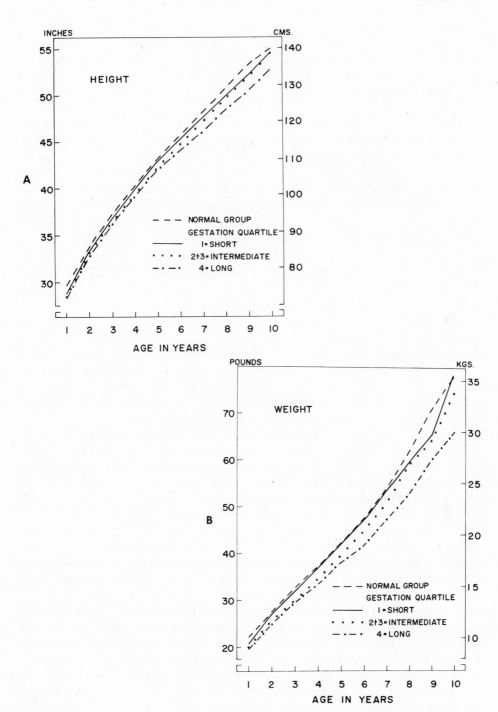

FIG. 3-1
A, Mean height for ages 1 to 10 of all infants in the quartiles for short, intermediate, and long gestation and in the normal group. **B,** Mean weight for ages 1 to 10 of all infants in the quartiles for short, intermediate, and long gestation and in the normal group. (From Beck, G. J., and van den Berg, B. J.: The relationship of the rate of intrauterine growth of low-birth-weight of infants to later growth, J. Pediatr. 86:504-511, 1975.)

during the first year of life. In the same period the small at birth attained a normal distribution curve for weight. There was a good correlation between placental and fetal weight at birth. However, this relationship between placental and infant weight did not continue after birth. It is inferred from such data that the influence of the placenta on infant size is temporary and is modified by extrauterine nutrition.

COMMENT: The importance of distinguishing between preterm and SGA babies in studying the subsequent growth of children who were small at birth is demonstrated clearly in the articles by Clarkson et al. and Beck et al. Both groups of investigators show that the preterm infant has, statistically speaking, a normal growth potential. In fact, a preterm baby who is small in absolute terms but relatively big for gestational age tends to be heavier than normal later in development. To the contrary, some SGA babies do not show adequate catch-up growth and tend to remain smaller, as shown in Fig. 3-1 of the article by Beck et al. Failure to classify newborn babies according to both weight and gestational age may partly explain why there are contradictory statements in the literature concerning growth of infants with small birth weight. As a recent example, Ratten et al. state in their article that children in the small-at-birth category attain a normal distribution curve for weight in the first year of life, but do not specify which type of small baby is under consideration.

The finding that SGA babies tend to remain smaller during subsequent development suggests the conclusion that fetal nutrition has a lasting effect on the whole growth of the human organism. This conclusion may be surprising to anyone who has observed so-called catch-up growth in children. As a rule, after a period of undernourishment, a growing organism tends to grow faster than the normal control until it regains the size that is appropriate for its age. However, experiments in animals have shown conclusively that this rule has important exceptions. In a recent, authoritative review Widdowson and McCance (A review: new thoughts on growth, Pediatr. Res. 9:154-156, 1975) summarize the results of their experiments on newborn rats. They show that rats undernourished before weaning do not become ravenously hungry when given food ad libitum and do not eat enough food to catch up to the weight of normal littermates. By contrast, rats undernourished for the same length of time but at a later period in life, become very hungry and catch up with the growth of controls when allowed food in adequate quantity. Widdowson and McCance postulate that there is a critical period of development in which the hypothalamic centers that regulate appetite are being integrated with the size of the developing organism. If the organism is on a low plane of nutrition during this critical period, the hypothalamus is permanently programed, so to speak, for an appetite level that sustains a relatively small organism.

It should be noted that experiments on the nutrition of newborn rats are relevant to the nutrition of the human fetus because rats are born at a less mature stage of development. Furthermore, the concept that nutritional deprivation in utero may negate subsequent catch-up growth has been shown to be correct in pigs and guinea pigs.

Whereas SGA babies are undernourished in utero, many preterm babies are not. It is perhaps this fundamental difference that underlies the statistical differences noted in their subsequent development.

Perinatal factors in adult obesity

■ Ravelli, G., Stein, Z. A., and Susser, M. W.: Obesity in young men after famine exposure in utero and early infancy, N. Engl. J. Med. **295:**349-353, 1976.

The authors of this article test the hypothesis that prenatal and early postnatal nutrition determines subsequent obesity. The study is on 300,000 19-year-old men exposed to the Dutch famine of 1944-1945 and examined at military induction. Obesity was defined as a value of weight for height equal to or greater than 120% of the standard. Exposure to famine during the last trimester of pregnancy and the first 3 to 5 months of postnatal life was associated with significantly lower obesity rates (p < .005). However, exposure to famine during the first half of pregnancy resulted in significantly higher obesity rates (p < .0005).

■ Charney, E., Goodman, H. C., McBride, M., Lyon, B., and Pratt, R.: Childhood antecedents of adult obesity. Do chubby infants become obese adults? N. Engl. J. Med. **295**: 5-9, 1976.

This study was designed to investigate whether there is a substantial correlation between weight attained in the first 6 months of life and obesity in the third decade of life. Records of subjects born between 1945 and 1955 were reviewed to select three groups of weight in the first 6 months of age—those that exceeded the 90th percentile at least once, those that ranged between 25th and 75th percentiles, and those below the 10th percentile at least once. Three hundred and sixty subjects, now between 20 and 30 years of age, were located and asked to provide present height and weight. Of those exceeding the 90th percentile as infants, 36% were overweight adults, as compared to 14% of the average and lightweight infants. A significantly higher incidence of adult obesity was evident when the infant exceeded the 75th percentile of weight, irrespective of height. Social class, educational level, and parental weight all correlated with adult weight. The data suggest that infant weight correlates strongly with adult weight independently of other factors considered.

■ Dugdale, A. E., and Payne, P. R.: Pattern of fat and lean tissue deposition in children, Nature (Lond.) **256**:725-727, 1975.

Published data on growth and body composition of normal children have been examined to calculate increments in body weight (ΔM), fat mass (ΔF), and lean mass (ΔL) from 13 weeks after conception to 17 years. Fig. 3-2 shows how lean tissue growth expressed as percentage of the increment in body mass ($100 \frac{\Delta L}{\Delta M}$) varies with age. It would appear that

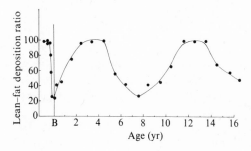

FIG. 3-2
Variations with age in the ratio between lean (ΔL) and fat (ΔF) deposition in normal males ranging in age from 26 weeks after gestation to 16 years. (From Dugdale, A. E., and Payne, P. R.: Pattern of fat and lean tissue deposition in children, Nature (Lond.) **256**: 725-727, 1975.)

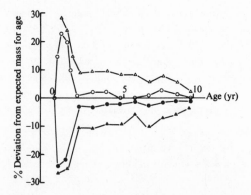

FIG. 3-3
Predicted changes in body mass in children who have been given a 20% deficit or excess in calories from birth to 1 year and then a normal calorie intake. Changes are shown as percentage of expected mass for age: fat mass (Δ) and total body mass (○) with excess calories; fat (▲) and total body mass (●) with calorie deficit. (From Dugdale, A. E., and Payne, P. R.: Pattern of fat and lean tissue deposition in children, Nature [Lond.] **256**:725-727, 1975.)

in early and midfetal life the deposited tissue is almost entirely lean, but fat deposition is favored nearer full-term and throughout the first year of life. The proportion of lean rises to a maximum again at about 4 years. This cycle is repeated again, with a peak of fat deposition between 6 and 10 years, and a peak of lean deposition between 12 and 14 years. Computer models that assume overfeeding or underfeeding by 20% during the first year after birth in an organism following the time sequence shown in Fig. 3-3 suggest marked effects on body composition that persist throughout the subsequent 9 years of normal feeding. Such models may provide a rationale for the importance of overfeeding or underfeeding during early life.

■ Kaplan, M. L., Trout, J. R., and Leveille, G. A.: Adipocyte size distribution in ob/ob mice during preobese and obese phases of development (39572), Proc. Soc. Exp. Biol. Med. **153**:476-482, 1976.

This study was on genetically obese mice that were identified in the preobese phase of development by measuring their oxygen consumption. The frequency distribution of adipose cell size was studied in the preobese (less than 4 weeks of age) and obese (greater than 4 weeks of age) state. Normal littermates were used as controls. Among the genetically obese animals there was an increase in the frequency of small adipocytes throughout development, which resulted in a biomodal frequency distribution after 10 weeks of age. During the preobese phase at week 3, the adipocyte size frequency distribution may be used to identify genetically obese animals during the preobese phase of development.

COMMENT: Experiments in laboratory animals and clinical observations have established that obesity has several etiologic factors. In laboratory animals there are forms of obesity that are inherited as a Mendelian trait, forms caused by hypothalamic lesions, and forms induced by the availability of appetizing food in excessive quantity. In recent years several investigations have been focused on the developmental aspects of obesity. The central theme of this research has been that in the growth of an organism there are "critical periods" in which a given organ or a system is susceptible to permanent injury. In the case of abnormalities of fat depositions, two possible critical periods have been identified. The first is represented by the time during which the hypothalamic centers that regulate food intake differentiate. The second coincides with the growth of adipocytes.

The article by Ravelli et al. explores the possibility that the incidence of obesity in young men could be related to nutrition in intrauterine and early postnatal life; that is, in a period that includes both hypothalamic differentiation and adipocyte growth. The study is in a population of 19-year-old men who were at different stages of fetal and neonatal development during the Dutch famine of 1944-1945. Significant differences with respect to a control group (higher incidence of obesity if exposed to undernutrition during the first half of pregnancy, lower incidence if exposed during the last trimester of gestation and the first month of life) support the concept that intrauterine nutrition has lasting effects on such variables as body composition and food intake in the adult. However, it is doubtful that more precise inferences could be drawn from the statistical evidence. For example, the paradoxical finding of obesity associated with food deprivation in the first half of pregnancy could be due to abnormal hypothalamic differentiation, as the authors suggest, or could be due to compensatory overeating by the mother immediately after the famine. The statistical study by Charney et al. provides evidence that obese infants tend to become obese adults. This finding could be due to the fact that the first year of life is characterized by a rapid rate of adipocyte multiplication (Brook et al.: Relation between age of onset of obesity and size and number of adipose cells, Br. Med. J. 2:25-27, 1972) and fat deposition, as shown in Fig. 3-2 from the article by Dugdale and Payne. Experiments in rats (Stern and Greenwood: A review of development of adipose cellularity in man and animals, Fed. Proc. 33:1952-1955, 1974) have shown that underfeeding or overfeeding in the period of adipocyte multiplication has a significant effect on the ultimate number of adipocytes. Furthermore, patients with an early onset of obesity tend to have a relatively high number of adipocytes. Therefore one can assume that the first year of life in man is a critical period of nutrition with respect to adult obesity and that a judicious restriction of overfeeding at this age could be beneficial. However, excessive fat deposition in early childhood is likely to have multiple etiology and to respond nonuniformly to dietary restrictions.

The article by Kaplan et al. on genetically obese mice suggests that the analysis of biopsies of adipose tissue will eventually play a crucial role in the differential diagnosis of obesity in infants. According to this article, the adipocyte size frequency distribution in a strain of genetically obese mice has unique characteristics that can be recognized even in the preobese state.

Maturation of the fetal lungs

■ Egan, E. A., Olver, R. E., and Strang, L. B.: Changes in non-electrolyte permeability of alveoli and the absorption of lung liquid at the start of breathing in the lamb, J. Physiol. 244:161-179, 1975.

The experiments described in this article were done on twenty-two mature fetal lambs, exteriorized from the uterus and maintained with the umbilical cord intact, and also on four newborn lambs at 12 to 60 hours' postnatal life. In the fetus, test substances were added to lung liquid and then spontaneous ventilation was induced or the lungs were statically inflated. In the newborn lambs the left lung was ventilated to maintain gas exchange, and fetal lung liquid taken from previous experiments and containing test substances was introduced into the right lung, which was then used for permeability measurements. In both fetuses and newborns, the gas used to inflate the lungs was oxygen or nitrous oxide. The test molecules used were labeled erythritol, sucrose, inulin, albumin, and the polymer PVP. Albumin or a large-molecule fraction of PVP was used as a volume marker. Spontaneous ventilation of the fetal lungs was associated with the absorption of liquid and with an alteration in the fetal pattern of nonelectrolyte permeability that could be characterized by postulating the opening up of water-filled cylindric pores to 34 to 56 Å in radius. In the newborn lambs the results suggested pores 7 to 14 Å in radius. Static inflation of the fetal lungs with gas to pressures of 25 to 35 cm H_2O gave permeabilities appropriate for pores 5.5 to 12 Å in radius. Static inflation with larger pressure, 41 to 49 cm H_2O, caused permeability changes that suggest the opening up of very large channels.

It is concluded that in the initial stages of pulmonary ventilation a change takes place in the alveolar walls that can be visualized as the opening up of water-filled channels between alveolar epithelial cells. The opened-up channels would be sufficiently large to allow for rapid liquid absorption by osmosis, but not large enough to permit significant penetration by plasma albumin. The results in the newborn lamb suggest that the permeability changes at birth are temporary because alveolar permeability returns toward the fetal pattern. The change in permeability of the alveoli at birth appears to depend on the degree of lung expansion with gas.

■ Mescher, E. J., Platzker, A. C. G., Ballard, P. L., Kitterman, J. A., Clements, J. A., and Tooley, W. H.: Ontogeny of tracheal fluid, pulmonary surfactant, and plasma corticoids in the fetal lamb, J. Appl. Physiol. **39:**1017-1021, 1975.

The aim of this study was to describe changes in flow rate, composition, and surfactant concentration of tracheal fluid in the fetal lamb during the last quarter of gestation and to correlate these changes with simultaneous measurements of fetal plasma corticoids. The ex-

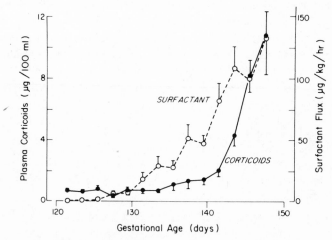

FIG. 3-4
Plasma corticoids and tracheal fluid surfactant flux in the fetal lamb as a function of gestational age. Each circle represents the mean of all the collections from all sheep over a 2-day interval. (From Mescher, E. J., Platzker, A. C. G., Ballard, P. L., Kitterman, J. A., Clements, J. A., and Tooley, W. H.: Ontogeny of tracheal fluid, pulmonary surfactant, and plasma corticoids in the fetal lamb, J. Appl. Physiol. **39:**1017-1021, 1975.)

periments were on chronic preparations equipped with catheters for the collection of fetal tracheal fluid and blood samples. From 120 to 148 days of gestation the rate of tracheal fluid production was 4.5 ml/kg of fetal body weight per hour. The pH (6.23), sodium (147.8 mEq/L), chloride (153.1 mEq/L), and calcium (2.2 mg/160 ml) of the fluid did not change in the period, but the potassium concentration increased from 4.3 to 8.9 mEq/L. The results of measurements of surfactant production (μg/kg/hr) and plasma corticoids concentration (μg/dl) are presented in Fig. 3-4 of the original. It can be seen that surfactant production is negligible up to 25 days prior to delivery, and then rises rapidly. A rapid rise in total plasma corticoids does not occur until about 10 days after the initial appearance of surfactant. This finding suggests that a rise in circulating glucocorticoids is not the physiologic trigger for the initial release of surfactant into the alveolus. However, in the last week before delivery, both cortisol and surfactant increase dramatically, which is consistent with the hypothesis that glucocorticoids and increase in surfactant synthesis and secretion are related.

COMMENT: The elegant experiments described in the article by Mescher et al. show that the fetal lungs produce a fluid which is excreted by way of the trachea at the rate of approximately 4.5 ml/kg/hr. This rate is remarkably high, being similar to the rate of production of fetal urine, which is ⌣ 8 ml/kg/hr. The lung fluid appears to be the result of a secretory process that involves the active transport of chloride ions (Olver and Strang: Ion fluxes across the pulmonary epithelium and the secretion of lung liquid in the foetal lamb, J. Physiol. 241:327-357, 1974). Early in gestation this fluid does not contain appreciable amounts of surfactant. In the sheep fetus, surfactant first appears in the fluid secreted by the lungs approximately 20 days before parturition; that is, at the same time in which production of fetal hemoglobin begins to be turned off (see abstract of article by Wood et al.: Nature [Lond.] 264:799-801, 1976, reviewed in Chapter 4). One wonders whether this is a mere coincidence or the expression of a common triggering mechanism. Of interest is the observation that the appearance of surfactant precedes the surge of corticoids in fetal blood. Since the administration of glucocorticoids to fetuses of several species accelerates the appearance of surfactant in the alveoli, several investigators had suggested that glucocorticoids may be the normal trigger for the production of surfactant. It would seem now that this suggestion is not supported by the experimental evidence. At birth the lungs must stop producing a net amount of fluid and must remove quickly the liquid present in the potential air spaces. According to the results obtained in Strang's laboratory, the distention of the lungs at birth opens up pores in the alveolar membrane through which the water present in the alveoli is rapidly removed, presumably by the oncotic pressure of interstitial proteins.

It is important to note that the diameter of such pores must be large enough for the rapid reabsorption of a salt solution but not so large that it permits the free diffusion of macromolecules. In the article by Egan et al. it is suggested that an excessive inflating pressure may indeed cause disruption of the alveolar epithelium and therefore allow the passage of proteins in the alveolar space.

Maturation of the gastrointestinal tract

■ Widdowson, E. M., Colombo, V. E., and Artavanis, C. A.: Changes in the organs of pigs in response to feeding for the first 24 hours after birth. II. The digestive tract, Biol. Neonate 28:272-281, 1976.

As part of a study of the rate of growth of individual organs in newborn piglets, these authors investigated 8 litters of piglets containing a total of thirty-eight infants. They were

TABLE 3-1

Weights and measurements of stomach and small and large intestines
(mean ± SD)*

	Unfed		Suckled	
	At birth	24 hr	24 hr	10 days
Stomach				
Weight, gm	4.75 ± 0.58	4.76 ± 6.57	6.09 ± 0.93	16.2 ± 2.6
Small intestine				
Weight, gm	27.7 ± 4.03	24.0 ± 3.6	44.5 ± 6.8	112 ± 8.5
Length, cm	358 ± 34.8	365 ± 36.5	440 ± 37.9	674 ± 64.4
gm/cm	77.2 ± 8.79	66.6 ± 9.90	102 ± 15.6	174 ± 8.71
Large intestine				
Weight, gm	6.05 ± 1.78	5.74 ± 1.29	8.60 ± 1.80	31.0 ± 6.96
Length, cm	74.4 ± 6.98	83.7 ± 11.1	99.7 ± 6.33	130 ± 10.3
gm/cm	78.0 ± 18.9	68.6 ± 11.3	87.3 ± 14.4	203 ± 24.6

*From Widdowson, E. M., Colombo, V. E., and Artavanis, C. A.: Changes in the organs of pigs in response to feeding for the first 24 hours after birth. II. The digestive tract, Biol. Neonate 28:272-281, 1976; S. Karger AG, Basel.

divided into four groups. Some were killed at once before being fed; a second group were killed after receiving 20 ml of water by stomach tube every 4 hours for 24 hours; a third group after being suckled for 24 hours; and a fourth group after being suckled for 10 days. The stomach and small and large intestines of the piglets were studied for changes in weight, length, protein, and DNA concentrations. Table 3-1 taken from their report shows that there was a striking increase in weight and length of the small and large intestine even after a short feeding period of 24 hours. These changes did not occur in the animals that were starved for 24 hours. The weight per unit length increased in both the small and large intestine. The striking increase in protein concentration in the tissues of the small intestine may at least in part be due to the absorption of protein from the intraluminal contents.

COMMENT: It is striking that the large intestine increased its weight by 40% and its length by 34% in the first 24 hours, a time in which there was very little material reaching the large intestine for absorption. This study clearly demonstrates the striking changes in the digestive tract initiated by the first feedings in a newborn animal and deserves confirmation in other newborn animals as well.

Cost of growth

■ Hommes, F. A., Drost, Y. M., Geraets, W. X. M., and Reijenga, M. A. A.: The energy requirement for growth: an application of Atkinson's metabolic price system, Pediatr. Res. 9:51-55, 1975.

In this article the investigators calculate the caloric equivalent required for synthetic activity in a 3-week-old "male reference baby." Calculations lead to the conclusion that approximately 2.2% of the total caloric intake would be required for the synthetic reactions involved in the synthesis of new tissue.

COMMENT: The growing organism requires a certain caloric intake to build new tissues. In theory, this intake can be subdivided into two parts: (1) the "raw material"—i.e., amino acids, carbohydrates, and lipids—which is incorporated into the new tissues, and (2) the "metabolic fuel," which provides the energy for producing the complex structures of living cells. The article by Hommes et al. shows, in agreement with other studies, that the calories incorporated into new tissue are a negligible quantity in comparison to the entire energy balance of a child. Implicit in this demonstration is that heat production and oxygen uptake by a growing child have essentially the same meaning that they have in the adult; they are an expression of the energy needed to maintain the integrity and function of the tissues that are already built. Although a child has a relatively high rate of oxygen consumption, there is no theoretical basis for assuming that this high rate is related to the energetic needs of growth.

Effect of aging on hormone responsiveness

■ Cooper, B., and Gregerman, R. I.: Hormone-sensitive fat cell adenylate cyclase in the rat, J. Clin. Invest. 57:161-168, 1976.

This article describes the effects of growth, maturation, and senescence on fat cell adenylate cyclase of the rat. Isolated cells were prepared from epididymal fat pads of rats of different ages, ranging from 1 month old to senescence (24 months old). Adenylate cyclase was assayed in cell membranes (ghosts). Enzyme activity was determined in the basal state and in the presence of varying concentrations of glucagon, ACTH, epinephrine, and fluoride. Basal activity per cell increased threefold between 1 and 2 months with a comparable increase in cell surface area. Epinephrine and fluoride stimulated adenylate cyclase throughout the life-span of the rat in constant proportion to the basal level. To the contrary, glucagon stimulated adenylate cyclase 4.5-fold relative to basal level in the 1-month-old rat, and then its effect rapidly decreased and was absent by 12 months. Similarly, the fourfold stimulation by ACTH noted in the 1-month-old animal decreased gradually with age but was still twice basal level in the senescent rat. Diminished hormone sensitivity with senescence was not related to changes of cell size. Loss of hormone receptors may partially explain the age-related decreases of glucagon and ACTH sensitivity, but decreased basal-, epinephrine-, and fluoride-stimulated responses suggest loss of some other component of the adenylate cyclase enzyme complex.

COMMENT: It has been recognized for some time that changes in the rate of secretion and metabolism of hormones play an important role in the aging of the organisms from embryonic life to senescence. Changes in the responsiveness of target cells to hormones are equally important. This article by Cooper and Gregerman provides an interesting illustration of age-related variations in the responsiveness of fat cells to hormones, which act by stimulation of cyclic AMP production. The study suggests that each cell can modify its responsiveness by several mechanisms, such as changes in the number of receptor molecules on the cell surface or changes in some catalytic component within the cell. The practical application of this knowledge is difficult because target cells are not as accessible to analysis as is blood. However, the concept that substantial modifications in the sensitivity of target cells are part of hormonal regulation is extremely important in understanding why hormonal levels in blood and physiologic action are often poorly correlated.

Relationship of function to structure in the developing kidney

■ Aschinberg, L. C., Goldsmith, D. I., Olbing, H., Spitzer, A., Edelmann, C. M., Jr., and Blaufox, M. D.: Neonatal changes in renal blood flow distribution in puppies, Am. J. Physiol. 228:1453-1461, 1975.

The intrarenal distribution of blood flow was studied in thirty-one newborn puppies from 18 hours to 70 days. The experiments were conducted under general ether anesthesia. Xenon washout tracings and autoradiography of tissue sections prepared at selected times after injection of krypton were used to measure blood flow and its distribution. Mean renal blood flow increased from 0.39 ± 0.05 ml/gm/min the first week to 2.06 ± 0.12 ml/gm/min at 6 weeks. During the first week the renal cortex was perfused homogenously by approximately 35% of the total renal flow. During the second week a narrow, rapidly perfused zone of outer cortex could be identified that was perfused at a relatively rapid rate and received 19.5% $\pm$ 5% of total renal flow. Outer cortical flow increased with age, reaching adult values by about 6 to 10 weeks when the rapidly perfused area represented approximately 40% of the cortex.

COMMENT: The development of nephrons is a gradual process that extends from fetal life well into extrauterine existence. The process is asynchronous; i.e., during most of its development the kidney contains nephrons at different stages of maturation. At birth, the most mature nephrons are found in the inner part of the cortex, whereas the outer cortex contains immature nephrons. In agreement with these histologic data are recent measurements of renal blood flow and its distribution in fetal and neonatal animals. According to such measurements, renal blood flow per gram of organ in fetal and early neonatal life is relatively small, probably reflecting the fact that a large fraction of the nephrons is underdeveloped. In addition, the more mature glomeruli of the inner cortex receive a large fraction of the total flow. As the nephrons in the outer cortex mature, renal blood flow increases markedly and tends to assume the distribution pattern of the adult kidneys. Although the physiologic observations appear to be in agreement with histologic data, it should be noted that most of the experiments on renal blood flow distribution have been performed in anesthetized animals under surgical stress. Therefore the normal quantitative relationship between function and structure in the developing kidney needs further investigation.

Patterns of fetal growth

■ Iffy, L., Jakobovits, A., Westlake, W., Wingate, M., Caterini, H., Kanofsky, P., and Menduke, H.: Early intrauterine development. I. The rate of growth of Caucasian embryos and fetuses between the 6th and 20th weeks of gestation, Pediatrics 56:173-186, 1975.

This study presents data on various body measurements of fetuses delivered following therapeutic abortions up to the twentieth week of gestation. The data were used to present certain standards for the rate of growth of the human fetus up to the twentieth week of gestation. Fig. 3-5 taken from their report points out that in the past, material from spontaneous abortions was used to provide standards of fetal growth in the early part of pregnancy. It is clear that in cases of early spontaneous abortion or cases following ectopic pregnancy, the fetuses were far too large to be consistent with the estimated gestational age. Data from the present report on crown-rump length were used to calculate mean infant weights at the various stages of gestation and were compared with 10th and 50th percentiles of the University of Colorado gestational age/birth weight charts, which terminate at the twenty-fourth week of gestation (Fig. 3-6). It is clear from Fig. 3-6 that additional information is required on human fetal growth between the twentieth and twenty-fourth weeks of gestation. Secondly, the growth rate of the fetus before the twentieth week of gestation indicates a slower overall rate of intrauterine growth than does the data after the twenty-fourth week of gestation. The authors suggest the possibility that this might be a reflection of some bias on

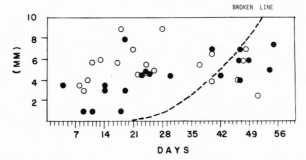

FIG. 3-5
Correlations between menstrual age, *abscissa*, and embryonic crown-rump length, *ordinate*, in twenty cases of early spontaneous abortion (●) and twenty cases of ectopic pregnancy (○) based on some of the youngest specimens in the Embryonic Collection of the Carnegie Institution of Washington. Broken line indicates the average rate of embryonic growth based on normal human specimens obtained by artificially induced abortion. Note that the majority of spontaneously aborted and ectopic embryos are far too well developed for their calculated ages. Embryonic size is obviously incompatible with the length of the amenorrhea in many cases. (From Iffy, L., Jakobovits, A., Westlake, W., Wingate, M., Caterini, H., Kanofsky, P., and Menduke, H.: Early intrauterine development. I. The rate of growth of Caucasian embryos and fetuses between the 6th and 20th weeks of gestation, Pediatrics **56**:173-186, 1975.)

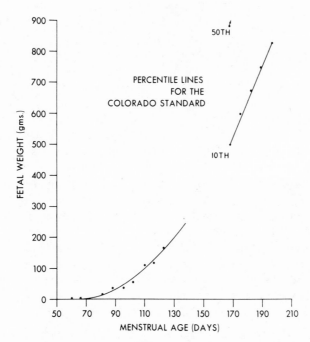

FIG. 3-6
A smoothed curve of fetal weight increase between 6 and 20 weeks' gestation in comparison with the lower 10th and 50th percentile lines of the Colorado standards. (From Iffy, L., Jakobovits, A., Westlake, W., Wingate, M., Caterini, H., Kanofsky, P., and Menduke, H.: Early intrauterine development. I. The rate of growth of Caucasian embryos and fetuses between the 6th and 20th weeks of gestation, Pediatrics **56**:173-186, 1975.)

the part of physicians to reject the possibility of large-for-gestational age (LGA) fetuses from the group of midtrimester abortions, thus tending to reduce the slope of the gestational age/birth weight plot for the fetal data.

■ Sabbagha, R. E., Barton, B. A., Barton, F. B., Kingas, E., Orgill, J., and Turner, J. H.: Sonar biparietal diameter. II. Predictive of three fetal growth patterns leading to a closer assessment of gestational age and neonatal weight, Am. J. Obstet. Gynecol. **126:**485-490, 1976.

A total of 375 measurements of fetal biparietal diameter (BPD) were performed in 142 gravidas between 20 and 40 weeks of pregnancy. The BPDs at any given age were classified into three groups: (1) greater than the 75th percentile, (2) ranging between the 25th and the 75th percentile, and (3) less than the 25th percentile. The results show that 90% of the fetuses maintained their cephalic growth within a percentile grouping. Eleven of the 142 fetuses dropped from the initial BPD rank into the next lower rank. Three of the 142 fetuses did the opposite. It is concluded that under normal conditions the BPDs of most fetuses tend to grow within the confines of a given percentile rank. This knowledge indicates that it is possible to estimate accurately fetal age by measuring BPD growth and that the technique is useful in detecting abnormal intrauterine growth patterns.

COMMENT: Reliable statistical data about the growth of the human fetus are essential for identifying cases of abnormal growth. In addition, they are important for an understanding of the physiology of pregnancy. Fig. 3-6, reproduced from the article by Iffy et al., shows how fetal mass increases rapidly from the fourteenth week on, thus imposing on the mother a progressively greater demand for the supply of oxygen and nutrients. On the other hand, the relative rate of growth of the human fetus, expressed as growth increment per unit of weight, is extremely high at the tenth week of gestation (70% per week) and then plateaus to about 13% per week from the twenty-fifth to the thirty-second week. The data in Fig. 3-6 are a composite of information derived from therapeutic abortion and premature birth. It is apparent that the data on early growth cannot be extrapolated to fit the data on growth from the twentieth week on, unless one assumes a large growth spurt between the twentieth and twenty-fourth week. It is more likely that errors in data collection account for the discrepancy. Thus more work is needed in providing a growth chart of the human fetus throughout gestation.

Important understanding about fetal growth will be obtained also by observing the growth patterns of individual fetuses. Growth retardation could be the result of different growth patterns. In some fetuses, a slow growth rate may have been present throughout the period of fetal development, whereas in others, growth may have decelerated in the late stages of pregnancy. It would be important to establish the occurrence and relative frequency of these patterns to identify types of growth retardation that have different etiologies. The article by Sabbagha et al. indicates that different patterns of fetal growth do in fact exist, even in a group of normal pregnancies. The predominant modality is that in which a certain growth rate is maintained from midgestation on. However, in some cases, there is marked deceleration or acceleration of growth after the twentieth week. In experimental animals it is possible to decelerate fetal growth by several means such as ligation of uterine or umbilical vessels, placental embolism, or maternal malnutrition. It would be interesting to know whether placental infarction or a sudden change in the nutritional state of the mother could account for some cases of fetal growth deceleration, as documented by the sonar technique.

CHAPTER 4

Fetal respiratory and cardiovascular physiology

Fetal respiratory center

■ Bahoric, A., and Chernick, V.: Electrical activity of phrenic nerve and diaphragm in utero, J. Appl. Physiol. **39:**513-518, 1975.

Phrenic nerve and diaphragmatic electrical activity and tracheal or pleural pressure changes were recorded in chronic fetal sheep preparations. Three patterns of fetal phrenic nerve activity were observed: (1) a single burst; (2) irregular nonryhthmic bursts; and (3) prolonged ryhthmic activity, seen only in two fetuses that died within 6 hours after its appearance. The single bursts appeared randomly during the quiescent periods of type 2 or 3 activity. Nonrhythmic bursts, irregular in both pregnancy and duration, were the most prevalent type of activity seen during these experiments. The total recording time was ~55 hours and the total duration of phrenic nerve activity was ~65 minutes (2.16%). Phrenic nerve activity was present in all fetuses and 97.5% of the time was coupled with diaphragmatic activity. Both diaphragmatic activity and pressure changes occurred in the absence of phrenic nerve activity. Tracheal pressure changes were seen in three fetuses with both phrenic nerves transected. Thus changes in fetal tracheal pressure or diaphragmatic activity do not necessarily represent the output of the fetal respiratory center. This study suggests that the fetal respiratory center is active in utero, but this activity is minimal and has a different pattern from that seen after birth.

■ Bystrzycka, E., Nail, B. S., and Purves, M. J.: Central and peripheral neural respiratory activity in the mature sheep foetus and newborn lamb, Respir. Physiol. **25:**199-215, 1975.

Activity from respiratory neurons in the medulla and the phrenic and intercostal nerves was recorded in twenty-five fetal lambs, exteriorized a few days before term from ewes sedated with ketamine and under spinal anesthesia. In twelve fetuses there was little or no sustained respiratory activity, and the electrical activity in the medulla consisted of tonically discharging expiratory and other neurons and silent inspiratory neurons. In the remaining thirteen fetuses, respiratory activity was periodic or continuous, and it was possible to confirm that apneic episodes were not due to a generalized medullary depression like that seen with barbiturate narcosis, severe hypoxia, or hypocapnia. Fetal respiration was unaffected by chemoreceptor stimulation, noise, light, and electrical stimulation of the sciatic nerve and only slightly by inflation or deflation of the lungs. All these stimuli were effective shortly after birth. Occlusion of the umbilical cord caused poorly sustained gasps in "nonbreathing" fetuses and in "breathing" fetuses caused abolition of inspiratory and expiratory activity in the medulla, as well as onset of gasps and flattening of the electroencephalogram. Rhythmic respiration resumed after release of the cord with a latency that varied with the duration and severity of the asphyxia. The respiratory depression following cord occlusion was due not to reflex but to a direct, central action of hypoxia.

■ Wyszogrodski, I., Taeusch, H. W., Jr., and Williams, R. L.: Spontaneous phrenic nerve activity in the exteriorized fetal lamb, J. Appl. Physiol. **39:**124-128, 1975.

Phrenic nerve activity and tracheal pressure changes were recorded in four exteriorized fetal lambs (120 to 135 days' gestation) from ewes anesthetized with sodium pentobarbital. Single- or few-fiber preparations of the phrenic nerve were prepared and placed on silver-wire, bipolar electrodes immersed in a pool of paraffin. Two types of spontaneous neural activity were found. The first consisted of high-frequency, multiunit bursts (mean duration, 820 msec; range, 450 to 2500 msec) that preceded a gasp. Individual units within these bursts reached peak discharge frequencies as high as 40 impulses/sec. The second type of neural activity consisted of single-unit, low-frequency (1 to 14 impulses/sec) irregular background discharges lasting up to several seconds without change in tracheal pressure. The data indicate that the neural correlate of a fetal gasp includes high-frequency and synchronized bursts of activity in the phrenic nerve. In addition, background phrenic activity can be detected in the exteriorized fetal lamb that reflects central nervous activity in the absence of tracheal pressure changes.

■ Condorelli, S., and Scarpelli, E. M.: Somatic-respiratory reflex and onset of regular breathing movements in the lamb fetus in utero, with the technical assistance of F. A. Taylor, Pediatr. Res. **9:**879-885, 1975.

Breathing activity of six mature lamb fetuses was monitored in utero from recordings of intraesophageal pressure, intratracheal pressure, and tracheal circumference from a mercury strain gauge before, during, and after stimulation of the central end of a cut sciatic nerve. No spontaneous breathing movements were recorded for about 60 minutes after the induction of anesthesia with sodium thiopental, nor was it possible to elicit breathing by stimulation of the sciatic nerve during this time. Thereafter, when not specifically stimulated, the fetus made spontaneous, irregular breathing efforts. After 60 minutes, breathing movements could be induced consistently in all fetuses by stimulation of the sciatic nerve with pulses of 15 V, 1.05 to 1.25 msec duration. In one third of the triads the "reflex" response was followed by spontaneous regular breathing movements which continued from 1 minute to 2 hours 30 minutes after the stimulation was stopped.

■ Jansen, A. H., and Chernick, V.: Site of central chemosensitivity in fetal sheep, J. Appl. Physiol. **39:**1-6, 1975.

Heart rate, blood pressure, and respiratory response to topically applied cyanide in the ventrolateral medullary surface and upper spinal cord was studied on twenty exteriorized fetal lambs under pentobarbital anesthesia. The respiratory response was measured by means of a liquid plethysmograph connected to the trachea. Peripheral chemoreceptor and pressoreceptor function was eliminated by bilateral section of the sinus and vagus nerves. On all sites tested, cyanide produced a rapid increase in heart rate and blood pressure, which was most pronounced from the area adjacent to the nerve roots lx to xl (pressure change from 67 ± 20.2 to 88 ± 21.8 torr and heart rate change from 184 ± 46.3 to 249 ± 44.5 beats/min). Respiratory efforts consisting of 1 to 8 gasps were induced in half the applications to the medulla, but never when the cyanide was applied to the spinal cord. After cautery of the chemosensitive areas, topical application of cyanide failed to stimulate gasping, whereas intravenous cyanide or cord clamping still produced a vigorous respiratory response. It is concluded that sympathetic stimulation of the heart and blood vessels can originate centrally in response to local histotoxic hypoxia of the ventral medulla and upper spinal cord. Furthermore, it is proposed that in the apneic fetus, histotoxic hypoxia of the medulla initiates respiration, possibly by stimulating a special "gasping center" that is separate from the respiratory center responsible for rhythmic breathing after birth and is located at least 2 mm beneath the ventral surface of the medulla. When the gasping center is stimulated by hypoxia, it can temporarily overcome the inhibition of the respiratory center but is incapable of maintaining prolonged rhythmic breathing.

COMMENT: The study by Bahoric and Chernick demonstrates that in an unanesthetized chronic fetal lamb preparation there are bursts of phrenic nerve activity. This activity differs from that observed in postnatal life: it occurs infrequently (approximately 2% of the time) and is irregular; i.e., periods of activity are interspersed with quiescent periods of varying duration. Presumably, the phrenic nerve activity reflects the synchronized firing of inspiratory neurons in the respiratory center of the fetal medulla. The fact that this firing is infrequent indicates that during fetal life the medullary respiratory center is under some inhibitory influence. It would be important to understand the nature and origin of such inhibition because the establishment of normal, regular breathing at birth depends on its removal. To study the respiratory center of the fetus, several investigators have used anesthetized, exteriorized fetal preparations. Since surgical stress, anesthetics, and exteriorization influence the physiologic state of the fetus, the general validity of the studies must be accepted with caution.

It would appear from the study of Bystrzycka et al. that the inhibition of the fetal medullary respiratory center is not due to a generalized state of depression like that seen with barbiturate narcosis, severe hypoxia, or hypocapnia. Tonic or irregularly discharging units are present in the medulla of the fetus even when the fetus is apneic. Furthermore, as demonstrated in the study by Wyszogrodski et al., single inspiratory units may show bursts of activity that are not associated with any breathing movement because their activity is not synchronous with that of other units. It is the rhythmic, massive firing of inspiratory units that is inhibited most of the time. A question then arises concerning the stimuli that may release such inhibition. In the preparation studied by Bystrzycka et al., external stimuli such as manipulation, noise, light, or electric stimulation of nerves failed to affect fetal breathing. To the contrary, the fetal lamb preparation investigated by Condorelli and Scarpelli showed a consistent association between sciatic nerve stimulation and breathing movements. The discrepancy in the results of the two studies is probably due to methodologic differences. For instance, in the study of Bystrzycka et al., the ewe was sedated with ketamine and the fetus was exteriorized, whereas in Condorelli's study only one fetal hindlimb was exteriorized, and the response to nerve stimulation was studied an hour after induction of anesthesia with sodium thiopental. Such discrepancy serves to emphasize the importance of the fetal physiologic state in determining the results of any one study.

The relationship of hypoxia to fetal and newborn breathing movements is complex. In the study by Bystrzycka et al., occlusion of the cord abolished inspiratory and expiratory activity in the medulla and stimulated the onset of gasping. In agreement with this finding, the study by Jansen and Chernick shows that a selective hypoxic stimulus to the fetal medulla (obtained by placing cyanide-soaked pledgets of filter paper on the ventrolateral medullary surface) stimulates gasping. Hence the suggestion of a gasping center in the medulla, separate from the respiratory center. The medullary respiratory center, which is responsible for rhythmic breathing after birth, is depressed by hypoxia. For this reason, the hypoxia that is often associated with birth should not be considered a direct stimulus for the onset of regular breathing. Hypoxia may act indirectly by stimulating gasping, which causes a temporary improvement of oxygenation and therefore creates a more favorable condition for the activation of regular breathing. On the other hand, hypoxia of sufficient severity and duration may depress the respiratory center to such an extent that its spontaneous activation is impeded.

Effects of carbon monoxide in pregnancy

■ Longo, L. D.: Carbon monoxide: effects on oxygenation of the fetus in utero, Science 194: 523-525, 1976.

Unanesthetized pregnant sheep with chronically implanted catheters for the sampling of maternal and fetal blood were exposed to carbon monoxide concentrations of 30, 50, or 100 parts per million (ppm) for 36 to 48 hours. During maternal-to-fetal carbon monoxide exchange after exposure, oxygen partial pressures decreased in the maternal uterine vein and in the fetal descending aorta and inferior vena cava. On the basis of these experiments, it is estimated (Fig. 4-1) that a human fetus with 10% of his hemoglobin converted to carbon carboxyhemoglobin would have a venous P_{O_2} substantially lower than normal (11 vs 16 torr). Decreases in oxygen tension may be a factor in the lower birth weights of infants born to women who smoke or are exposed to severe air pollution.

■ Dow, T. G. B., Rooney, P. J., and Spence, M.: Does anaemia increase the risks to the fetus caused by smoking in pregnancy? Br. Med. J. 4:253-254, 1975.

Three groups of women were selected for this study. All were regular cigarette smokers. The first group consisted of ten normal women late in the second trimester of pregnancy, with hemoglobin levels of over 11 gm/dl. The second group consisted of ten women at the same stage of pregnancy, but whose hemoglobin was less than 10 gm/dl. The third group consisted of ten normal nonpregnant women with hemoglobin levels >11 gm/dl. The carboxyhemoglobin in maternal venous blood (HbCO) was measured before and 2 minutes after smoking one cigarette. A significantly greater rise in HbCO was shown in pregnant (3.9% increase) as opposed to nonpregnant (2.1% increase) women. The increase was more pronounced when anemia was present (from 1.68 ± 0.22 to 6.7 ± 0.22) and appeared to be inversely related to the hemoglobin concentration. It is suggested that the risks to the fetus may be particularly increased when anemia complicates pregnancy in women who smoke cigarettes.

COMMENT: The study by Longo provides valuable data about the effect of maternal CO inhalation on fetal oxygenation. Increasing HbCO in maternal blood decreases the maternal O_2 capacity (that is, the amount of hemoglobin capable of combining reversibly with O_2) and shifts the oxyhemoglobin saturation curve to the left. These two changes cause a decrease of the P_{O_2} in the maternal blood that perfuses the intervillous space. The CO diffuses across the placenta and combines with fetal hemoglobin, causing in fetal blood also a decrease of O_2 capacity and a leftward shift of the oxyhemoglobin saturation curve. The cumulative effect of these changes in the maternal and fetal organism is that a relatively modest level of HbCO in maternal blood is associated with a substantial decrease of fetal arterial P_{O_2}. Fig. 4-1 illustrates the effect of 9.4% maternal HbCO in fetal oxygenation. Concentrations of HbCO between 5% and 10% are common in persons who smoke one to two packs of cigarettes a day and therefore CO-induced hypoxia is one of the effects of maternal smoking on the fetus.

It would seem that the association of smoking and anemia should be of particular con-

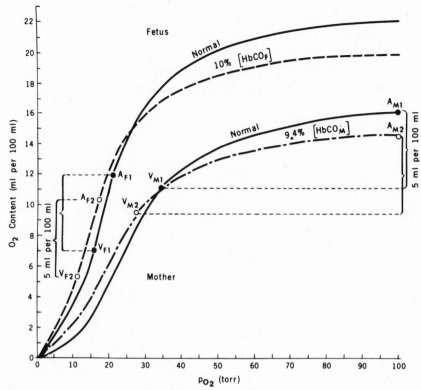

FIG. 4-1

Oxyhemoglobin saturation curves of human maternal and fetal blood under control conditions and during steady state conditions with 10% fetal and 9.4% maternal HbCO concentrations. The maternal and fetal hemoglobins contents were assumed to equal 12 and 16.3 gm/100 ml of blood, respectively. A normal oxygen consumption of 5 ml/100 ml of blood was assumed for both the uterus and its contents and the fetus. (See text for details.) (From Longo, L. D.: Carbon monoxide: effects on oxygenation of the fetus in utero, Science **194:**523-525, Oct. 29, 1976; copyright 1976 by the American Association for the Advancement of Science.)

cern in this regard. Presumably, the same level of HbCO tends to cause a greater degree of hypoxia in the fetus of an anemic mother. In addition, the statistical study by Dow et al. shows that patients with anemia have a significantly greater rise in HbCO concentration in response to smoking a single cigarette. The reasons for this phenomenon are not clear.

For a discussion of other effects of smoking on fetal growth, see Chapter 3.

Relationship of placental blood flow to blood pressure and catecholamines

■ Venuto, R. C., Cox, J. W., Stein, J. H., and Ferris, T. F.: The effect of changes in perfusion pressure on uteroplacental blood flow in the pregnant rabbit, J. Clin. Invest. **57:**938-944, 1976.

The effect of arterial pressure on uterine blood flow was studied in pregnant rabbits by means of the microsphere technique. The animals were between the twenty-third and

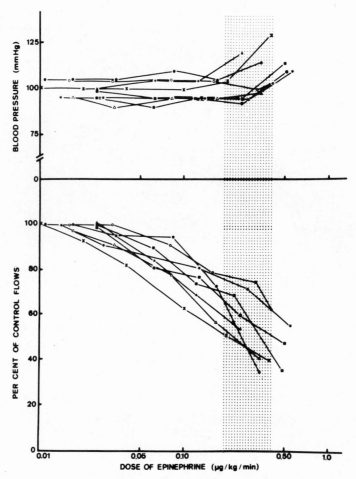

FIG. 4-2

The responses of uterine blood flow, as measured with the flowmeters, and mean systemic blood pressure to increasing doses of epinephrine. The shaded area represents the dose range employed in the microsphere portion of the study (0.2 to 0.4 gm/kg/min). Uterine blood flow is presented as percent of control flows. (From Rosenfeld, C. R., Barton, M. D., and Meschia, G.: Effects of epinephrine on distribution of blood flow in the pregnant ewe, Am. J. Obstet. Gynecol. **124:**156-163, 1976.)

twenty-ninth day of gestation and under pentobarbital anesthesia. In one group of rabbits control mean pressure of 93 torr ± 2.6 SEM was raised by carotid ligation to 109 ± 4.1 torr and then reduced with antihypertensive drugs to 74 ± 1.3 torr. Over this range of pressure there was no significant change in cardiac output or uteroplacental blood flow. Similar results were obtained in a second group of animals treated with meclofenamate, a prostaglandin synthesis inhibitor. In a third group in which the mother was made severely hypotensive by means of an intravenous infusion of trimethaphan, arterial pressure fell from 92 to 39 torr, cardiac output fell from 514 to 407 ml/min (p < .025), and uterine blood flow fell from 32.4 to 10.6 ml/min (p < .025). There was no significant change in renal blood flow with trimethaphan infusion. According to these studies uteroplacental blood flow

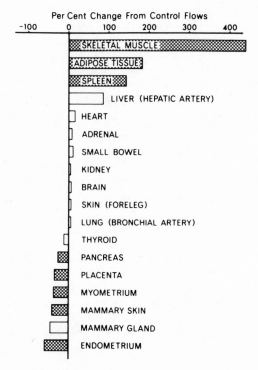

FIG. 4-3

The percent change in organ and tissue blood flows during a systemic infusion of epinephrine (0.2 to 0.4 gm/kg/min) in pregnant ewes. The shaded bars are statistically significant at $p < .05$. (From Rosenfeld, C. R., Barton, M. D., and Meschia, G.: Effects of epinephrine on distribution of blood flow in the pregnant ewe, Am. J. Obstet. Gynecol. **124:**156-163, 1976.)

in pregnant rabbits is maintained relatively constant over a range of perfusion pressure of 60 to 140 torr. However, with reduction of pressure to 40 torr, uteroplacental blood flow falls significantly.

■ Rosenfeld, C. R., Barton, M. D., and Meschia, G.: Effects of epinephrine on distribution of blood flow in the pregnant ewe, Am. J. Obstet. Gynecol. **124:**156-163, 1976.

Nonanesthetized pregnant sheep in the last 2 months of gestation were infused with systemic doses of epinephrine to measure the response of the circulatory system to this hormone. Electromagnetic flow probes that had been implanted around both uterine arteries were used for the continuous measurement of uterine blood flow. The injection of microspheres at selected times before and during the infusion was used to measure flows to other regions of the body and to analyze uterine blood flow in its three major components—placental, myometrial, and endometrial flows. The response of systemic blood pressure and uterine blood flow to increasing doses of epinephrine is shown in Fig. 4-2. Note that a significant decrease in uterine flow begins at doses that have no significant effect on blood pressure. The general effect of epinephrine at doses that cause a reduction of approximately 40% in uterine flow is shown in Fig. 4-3. It is apparent that the placenta, myometrium, and endometrium are all rather sensitive to the vasoconstrictive effect of epinephrine.

■ Greiss, F. C., Jr., Anderson, S. G., and Still, J. G.: Uterine pressure-flow relationships during early gestation, Am. J. Obstet. Gynecol. **126:**799-808, 1976.

Placental and myoendometrial pressure/flow relationships were studied in 17 gravid ewes between 29 and 110 gestational days with the use of radioactive-labeled microspheres. The uterine perfusion pressure was varied by means of an occluding device around the abdominal aorta. The relationship between myoendometrial flow and pressure was consistently curvilinear with convexity toward the flow axis, thus indicating autoregulation in this portion of the uterine blood flow. After 50 days of gestation, the relationship between placental flow and pressure was slightly but significantly curvilinear with convexity toward the pressure axis. This finding indicates that there is no autoregulation of placental blood flow. From 29 to 40 days, the blood flow to the sites of implantation (caruncles) behaved similarly to myoendometrial flow. From 42 to 50 days, at the time when placental cotyledons are formed, the pressure-flow relationship of the placental flow was intermediate to that observed in the preimplantation and postimplantation stages.

COMMENT: **Several organs, notably the kidney, show autoregulation of blood flow; i.e., they respond to variations of blood pressure by changing the diameter of the arterioles so that the rate of perfusion remains constant over a wide range of blood pressure. The experiments by Greiss et al. lead to the concept that there is no autoregulation of placental blood flow. This is a concept of practical importance in obstetrics because it implies that acute hypotension causes a decrease of placental blood flow below normal and therefore endangers fetal life.**

It should be noted that to have a compensatory dilation of the placental arterioles in response to hypotension, it would be necessary for these arterioles to be partially constricted in the normal state. Thus far, studies in sheep have failed to demonstrate the existence of a substantial normal tone of the placental arterioles. Although the placental vascular bed may be near full dilation normally, it can readily constrict in response to sympathetic stimuli. In fact, the article by Rosenfeld et al. demonstrates that the placental vascular bed is among the most sensitive to the constrictive effect of epinephrine. However, there is an apparent species difference if one considers the report by Venuto et al. in pregnant rabbits. Their results suggest that the rabbit uterus is endowed with autoregulation over a blood pressure range between 60 and 140 torr. However, the discrepancy between the results obtained in rabbits versus sheep may be only apparent.

First, it is important to realize that the regulation of blood flow to uterine muscle versus that to the placenta is extremely different, as demonstrated in the article by Greiss et al. Therefore some degree of autoregulation by the uteroplacental blood flow may reflect properties of the myometrial vascular bed and mask the true effect of blood pressure on placental blood flow.

Second, it is not clear whether the control uteroplacental flows in the anesthetized rabbit studied by Venuto et al. were normal or representative of a vascular bed partially constricted in response to the stress of anesthesia and surgery. If the latter were the case, it would be easy to see how the injection of antihypertensive drugs may release the existing constriction and give the appearance of autoregulation by maintaining the blood flow at an abnormally low, but constant, level.

In the absence of more definitive data, caution dictates that to all practical purposes, placental blood flow should be considered as incapable of autoregulation and very sensitive to the vasoconstrictive effect of catecholamines.

Comparative fetal respiratory physiology

■ Silver, M., and Comline, R. S.: Transfer of gases and metabolites in the equine placenta: a comparison with other species, J. Reprod. Fert. **23**(supp.):289-594, 1975.

Pregnant mares with indwelling catheters in the uterine and umbilical vessels were used to measure oxygen and carbon dioxide tensions on the maternal and fetal sides of the placenta and pH and oxyhemoglobin dissociation curves of maternal and fetal blood. Simultaneous measurements of umbilical and uterine blood flows and arteriovenous differences were performed to estimate the uptakes of oxygen and glucose by the fetus. The umbilical venous P_{O_2} in the mare is rather high (50 to 54 torr) in comparison to that in sheep or primates. The P_{CO_2} difference across the equine placenta is virtually zero. The umbilical blood flow in the conscious mare is 171 ± 21 ml/kg of fetal body weight. The oxyhemoglobin dissociation curve of the equine fetus is shifted to the left of the maternal curve, but the shift is much less than that in other species. The oxygen uptake by the fetal horse is 7.4 ± 0.3 ml/kg/min; i.e., similar to that measured in the cow, sheep, and rhesus monkey. In the mare the glucose/oxygen quotient across the umbilical circulation is 0.7.

COMMENT: **Pronounced differences in placental morphology and growth rates make hazardous the extrapolation of physiologic data from the fetus of any one species to the human fetus; hence the unique importance of a comparative approach in fetal physiology. Measurements performed in mammals that differ widely as to placental structure and fetal size and growth may reveal eventually a meaningful pattern and therefore provide a more solid ground for inferences about human fetal physiology. The article by Silver and Comline on the equine placenta is an important contribution to the development of such a pattern. Differences as well as similarities among species begin to emerge. The high oxygen pressure in the umbilical venous blood of the fetal foal presents a striking contrast to the umbilical venous oxygen pressure observed in ruminants and primates. The structural differences of the placenta that create this discrepancy of umbilical P_{O_2} among species are not yet clear. The observation that fetal oxygen consumption per kilogram of body weight is similar to that measured in other species is also of interest. If further comparative studies will confirm that fetal oxygen uptake per unit of body weight varies within a narrow range despite a wide variability of fetal sizes and growth rates, it may be possible to estimate the normal oxygen requirements of the human fetus with some degree of confidence.**

Effects of variations of maternal arterial Po_2, Pco_2, and pH on placental blood flow

■ Buss, D. D., Bisgard, G. E., Rawlings, C. A., and Rankin, J. H. G.: Uteroplacental blood flow during alkalosis in the sheep, Am. J. Physiol. **228**:1497-1500, 1975.

Eight ewes in the last 30 days of gestation were utilized for a study of uteroplacental blood flow before and during metabolic alkalosis. The flows were measured by means of the radioactive microsphere technique in awake, unanesthetized animals. Alkalosis was produced by the intragastric administration of 3 gm of sodium bicarbonate per kilogram of body weight. This procedure resulted in a gradual rise of maternal plasma pH, which reached maximal levels approximately 90 minutes after the administration. For the purpose of this study, alkalosis was defined as an arterial pH of 7.6 or greater. The rise in pH did not cause significant changes in blood pressure and cardiac output but did produce a slight increase of P_{CO_2} (from 31 to 34.8 torr). Placental blood flow declined from a control flow of 1177 ml/min to 1025 ml/min during alkalosis. This decline of 13% was statistically significant (p < .02). Blood flow to other tissues within the pregnant uterus did not change significantly. It is concluded that maternal metabolic alkalosis causes a small increase in the resistance of the uteroplacental circulation.

■ Hanka, R., Lawn, L., Mills, I. H., Prior, D. C., and Tweeddale, P. M.: The effects of maternal hypercapnia on foetal oxygenation and uterine blood flow in the pig, J. Physiol. **247:**447-460, 1975.

The purpose of this investigation was to determine the effects of maternal hyperoxia and hypercapnia on uterine blood flow and fetal oxygenation in the sow at 80 to 90 days' gestation. When the sows were ventilated with 100% O_2, there was a significant rise in maternal arterial P_{O_2}, but no other statistically significant changes in blood gases or blood flow were observed. When the mother was ventilated with O_2 plus 6% CO_2, the maternal arterial P_{CO_2} rose to 84.3 ± 5.8 torr, and the P_{O_2} and O_2 saturation of both uterine and umbilical venous blood were significantly increased. Similar but more pronounced changes were found by ventilating the mother with O_2 plus 50% CO_2. When hypercapnia was induced by inhalation of 5% CO_2 in air, significant increases were recorded in P_{O_2} and O_2 saturation of uterine and umbilical venous blood. The maternal arterial blood pressure rose 49%, the uterine blood flow increased 117%, and uterine vascular resistance fell 25%. It would seem that the P_{CO_2} of maternal arterial blood plays an important role in determining blood flow through the pregnant uterus of the sow.

COMMENT: Variations in the partial pressure of respiratory gases have a considerable effect on the circulation of some organs (for example, the brain). Therefore several investigators have sought to define the effect that changes of maternal P_{O_2} and P_{CO_2} might have on the placental circulation. At the moment there is general agreement that acute variations of P_{O_2} do not have any direct effect on placental blood flow. Severe degrees of acute hypoxia may cause a decrease of placental blood flow, but such a decrease is probably secondary to sympathetic stimulation. Whether or not there is a direct effect of P_{CO_2} on placental perfusion is much less clear. Several investigators have inferred an effect because they have observed changes of fetal oxygenation that were associated with variations of maternal P_{CO_2}. However, changes of maternal blood pH can change fetal P_{O_2} in the absence of any circulatory effect because the equilibrium between free and hemoglobin-bound oxygen depends on pH.

The article by Hanka et al. reports that inhalation of 5% carbon dioxide in air by a pregnant sow tranquilized with phencyclidine and anesthetized with pentobarbital has rather spectacular effects on blood pressure and uterine blood flow. The blood pressure rose 49%, and uterine flow more than doubled. The unusually large effect on blood pressure suggests that the phenomenon may be peculiar to that species under a particular type of anesthesia. Much more evidence is needed before one can generalize from this observation. If indeed maternal hypercapnia (that is, high P_{CO_2}) increases uterine blood flow, then one may expect maternal hypocapnia (that is, low P_{CO_2}) to have the opposite effect. A fair amount of evidence, mostly indirect, which is summarized in the article by Buss et al., suggests that hypocapnia decreases uterine blood flow. However, there is no agreement as to the magnitude of the phenomenon, whether it is a direct effect of P_{CO_2} on the uterine vascular bed, and whether a change in maternal pH rather than hypocapnia is responsible for altering uterine blood flow. The article by Buss et al. demonstrates that in sheep a pronounced metabolic alkalosis (pH > 7.6) decreases placental blood flow by 13%. This relatively small effect by itself could not explain the severe fetal hypoxia that has been reported in some animals as a consequence of maternal hyperventilation, but could be a contributing factor.

Relationship of fetal and maternal acid-base balance

■ Chang, A., and Wood, C.: Fetal acid-base balance. 1. Interdependence of maternal and fetal P_{CO_2} and bicarbonate concentration, Am. J. Obstet. Gynecol. 125:61-64, 1976.

Maternal capillary and fetal scalp blood measurements of pH, P_{CO_2}, base excess, bicarbonate, and total carbon dioxide were made in patients between 38 and 42 weeks of pregnancy. The patients were not in labor at the time of sampling. There was a highly significant correlation between maternal and fetal base excess, bicarbonate and total carbon dioxide (correlation coefficient, 0.54 to 0.67) and a lesser but significant correlation between maternal and fetal P_{CO_2} (correlation coefficient, 0.31). From the results obtained and from a review of the literature, it is proposed that bicarbonate concentrations equilibrate across the placenta.

COMMENT: The relationship between fetal and maternal acid-base balance is of interest for two reasons: (1) in the study of the physiology of intrauterine life, it is important to know the degree of autonomy that the fetus has in regulating its own acid-base balance; (2) the correct interpretation of clinical measurements of fetal pH require an understanding of this relationship. In fetal plasma, fetal pH is related to the ratio bicarbonate concentration/P_{CO_2}. There is no doubt that fetal P_{CO_2} is closely related to maternal uterine venous P_{CO_2} throughout gestation, as long as the perfusion of the placenta by maternal and fetal blood is maintained. This is true even with rapid changes in maternal P_{CO_2}.

It should be noted that the relatively small correlation between maternal and fetal P_{CO_2} shown in the article by Chang and Wood does not contradict this statement. The physiologic range of variability of P_{CO_2} is rather small, and there are several sources of error in the measurement of fetal scalp blood P_{CO_2}. Furthermore, a much better correlation would be obtained by comparing umbilical and uterine venous P_{CO_2}. Therefore the degree of autonomy of fetal pH from maternal pH depends on one factor—the ability of the placenta to exchange between mother and fetus small negative ions such as lactate, chloride, and bicarbonate. If this exchange could not take place, fetal pH could be regulated independently of maternal pH. On the other hand, a rapid exchange would prevent the fetus from regulating its own pH. In the extreme case of a very rapid exchange, the fetal extracellular fluid would be simply an extension of maternal extracellular fluid and follow passively any change of maternal pH. In some animals (for example, sheep and goats) the placenta does not exchange chloride and bicarbonate rapidly. In these animals, it is possible to create a severe maternal acidosis by means of an ammonium chloride infusion and to observe no appreciable decrease of fetal pH for at least 24 hours. However, the placenta of the rhesus monkey is more permeable to chloride ions than is the ovine placenta (Battaglia et al.: Clearance of inert molecules, Na, and Cl ions across the primate placenta, Am. J. Obstet. Gynecol. 102:1135-1143, 1968). Thus it seems probable that the human placenta does not permit the degree of fetal pH autonomy that is observed in sheep and goats. Unfortunately, the experimental evidence is conflicting, as pointed out in the article by Chang and Wood, and uncertainty is therefore considerable about the time course of equilibration of chloride and bicarbonate ions across the human placenta.

Effects of maternal oxygen therapy on fetal oxygenation

■ Morishima, H. O., Daniel, S. S., Richards, R. T., and James, L. S.: The effect of increased maternal Pa_{O_2} upon the fetus during labor, Am. J. Obstet. Gynecol. 123:257-264, 1975.

The effect of increased maternal arterial oxygen pressure (Pa_{O_2}) on the fetus during labor was studied in thirty-six subhuman primates. The results were analyzed by dividing the animals into two groups: one in which the fetus was not asphyxiated and showed no evidence of distress (group I) and another in which the fetus was acidotic, hypoxic, and exhibited the pattern of late deceleration of the heart rate (group II). Elevation of maternal Pa_{O_2} to 430 torr increased fetal arterial P_{O_2} and saturation in group I and in most instances in group II, without significant changes in the acid-base state. In group II, maternal hyperoxia also abolished or reduced the frequency of late deceleration of fetal heart rate in most fetuses. Termination of oxygen therapy resulted in a fall in maternal and fetal oxygen levels to their original values and the reappearance of late decelerations.

COMMENT: The effect of maternal oxygen inhalation on the fetus has been investigated extensively, both from the experimental and thoretical points of view. The results of these investigations lead to the conclusion that administration of oxygen to the mother is a potentially useful, important measure in correcting acute fetal hypoxia. It should be noted that there has been some reluctance in accepting the validity of this conclusion because of the observation that in fetuses of several species, including the human fetus, a very large increase of oxygen pressure in maternal arterial blood causes what appears to be a modest increase of oxygen pressure in fetal arterial blood.

The article by Morishima et al. shows that in the fetuses of subhuman primates, the arterial O_2 pressure increased only 4 to 8 torr when maternal arterial O_2 pressure increased from 116 to 429 torr. Similar results have been obtained in humans (Wulf et al.: Clinical aspects of placental gas exchange. In Longo, L. D., and Bartels, H., editors: Respiratory gas exchange and blood flow in the placenta, Bethesda, Md., 1972, HEW Pub. No. [NIH] 73-361). However, a large discrepancy between maternal and fetal arterial O_2 pressure changes does not justify the inference that O_2 therapy is not beneficial, or minimally beneficial, to the fetus. It is important to recognize that the survival of the organism depends on an adequate total amount of O_2 in arterial blood (i.e., free O_2 plus hemoglobin-bound O_2) rather than on any specific value of arterial O_2 pressure, which is a measure of the free O_2 alone. The important data in the article by Morishima et al. are the changes in O_2 content, which show that O_2 therapy more than doubled the O_2 saturation of fetal blood in the group of asphyxiated fetuses; i.e., that the O_2 content of fetal arterial blood increased dramatically. Large changes of O_2 content associated with relatively small changes of O_2 pressure are made possible in fetal blood by the high O_2 affinity of fetal red cells. The opinion that a substantial increase of arterial O_2 content can be extremely beneficial to the fetus is supported by the observation that it can abolish the late deceleration of the fetal heart during labor. Needless to say, administration of oxygen to the mother cannot be of any value to the fetus if there is no, or minimal, communication between the two organisms, for example, in cases of placental detachment or cord compression.

Switchover from fetal to adult hemoglobin

■ Wood, W. G., Pearce, K., Clegg, J. B., Weatherall, D. J., Robinson, J. S., Thorburn, G. D., and Dawes, G. S.: Switch from foetal to adult haemoglobin synthesis in normal and hypophysectomised sheep, Nature (Lond.) **264:**799-801, 1976.

Blood samples were drawn from eight normal and three hypophysectomized sheep fetuses by means of chronically indwelling catheters in the fetal carotid or femoral artery. The red cells were used for measurements of globin chain synthesis by incubation with tritium-labeled leucine, followed by separation of the individual globin chains by carboxymethylcellulose chromatography and determination of the radioactivity incorporated into each chain. Up to day 127 of gestation the beta chains of adult hemoglobin accounted for approximately 4% of the total non-alpha chains synthesized. However, in the normal fetus the proportion had risen to 43% by 143 days and by 150 days the switchover was complete. In the three hypophysectomized fetuses, an increase in beta chain production was observed at about the same time as in the normal fetuses, but the rate of increase was much reduced. In two of the fetuses that survived to 170 days, the changeover was virtually completed by this time.

These results suggest that the initial event in increasing adult hemoglobin synthesis is independent of an intact pituitary but that the process is accelerated in its presence. The role of the pituitary-adrenal axis in preparing the fetal lamb for extrauterine life may include acceleration of the replacement of fetal hemoglobin by the adult form.

■ Bard, H.: The postnatal decline of hemoglobin F synthesis in normal full-term infants, J. Clin. Invest. 55:395-398, 1975.

Studies were carried out in normal infants born at term to determine the proportion of fetal hemoglobin and adult hemoglobin being synthesized at different ages. Fifty-three blood samples from thirty-seven infants were incubated in an amino acid mixture containing ^{14}C-labeled leucine and chromatographed for separation of fetal and adult hemoglobin. There was a decline in fetal hemoglobin synthesis postnatally until 16 to 20 weeks of age when levels of 3.2% ± 2.1 SD were reached. By combining these data with fetal data already published, the complete switchover from hemoglobin F to hemoglobin A synthesis can be described. (See Fig. 4-4 of the original.) The whole process is represented by a sigmoid

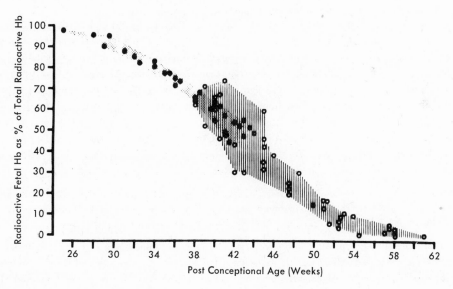

FIG. 4-4
The decline of Hb F synthesis during the prenatal period; ● represents cord blood data obtained from Bard et al. (The relative rates of synthesis of hemoglobin A and F in immature red cells of newborn infants, Pediatrics 45:766-772, 1970) from preterm newborn infants appropriate in weight for gestational age; ○ represents data on the postnatal blood samples in infants obtained from the present study. (From Bard, H.: The postnatal decline of hemoglobin F synthesis in normal full-term infants, J. Clin. Invest. 55:395-398, 1975.)

curve, with the middle centered at about 42 weeks and a steep portion extending from 32 to 52 weeks after conception.

COMMENT: There are several reasons for the current interest in the mechanisms underlying the switchover from fetal to adult hemoglobin. It is a model of differentiation that involves two important molecules, hemoglobin F and A, whose structure, function, and mechanisms of inheritance have been extensively studied. The time course of the process can be followed in the same individual by drawing blood samples at different times during development. In addition, as Wood et al. pointed out, there is evidence that if it were possible to prevent even partially the switch from fetal to adult hemoglobin, it might be possible to improve the condition of patients with sickle cell anemia and other disorders of beta chain structure.

A comparison of the articles by Wood et al. and by Bard shows that the process is rather similar in both man and sheep. The only clear difference—a shorter time course in sheep than in man—is not indicative of any fundamental difference in mechanisms. What seems much more important is that in both species the switchover to adult hemoglobin begins in utero at a fairly precise time; hence the possibility of using the fetal lamb as an appropriate animal model for studying the control of fetal and adult hemoglobin synthesis.

Effects of inhibitors of prostaglandin synthesis on the fetal circulation

■ Heymann, M. A., and Rudolph, A. M.: Effects of acetylsalicylic acid on the ductus arteriosus and circulation in fetal lambs in utero, Circ. Res. 38:418-422, 1976.

Catheters were placed in the inferior vena cava, abdominal aorta, carotid artery and vein, main pulmonary trunk, and stomach of six fetal lambs at 125 to 130 days' gestation. On the following day, fetal arterial pressure, P_{O_2}, P_{CO_2}, and pH were recorded, and fetal cardiac output and its distribution were measured by injection of radionuclide-labeled microspheres. Acetylsalicylic acid, 55 to 90 mm/kg, then was administered into the fetal stomach. Fetal pulmonary arterial pressure rose significantly after an average of 58 minutes, increasing the pressure difference between pulmonary artery and aorta from 2 ± 0.3 to 11.2 ± 1.6 mm Hg. Resistance across the ductus arteriosus rose from 4.2 ± 0.5 to 27.4 ± 4.0 units and flow fell from 495 ± 44 to 409 ± 20 ml/min. In two fetuses, infusion of prostaglandin E_1 reversed the pulmonary hypertension. It is concluded that inhibition of prostaglandin synthesis in fetal lambs causes constriction of the ductus arteriosus.

■ Sharpe, G. L., Larsson, K. S., and Thalme, B.: Studies on closure of the ductus arteriosus. XII. In utero effect of indomethacin and sodium salicylate in rats and rabbits, Prostaglandins 9:585-596, 1975.

Administration of prostaglandin synthesis inhibitors (indomethacin or sodium salicylate) to pregnant rats and rabbits in late gestation was followed by constriction of the fetal ductus arteriosus. The degree of constriction was studied by the whole-body freezing method. In the rat the constriction was well established 6 hours after administration by gavage of 15 mg/kg of indomethacin to the mother and persisted up to 36 hours. The same treatment earlier in pregnancy (18 days) had no effect, but fetuses at 20 and 22 days responded significantly to indomethacin. Fetuses in late pregnancy, 22 days, responded significantly to a relatively small dose of indomethacin—2.5 mg/kg. Both the rat and the rabbit were found to be sensitive also to sodium salicylate.

■ Manchester, D., Margolis, H. S., and Sheldon, R. E.: Possible association between maternal indomethacin therapy and primary pulmonary hypertension of the newborn, Am. J. Obstet. Gynecol. **126:**467-469, 1976.

This is a report of two cases of neonatal primary pulmonary hypertension following prenatal exposure to indomethacin. The indomethacin was administered to the mother in an attempt to prevent premature labor.

COMMENT: **There is good experimental evidence, both in vivo and in vitro, that the increase of arterial P_{O_2} at birth promotes closure of the ductus arteriosus. However, it seems unlikely that P_{O_2} would be the only controlling factor; thus there has been a continuous search for other physiologic or pharmacologic agents of ductus constriction and relaxation. Studies in vitro have shown that prostaglandin E can relax the ductus. Hence the hypothesis that inhibitors of prostaglandin synthesis may constrict the ductus in vivo. The studies by Sharpe et al. in rats and rabbits and by Heymann and Rudolph in sheep support this hypothesis by showing an effect of prostaglandin synthesis inhibitors on the ductus in utero. Since these inhibitors can cross the placenta, their possible harmful effect on the fetal circulation should be kept in mind whenever they are administered to the mother. The report by Manchester et al. suggests that indomethacin, a prostaglandin synthesis inhibitor given to pregnant patients to prevent premature labor, may in fact cause a temporary but severe pulmonary vasoconstriction in the newborn.**

Growth of the heart

■ Hollenberg, M., Honbo, N., and Samorodin, A. J.: Effects of hypoxia on cardiac growth in the neonatal rat, Am. J. Physiology **231:**1445-1450, 1976.

The aim of this article was to observe whether a low arterial oxygen pressure (Pa_{O_2}) enhances cardiac cell division in the neonatal period. Newborn rat pups were reared for 21 days in 12% to 15% oxygen. Left ventricle and right ventricle weights were 30% and 180% greater than controls matched for body weight. Left ventricular total DNA and DNA concentration were 95% and 48% greater than controls ($p < .001$). Labeling of nuclei with tritiated thymidine at day 1 and autoradiographic analysis at day 21 showed an increased dilution of the label in the cardiac muscle cells, fibroblasts, and endothelial cells—in agreement with the hypothesis that hypoxia in the neonatal period augments the rate of division and ultimate number of cardiac muscle cells.

COMMENT: **In the fetal rat the heart grows mainly by increasing its number of cells (hyperplasia). After birth there is a rapid loss of mitotic activity, and growth of the heart continues primarily because of hypertrophy of existing cells. Previous experiments by Hollenberg (Effect of oxygen on growth of cultured myocardial cells, Circ. Res. 28:148-157, 1971) had shown that the rate of division of cardiac cells grown in tissue culture is inversely related to the P_{O_2} of the medium. This observation has suggested the hypothesis that the decline of cardiac mitotic activity after birth is due, at least in part, to the increase of arterial P_{O_2} that characterizes the transition from fetal to neonatal life. Exposure of newborn rats to hypoxia appears to agree with the suggested hypothesis by showing that prolonging a low P_{O_2} environment past fetal life prolongs the phase of hyperplastic growth. An interesting implication of Hollenberg's hypothesis is that premature birth may result in a myocardium with a relatively small number of cells.**

CHAPTER 5

Placental growth and function

Glucose transfer across the placenta

- Boyd, R. D. H., Haworth, C., Stacey, T. E., and Ward, R. H. T.: Permeability of the sheep placenta to unmetabolized polar non-electrolytes, J. Physiol. **256**:617-634, 1976.

The rate of appearance in uterine venous blood of radioactively labeled, polar, nonelectrolytes was measured following their injection into the fetal circulation in the chronically catheterized sheep near term. Estimates of placental permeability to urea, erythritol, and mannitol were made, and the results were analyzed in terms of restricted diffusion by cylindric, water-filled pores. The results suggest the presence of a placental barrier having epithelial aqueous channels traversing it of a size comparable to those proposed for some cell membranes and some ten times smaller than those suggested for capillary walls.

- Schröder, H., Leichtweiss, H. P., and Madee, W.: The transport of D-glucose, L-glucose and D-mannose across the isolated guinea pig placenta, Pflügers Arch. **356**:267-275, 1975.

An isolated guinea pig placenta artificially perfused by means of the uterine and umbilical arteries was used to investigate whether there is a specific transport system for D-glucose. Rates of transfer from maternal to fetal circulation of D-glucose, L-glucose, and D-mannose were compared in sixteen experiments. Five additional experiments were performed to study the effect of phloretin (10^{-3}M) on transfer rates. In ten out of thirteen placentas, the transfer rates of D-glucose and D-mannose exceeded the transfer rate of L-glucose. In four out of five placentas, phloretin decreased significantly the transfer rates of D-glucose and D-mannose, without decreasing the transport of L-glucose. The placentas that could not discriminate between D- and L-hexoses had a relatively high transfer rate of L-glucose and showed a rapid washout of the sugar molecules by the fetal circulation after stopping the perfusion of the maternal side of the placenta. On the basis of these observations, it is assumed that in some placentas the carrier-mediated transport of glucose was masked by a nonspecific, diffusional transfer.

COMMENT: A prerequisite to an understanding of the physiologic regulation of glucose transfer across the placenta is to know the mechanism by which the transfer takes place. Investigators interested in elucidating this mechanism are using placentas perfused in vitro, as well as an in vivo approach. Although it may seem that the perfused placenta is easier to investigate, the experiments on the guinea pig placenta described by Schröder et al. demonstrate how difficult it is to obtain reproducible, quantitative information in experiments with artificial placental perfusion. Thus only some of the placentas could transfer D-glucose more rapidly than L-glucose, and among those that did there was considerable variability in the degree of discrimination. The studies in sheep by Boyd et al. were in vivo, in presumably normal animals. It would appear from such studies that the permeability of the ovine placenta to substances with physicochemical characteristics and molecular weights similar to those of D-glucose is rather low. Implicit in this finding is that the placenta has a specialized system for the rapid transfer of glucose from mother to fetus. Preliminary experiments by the same authors (Boyd et ai.: Permeability of sheep placenta to unmetabolized polar nor. electrolytes, J. Physiol. 254:16P-18P, 1976) show, in fact, that the sheep placenta transports one glucose analogue (3-o-methyl glucose) much faster than mannitol and that this transport is subject to competitive inhibition by glucose. We may conclude that the v.eight of the evidence favors the concept that glucose transfer from mother to fetus is mediated by a specific carrier. However, the evidence is scanty, and the physiologic implications of this knowledge have not been explored.

Factors that influence placental growth

- Lechtig, A., Yarbrough, C., Delgado, H., Martorell, R., Klein, R. E., and Béhar, M.: Effect of moderate maternal malnutrition on the placenta, Am. J. Obstet. Gynecol. **123**:191-201 1975.

The results of two studies on the influence of malnutrition on placental weight and chemical composition are presented. In the first study, two groups of pregnant women of high and low socioeconomic status from Guatemala City were compared. Both groups were similar with respect to age, parity, gestational age, and absence of severe diseases during pregnancy. The average placental weight in the low socioeconomic group was 15% below that of the high socioeconomic group. Placental weight was significantly correlated to postpartum maternal weight. There were no significant differences in the placental concentration of protein, water, ash, hemoglobin, and DNA; there was significantly less hydroxyproline and fat in the placentas of the low socioeconomic group. The second study compared groups in four rural villages in Guatemala. Two of the villages received a protein-calorie preparation, whereas the other two received a calorie supplement with no proteins. Placental weight was higher among women with high levels of supplemental calories during pregnancy, independently of the type of food supplement. On the average, the group with low-caloric supplementation had placental weight 11% below those with high-caloric supplementation. No significant differences in chemical composition were observed. It is concluded that moderate malnutrition during pregnancy leads to lower placental weight.

- Csapo A., Dray, F., and Erdos, T.: The biological effects of injected antibodies to estradiol-17 beta and to progesterone in pregnant rats, Endocrinology **97**:603-614, 1975.

Antibodies that bind 17-beta-estradiol (E_2) or progesterone (P) were injected intropperitoneally in pregnant rats, at day 6 or 10 of gestation. Before and at daily intervals after treatment, blood was collected from the tail vein, and the levels of circulating antibodies, total E_2, and P were measured. These data were used to calculate the plasma concentrations of unbound $E_2(E_{2u})$ and unbound $P(P_u)$. Treatment with anti-E_2 and anti-P antibodies lowered E_{2u} and P_u significantly ($p < .001$). In comparison with controls, the anti-E_2 treated animals showed significant increases in placental weight ($p < .001$). This effect was prevented by replacement therapy with diethylstilbestrol (DES), since anti-E_2 antibodies do not bind DES. Treatment at day 10 of gestation with anti-P antibodies (total "binding capacity" = 6 μg of P) provoked abortion. In contrast, the same treatment at day 6 (when the P levels are higher than at day 10) failed to induce abortion.

- Pijnenborg, R., Robertson, W. B., and Bronsens, I.: The role of ovarian steroids in placental development and endovascular trophoblast migration in the golden hamster, J. Reprod. Fertil. **44**:43-51, 1975.

Pregnant hamsters were ovariectomized (oophorectomized) on day 7 of gestation and daily supplemented with progesterone or progesterone plus estradiol benzoate. Fetal development and survival was 14% and 62%, respectively. Histologic examination indicated that fetal death was mainly due to inadequate development of the placental labyrinth, which resulted in failure to form an adequate number of maternal arterial spaces communicating with the base of the trophospongium. Progesterone was essential at all stages of gestation to sustain decidual tissue and allow survival of a minority of fetuses. Estradiol supplementation (1 μg/24 hr) significantly increased fetal survival but not to normal levels, suggesting that other substances or modalities of administration may be essential for the maintenance of normal pregnancy.

■ Abdul-Karim, R. W., Pavy, M., Beydoun, S. N., and Haviland, M. E.: The regulatory effect of estrogens on fetal growth. IV. Brain development in growth accelerated fetuses in rabbits, Biol. Neonate **29**:89-95, 1976.

It was shown earlier that oophorectomy and progesterone treatment in rabbits causes acceleration of growth of both fetus and placenta. In the experiments reported here, fetal brain DNA, RNA, and total protein were measured in similarly treated rats, and it was found that the treatment did not affect these parameters of growth.

COMMENT: It is well known that in several species, man included, the weight of the placenta varies over a considerable range among fetuses of the same age. In multiple pregnancies, placental weight is inversely related to the number of fetuses. The latter observation indicates that placental growth rate is not rigidly predetermined by the fetal genome, but depends on the response of the maternal environment.

The site of implantation is by itself an important determinant of placental growth. In the rat, conceptuses in the middle of the uterine horns tend to be heavier (Barr et al.: Fetal weight and intrauterine position in rats, Teratology 2:241-246, 1969). In species in which the formation of placental cotyledons can take place only in specialized areas of the uterine mucosa, the number of available areas influences placental weight (Alexander: Studies on the placenta of sheep [Ovis aries L.]. Placental size, J. Reprod. Fertil. 7:289-305, 1964). The mechanisms by which the sites of implantation influence placental growth are unknown.

There are also several components of the maternal environment that influence placental development. They can be subdivided into immunologic, nutritional, and endocrinologic factors. The importance of immunologic stimuli has been revealed by the observation that antigenic dissimilarity between fetus and mother favors the growth of a larger placenta (James, D. A.: Some effects of immunologic factors on gestation in mice, J. Reprod. Fertil. 14:265-275, 1967). The study by Lechtig et al. in Guatemala shows that maternal malnutrition tends to reduce placental weight. As to endocrinologic factors, the article by Csapo et al. describes an experimental situation in which the reduction of free estradiol concentration in the plasma of pregnant rats causes a significant increase of placental weight. Hence the suggestion that estradiol is an inhibitor of placental growth. Although this suggestion appears to be an appropriate explanation of data of Csapo et al., the role of estrogens in placental growth is probably more complex than that of an inhibitor. For example, according to the observations by Pijnenborg et al. estradiol plays a positive role in the vascularization of the placenta in hamsters. Judging from the report of Abdul-Karim et al., the previously described estrogen stimulation of fetal growth would now appear to be a hypertrophic rather than hyperplastic effect.

Placental clearance of dehydroisoandrosterone sulfate

■ Gant, N. F., Madden, J. D., Siiteri, P. K., and MacDonald, P. C.: The metabolic clearance rate of dehydroisoandrosterone sulfate. III. The effect of thiazide diuretics in normal and future pre-eclamptic pregnancies, Am. J. Obstet. Gynecol. **123:**159-163, 1975.

The metabolic clearance rate (MCR) of dehydroisoandrosterone sulfate (DS) was measured before, during, and after administration of oral hydrochlorthiazide (50 mg/24 hr for 7 days). The patients selected for the study were ten clinically normal but high-risk teenage primigravidas. Five patients were resistant to the pressor effects of infused angiotensin II, and five were angiotensin sensitive. The latter subsequently developed pregnancy-induced hypertension. In both groups the thiazide diuretic therapy caused a statistically significant decrease of MCR_{DS} (from 48.6 to 39.6 L/24 hr in the angiotensin-resistant group and from 73.4 to 67.2 L/24 hr in the preeclamptics). This observation appears to support the thesis that diuretics represent a potential hazard to the fetus by decreasing placental perfusion.

■ Clewell, W., and Meschia, G.: Relationship of the metabolic clearance rate of dehydroisoandrosterone sulfate to placental blood flow: a mathematical model, Am. J. Obstet. Gynecol. **125:**507-508, 1976.

It has been postulated that variations of the placental clearance of DS may reflect variations of placental blood flow. This hypothesis was tested by means of a mathematical model of the placenta that assumes normal placental blood flow in the last month of pregnancy is at least 500 ml/min. According to such a model, placental blood flow cannot be a limiting factor of DS clearance either normally or in pathologic states, due to the fact that DS clearance is much smaller (approximately one twentieth) than placental blood flow. It is concluded that changes in the clearance of DS, which have been observed in complicated pregnancies, imply a metabolic change within the placenta.

■ Singley, T., Madden, J. D., Chand, S., Worley, R. J., MacDonald, P. C., and Gant, N. F.: Metabolic clearance rate of dehydroisoandrosterone sulfate. VII. Effect of lateral versus supine recumbency, Obstet. Gynecol. **47:**419-422, 1976.

This study is based on the assumption that the MCR_{DS} reflects alterations in uteroplacental perfusion. Hence the effect of supine position on the MCR_{DS} of gravid women was studied, in the hope of gaining information about the effect of maternal position on uterine blood flow. No significant changes of MCR_{DS} could be detected in moving the patients from the lateral recumbent to the supine position.

■ Madden, J. D., Siiteri, P. K., MacDonald, P. C., and Gant, N. F.: The pattern and rates of metabolism of maternal plasma dehydroisoandrosterone sulfate in human pregnancy, Am. J. Obstet. Gynecol. **125:**915-920, 1976.

The purpose of this study was to measure the rates of the various metabolic pathways of plasma clearance of DS (MCR_{DS}) in pregnancy. The clearance of DS was largely accounted for by two major pathways that were not prominent in the nonpregnant woman. The first was clearance of maternal plasma DS by placental aromatization of DS to form estradiol (E_2). This pathway accounted for approximately 35% of the total clearance. The second major pathway was by 16-alpha-hydroxylation within the maternal organism. This pathway accounted for about 32% of MCR_{DS}. Loss to the fetus and excretion as unaltered DS into urine accounted for less than 1% of the total metabolic rate. The final pathway of DS metabolism was excretion as neutral steroid such as urinary 17-ketosteroids and other undefined losses. From measurements of MCR_{DS} and of the fraction of DS that is converted to

E_2, the placental clearance (PC) of DS ($PCDS_{E2}$) may be measured. The authors of this article postulate that $PCDS_{E2}$ reflects uteroplacental perfusion.

COMMENT: The development of tests of placental function is a fundamental goal of research in obstetrics. One of the most promising approaches to this goal is that of measuring the clearance of substances that are exclusively, or primarily, metabolized by the placenta. In this context, the study by Madden et al. is of particular interest because it represents the first major effort in searching for a substance that is cleared by the placenta. The test substance selected for the study, DS, has several routes of metabolism. However, its conversion of estradiol is unique to the placenta and represents a fairly large fraction (35%) of the total clearance. The reports by Singley et al. and Gant et al. are two examples of investigations in which measurements of DS clearance have been applied to the study of clinical problems. The former shows that changing the position of the mother from lateral recumbent to supine does not alter DS clearance, whereas the latter shows a decrease of DS clearance after thiazide diuretic therapy.

Unfortunately, the results of these studies are difficult to interpret for the following reasons. Any change of DS clearance could represent a change of either its placental or nonplacental components. In addition, the physiologic mechanisms that may cause a change of the placental component of the DS clearance have not been elucidated. Singley et al. and Gant et al. assume that variations of the DS clearance reflect variations of placental blood flow. It is difficult to visualize how this could be possible, since placental blood flow is at least ten times larger than the placental component of the DS clearance. This conceptual difficulty is pointed out in the article by Clewell et al.

Relationship of placental function to placental size and age

■ Rosso, P.: Changes in the transfer of nutrients across the placenta during normal gestation in the rat, Am. J. Obstet. Gynecol. 122:761-766, 1975.

At days of gestation ranging from the fourteenth to the twenty-first, rats were anesthetized with urethane and injected intravenously with either labeled glucose or labeled AIB (α-aminoisobutyrate), a nonmetabolizable amino acid. At elected times after the injection, samples of maternal plasma, one placenta, and one fetus were taken and analyzed for radioactivity. The data show that the rate of transfer of labeled AIB per gram of placenta (μmol/min/gm) rises exponentially from the fourteenth to the twentieth day of gestation, concomitant with a thirty-twofold increase of fetal weight. The data on the transfer of radioactive label after the injection of tritiated glucose show a similar phenomenon.

■ Pryse-Davies, J.: Fetal maturity and morbidity as related to placental weight and secondary ossification, Postgrad. Med. J. 51:727-730, 1975.

A normal range of trimmed placental weights was determined for a hospital population from a consecutive series of 202 uncomplicated deliveries near term (38 to 43 weeks' gestation). The mean placental weight and standard deviation (SD) was 489 ± 97 gm, range 295 to 683 gm. The mean placental/fetal weight ratio and SD was 14.6 ± 2.3%. An estimate of the range of placental weights for the last trimester of pregnancy was obtained from perinatal necropsies: 402 placentas were available for assessment, and 108 least likely to be affected by growth abnormalities or pathologic lesions were selected. In this group the correlations between placental weight and placental/fetal weight ratios according to gestation are highly significant statistically, as shown in Table 5-1. Using Table 5-1, very small pla-

TABLE 5-1

Trimmed placental weights and placental/fetal (P/F) weight ratios according to gestation in 108 selected fresh necropsies*

Gestation (wk)	Number of cases	Mean placental weight ± SD with 2 SD range (gm)	Mean P/F weight ratio ± SD with 2 SD range (%)
25–26	14	204 ± 43 (118–290)	23.5 ± 3.4 (16.7–30.3)
27–28	18	240 ± 31 (178–302)	23.5 ± 3.8 (15.9–31.1)
29–30	14	256 ± 38 (180–332)	20.2 ± 2.9 (14.4–26.0)
31–32	9	306 ± 57 (192–420)	18.4 ± 2.5 (13.4–23.4)
33–34	7	345 ± 40 (265–425)	17.0 ± 1.7 (13.6–20.4)
35–36	7	395 ± 66 (263–527)	16.5 ± 1.7 (13.1–19.9)
37–38	8	396 ± 79 (238–554)	13.4 ± 2.4 (8.6–18.2)
39–40	21	476 ± 71 (334–618)	14.0 ± 2.2 (9.6–18.4)
41–42	10	484 ± 87 (310–658)	13.9 ± 2.9 (8.1–19.7)

*From Prysi-Davies, J.: Fetal maturity and morbidity as related to placental weight and secondary ossification, Postgrad. Med. J. **51**:727-730, 1975.

cental weights and placental/fetal ratios were defined as values below the 2 SD range. According to this definition in a 276 necropsy series, the incidence of very small placenta/birth weight ratios was 3%; of very small placentas, 13%; and of very small birth weight, 22%. In 164 selected necropsies, the number of secondary ossification centers, total center diameter, and both os calcis diameters were correlated with gestational age. This correlation was then used to classify 379 perinatal cases as normal, advanced, or retarded in ossification. There were significant differences according to sex, growth retardation, congenital malformations, and multiple pregnancy. Anencephaly was associated with advanced, secondary ossification.

■ Teasdale, F.: Numerical density of nuclei in the sheep placenta, Anat. Rec. **185**:187-196, 1976.

Morphometric analysis was used to study six ovine placentas of different ages, and the results were correlated with physiologic and biochemical data. In agreement with studies of placental DNA content, there was no demonstrable increase in the total number of placental nuclei in the last 2 months of gestation. However, the number of fetal mesenchymal nuclei decreased, and there was a concomitant increase of fetal endothelial nuclei from 80 days to term. This increase correlates with a progressive increase of umbilical blood flow per gram of placenta (Fig. 5-1) and a decrease in volume of the core of the placental villi. During the last part of gestation there is also a marked increase in maternal placental blood flow per gram of placenta. However, the histologic analysis failed to demonstrate a morphologic basis for this phenomenon (Fig. 5-2).

COMMENT: The transfer of amino acids and glucose from mother to fetus is an important function of the placenta. The precise quantitative analysis of this function is a difficult task because it requires measurements of rate of transfer in relation to concentration gradients. The experiments described by P. Rosso about the transfer of glucose and one nonmetabolizable neutral amino acid across the placenta of rats follow a much simpler design. Nevertheless, their precision is adequate in demonstrating once again an important phenomenon: the transport properties per gram of placenta are radically different at different gestational ages. Because of this fact, the progressive decrease in placental/fetal weight ratio from 23.5% to 14%, which is observed in the last 15 weeks of human gestation (see Table 5-1

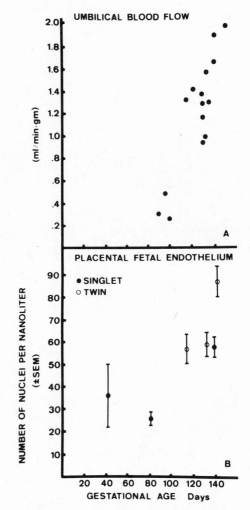

FIG. 5-1

Comparison of umbilical blood flow per gram of placenta with the numerical density of fetal endothelial nuclei (mean ± SEM). Data on umbilical flow from Makowski et al. (Measurement of umbilical arterial blood flow to the sheep placenta and fetus in utero, Circ. Res. 23: 623-631, 1968) and unpublished observations. (From Teasdale, F.: Numerical density of nuclei in the sheep placenta, Anat. Rec. 185:187-196, 1976.)

from the article by Pryse-Davies), does not have the functional significance that was attributed to it in the past; i.e., that the older fetus tends to outgrow the functional capacity of its placenta. As gestation progresses, the exchange function of the placenta "matures"; that is to say 1 gm of placenta can transfer progressively larger amounts of metabolic substrates between mother and fetus. In part this is due to increased rates of perfusion of the placenta by maternal and fetal blood, as shown in Figs. 5-1 and 5-2 from Teasdale's article: in part it is due to changes in permeability and transfer functions of the cells that constitute the placental barrier. Despite this process of functional maturation, at any given age placental function is related to placental weight. Therefore a small placenta or a placenta whose func-

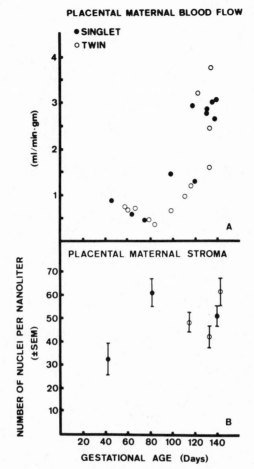

PLACENTAL MATERNAL BLOOD FLOW

FIG. 5-2

Comparison of maternal placental blood flow per gram of placenta with the numerical density of nuclei of the placental maternal stroma. Data on placental flow from Rosenfeld et al. (Circulatory changes in the reproductive tissues of ewes during pregnancy, Gynecol. Invest. 5:252-268, 1974). (From Teasdale, F.: Numerical density of nuclei in the sheep placenta, Anat. Rec. 185:187-196, 1976.)

tioning mass is decreased by infarction represents a handicap for the fetus. This handicap may express itself in the form of growth retardation and/or a decreased ability to withstand successfully the stress of labor.

Placental blood flow during contractions

■ Novy, M. J., Thomas, C. L., and Lees, M. H.: Uterine contractility and regional blood flow responses to oxytocin and prostaglandin E_2 in pregnant rhesus monkeys, Am. J. Obstet. Gynecol. 122:419-433, 1975.

The effects of oxytocin and prostaglandin E_2 (PGE_2) on the distribution of cardiac output and myometrial activity were studied in eighteen pregnant rhesus monkeys near term.

The animals were restrained supine on a padded board, which was then tilted to the left lateral position. Under local anesthesia, vascular catheters were advanced to the left ventricle, the left common iliac artery, and the right atrium. A catheter was inserted into the amniotic cavity for measuring intrauterine pressure. Cardiac output was estimated by indocyanine green dilution curves and its distribution by means of microspheres injected in the left ventricle for 20 to 35 seconds. In each animal these sets of measurements were performed three times: (1) during a control period, (2) at the height of a contraction, and (3) in the period of relaxation between contractions. The labor pattern was induced either by the infusion of oxytocin (0.4 to 4.5 mU/min) or PGE_2 (0.5 to 1.5 µg/min).

No significant difference was observed between PGE_2 and oxytocin with respect to their effect on cardiac output or uterine activity. The gastrointestinal tract received an increased percentage of cardiac output after PGE_2. During uterine contraction (average amniotic pressure 42 torr with oxytocin and 40 torr with PGE_2), there was a large reduction (average 73%) in placental blood flow, whereas myometrial blood flow was maintained or sometimes increased. A significant negative correlation was observed between intra-amniotic pressure and placental blood flow. During uterine relaxation, placental blood flow partially recovered, whereas myometrial flow nearly doubled with respect to prelabor values.

■ Bleker, O. P., Kloosterman, G. J., Mieras, D. J., Oosting, J., and Sallé, H. J. A.: Intervillous space during uterine contractions in human subjects: an ultrasonic study, Am. J. Obstet. Gynecol. **123:**697-699, 1975.

The dimensions of the placenta in six patients at term were examined by ultrasound scanning during uterine contraction and relaxation. The length, thickness, and surface of the placenta were found to increase during uterine contraction. This finding suggests that during uterine contractions the intervillous space is distended because of an imbalance between arterial inflow and venous outflow.

COMMENT: The experiments by Novy et al. provide direct evidence that uterine contractions cause a reduction in placental blood flow. The magnitude of the reduction is correlated to amniotic pressure. Extrapolation of the data on which this correlation is based shows that zero placental flow would occur at approximately 40 to 50 torr of amniotic pressure. This shut-off pressure, being considerably lower than the arterial pressure, suggests that compression of a portion of the placental circulation which is distal to the arteries is responsible for the decreased flow. The observations by Blecker et al., according to which the intervillous space is distended during contractions, place the site of compression at the level of the veins draining the intervillous space. If contraction were to continue indefinitely at a pressure of 40 to 50 torr, the higher arterial pressure should eventually reestablish some small flow through the placenta. However, the inertia of the system may be such that in the short period of a strong contraction of normal duration, a pressure below the arterial is sufficient to create a temporary but virtually complete interruption of placental flow.

It should be noted that a purely mechanical explanation of the events that lead from contraction to reduction in placental blood flow neglects to consider the possibility of changes in the tone of the uterine arteries, which are synchronous with contraction and relaxation.

Relationship of prostaglandin E to uterine blood flow

■ Venuto, R. C., O'Dorisio, T., Stein, J. H., and Ferris, T. F.: Uterine prostaglandin E secretion and uterine blood flow in the pregnant rabbit, J. Clin. Invest. **55:**193-197, 1975.

The experiments were performed in ten pregnant rabbits between the twenty-third and twenty-ninth day of gestation to assess the effect of inhibition of prostaglandin synthesis on uterine blood flow. The animals were nephrectomized 24 hours before the experiment and anesthetized with pentobarbital. In each experiment uteroplacental blood flow was measured twice by means of the microsphere technique, before and 30 minutes after intravenous infusion of meclofenamate or indomethacin (2 mg/kg). These drugs are inhibitors of prostaglandin synthesis. Systemic arterial pressure increased significantly after prostaglandin inhibition (from 86 to 98 torr). Cardiac output was unchanged while uteroplacental blood flow fell from 16.5 to 7.8 ml/min (p < .01). Uterine venous concentrations of prostaglandin E (PGE) were extremely high in the control period, 172.4 ng/ml ± 48.3 SEM, and fell to 23 ng/ml ± 9.8 SEM after administration of either meclofenamate or indomethacin. Studies in four nonnephrectomized pregnant rabbits demonstrated that PGE production is considerably greater in the gravid uterus than in the kidney. It is suggested that the production of PGE may play a key role in the regulation of uteroplacental blood flow.

COMMENT: The observations by Venuto et al. show that uterine venous blood in the anesthetized pregnant rabbit contains extremely large amounts of PGE in comparison to peripheral blood. This very large output of a vasoactive compound by the pregnant uterus suggests that it plays a role in the regulation of uterine blood flow. Presumably, the role of PGE is that of a uterine vasodilator because the administration of prostaglandin synthesis inhibitors was associated with a decrease in uteroplacental blood flow. The authors of this article point out that the vasodilator effect of PGE may be indirect, by attenuation of the effects of norepinephrine or some other vasoconstrictor. To place the above information in proper perspective, it would be important to measure the output of prostaglandins by the pregnant uterus of the normal, unanesthetized, stressed rabbit. In addition, attention should be given to the effect that PGE and the inhibitors of prostaglandin synthesis may have on uterine contractions because of the ability of PGE_2 to promote contractions in primates and because of the relationship between contractions and placental blood flow. (See article by Novy et al.) At the moment, it is not clear whether the observed output of PGE by the uterus of the pregnant rabbit is part of the parturition mechanism activated by severe surgical stress or is part of the normal mechanisms that cause and maintain an adequate flow of blood through the pregnant uterus of this species.

Proteins of trophoblastic origin in maternal plasma

■ Lin, T. M., Halbert, S. P., and Spellacy, W. N.: Relation of obstetric parameters to the concentrations of four pregnancy-associated plasma proteins at term in normal gestation, Am. J. Obstet. Gynecol. **125:**17-24, 1976.

The relationship between obstetric parameters (placental weight, newborn sex, newborn weight, 1- and 5-minute Apgar scores, maternal age, maternal weight, parity, maternal blood pressure) and the maternal levels of four pregnancy-associated plasma proteins (PAPPs) were studied in 187 normal pregnant women within 7 days before delivery. The levels PAPP-A were correlated with placental and newborn weights. Women with very high levels of PAPP-A were likely to have very large placental weights and to be primigravid. On the other hand, an extremely large placental weight was not associated with a high PAPP-A level. The PAPP-C (also known as protein Sp-1 of Bohn) was not correlated with placental or newborn weight. Human chorionic somatomammotropin (HCS, or PAPP-D, in the nomenclature adopted in this article) was significantly related to placental weight and in-

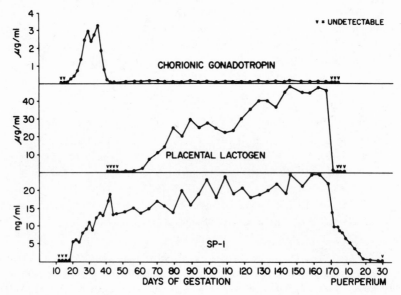

FIG. 5-3
Patterns of serum Sp-1, baboon chorionic gonadotropin, and baboon placental lactogen
during a normal baboon pregnancy. Parturition in this animal was at 170 days of gestation.
(From Stevens, V. C., Bohn, H., and Powell, J. E.: Serum levels of a placental protein
during gestation in the baboon, Am. J. Obstet. Gynecol. **124:**51-54, 1976.)

versely related to maternal weight. In addition to the above proteins, the pregnancy zone protein (PZP) was measured in the same group of patients. This protein was correlated with
parity and showed an inverse correlation with placental weight in primigravidas.

■ Stevens, V. C., Bohn, H., and Powell, J. E.: Serum levels of a placental protein during
gestation in the baboon, Am. J. Obstet. Gynecol. **124:**51-54, 1976.

A placental specific protein (Sp-1) isolated from human placentas was used to establish
a radioimmunoassay for measurement of a similar protein in the sera of pregnant baboons.
No reaction was observed with any other known pituitary or placental hormone in this assay
system. Significant levels of Sp-1 were detectable at 17 to 18 days of gestation and reached
high levels by the end of the first third of pregnancy. A slow increase in serum levels continued thereafter until parturition. Disappearance of Sp-1 postpartum was slow and required 26 to 34 days to become undetectable in the serum. The concentration pattern of
Sp-1 during gestation is different from that of chorionic gonadotropin and placental lactogen.
(See Fig. 5-3 from the original.)

■ Badger, K. S., and Sussman, H. H.: Structural evidence that human liver and placental
alkaline phosphatase isoenzymes are coded by different genes, Proc. Natl. Acad. Sci. USA
73:2201-2205, 1976.

Human liver and placental alkaline phosphatases were purified and compared. The
results indicate a totally different pattern of peptide structure. Other molecular properties
differentiating the two enzymes are a higher apparent molecular weight for the liver enzymes,
different sedimentation patterns in a sucrose gradient, different carbohydrate content, and a

different isoelectric point. The immunochemical specificity of each enzyme was not affected by removal of sialic acid groups. These data indicate that the enzymes are synthesized by different structural genes.

■ Sammour, M. B., Ramadan, M. A., Khalil, F. K., and Abd-El-Fattah, M. M.: Serum and placental lactic dehydrogenase and alkaline phosphatase isoenzymes in normal pregnancy and in pre-eclampsia, Acta Obstet. Gynecol. Scand. **54:**393-400, 1975.

Lactate dehydrogenase (LDH) isoenzymes and heat-stable alkaline phosphatase were measured in the serum and placental extracts of twenty cases of preeclampsia and ten normal pregnancies. LDH_4 and LDH_5 were the main isoenzymes in the placenta, whereas LDH_1 and LDH_2 were the main isoenzymes in the serum. Heat-stable alkaline phosphatase concentration was significantly higher in patients with mild and severe eclampsia than in the normal pregnant patients.

COMMENT: In the plasma of pregnant women there are numerous proteins of trophoblastic origin. Some of these—for example, human chorionic gonadotrophin (HCG), placental lactogen (HCS), and chorionic thyrotropin (HTS)—appear to be hormones in the classic sense of the word. Others are recently discovered entities whose functional meaning is obscure. Lin et al. have identified two new pregnancy-associated plasma proteins that they have named PAPP-A and PAPP-B. In addition, they have confirmed the existence of a third protein (PAPP-C) that was discovered by Bohn and named by him Sp-1. The latter molecule, a glycoprotein with molecular weight circa 110,000, is particularly interesting for the following reasons: (1) it is present in relatively large amounts in human pregnancy serum (2 mg/ml at midpregnancy), (2) its concentration pattern during gestation is distinctly different from that of HCG and HCS, and (3) antisera produced against this protein cause abortion in pregnant cynomolgus monkeys. Two different approaches are being pursued in the hope of identifying a physiologic role for protein Sp-1. The first, which is exemplified in the article by Lin et al., consists of seeking a correlation between so-called obstetric parameters and plasma concentration of PAPPs. The second consists of experimenting on subhuman primates that also possess this protein, as clearly demonstrated in the article by Stevens et al.

Although it seems likely that the placental proteins recently found in the maternal plasma of primates are hormones secreted by the trophoblast, we cannot exclude at present other possibilities. The first is that they may play a role in suppressing the rejection of the placenta by the maternal immunologic system. The second is that some of these proteins may simply represent products of trophoblastic degradation and have no hormonal function. In the hemochorial placenta of man and other primates there is an enormous surface of direct contact between trophoblast and maternal plasma. Thus it is reasonable to postulate a certain leakage of trophoblastic proteins in the medium. The possibility that degenerating placental cells release into maternal blood trophoblast-specific proteins is usually raised in a discussion of placental enzymes that are found in maternal serum. Among these, one of the better characterized is the heat-stable alkaline phosphatase, which is known also as Regan isoenzyme. As shown in the article by Badger and Sussman, the placental alkaline phosphatase is distinctly different from liver alkaline phosphatase. It is one of many proteins coded by genes that are expressed only during fetal life and may be reactivated in neoplastic tissue (so-called carcinoplacental proteins). A rare variant of Regan isoenzyme that occurs in ovarian tumors has been identified in normal placentas also. (Doellgast and Fishman: L-leucine, a specific inhibitor of a rare human placental alkaline phosphatase phenotype, Nature [Lond.] 259:49-51, 1976.) The article by Sammour et al. confirms the observation that placental alkaline phosphatase is significantly increased above normal in the serum of preeclamptic patients. Such an observation seems to favor the idea that "placental damage" is responsible for the presence of this enzyme in maternal plasma.

Effect of estrogens on uterine blood flow

■ Rosenfeld, C. R., Morriss, F. H., Jr., Battaglia, F. C., Makowski, E. L., and Meschia, G.: Effect of estradiol-17β on blood flow to reproductive and nonreproductive tissues in pregnant ewes, Am. J. Obstet. Gynecol. 124:618-629, 1976.

The effect of estradiol on regional blood flow and cardiac output was studied by means of radioactive microspheres in six nonpregnant and thirteen pregnant ewes 5 to 7 days after surgery. Each animal was equipped with electromagnetic flow probes around both uterine arteries for the continuous measurement of uterine blood flow. Estradiol caused vasodilation in myometrium, endometrium, and placental cotyledons throughout pregnancy, but these responses were much less than the fifteenfold increase seen in nonpregnant oophorectomized ewes. In sheep between 120 and 139 days of pregnancy uterine blood flow increased from 1099 to 1575 ml/min (p < .005). However, the major portion of this increase was in the myometrial and endometrial flows. Placental blood flow increased only 25%. Under estrogen stimulation, significant increases of blood flow occurred also in the ovaries, cervix, vagina, uterine tubes, mammary glands, skin, and adrenal glands of the pregnant animals. Cardiac output increased by 14%. No significant changes in uterine oxygen consumption were associated with the increase in blood flow to the pregnant uterus.

■ Nuwayhid, B., Brinkman, C. R., III, Woods, J. R., Jr., Martinek, H., and Assali, N. S.: Effects of estrogens on systemic and regional circulations in normal and renal hypertensive sheep, Am. J. Obstet. Gynec. 123:495-504, 1975.

The effect of estrogen administration on blood pressure, cardiac output, and uterine, renal, superior mesenteric, and iliac blood flows was studied in nonpregnant and pregnant ewes at 100 to 140 days' gestation. Some of the nonpregnant animals and one of the pregnant ewes were made hypertensive by means of renal artery constriction and removal of one kidney. The cardiac output was measured by the dye dilution technique and the regional blood flows by means of electromagnetic flow probes. The probe for measuring uterine blood flow was placed around the common artery that supplies both uterine horns. In all animals, intravenous administration of either conjugated estrones (Premarin) or estradiol produced an increase in uterine blood flow without significant change in arterial pressure, heart rate, and the other regional blood flows. The average increase of uterine flow in the pregnant ewes was 92%. In response to estrogen, uterine blood flow increased 184% in the nonpregnant normotensive group and 223% in the nonpregnant hypertensive group. In the one pregnant ewe made hypertensive, the percent change of uterine flow in response to estrogens was greater than during the normotensive state, and there was an increase of approximately 70% in uterine oxygen uptake following estrogen administration. The use of several autonomic blockers failed to alter the magnitude of the estrogen-induced uterine vasodilatation.

COMMENT: It is well established that estrogens cause a marked vasodilatation of the nonpregnant uterus in normal, unstressed animals. The action of estrogens on the blood flow to the pregnant uterus has been much more difficult to define. The article by Rosenfeld et al. shows that in early pregnancy, around the time of formation of placental cotyledons, estrogens are still capable of producing a marked uterine vasodilatation. However, as pregnancy progresses, the effect of estrogens on uterine blood flow is much less noticeable and is limited primarily to myometrium and endometrium.

It can be argued that this observation is valid for normal pregnancies only. Under normal conditions the placental arterioles may be already dilated and therefore incapable of responding to a vasodilating agent. Under certain pathologic conditions in which the placental arterioles are constricted, estrogen administration could improve dramatically placental blood flow. The observations described in the article by Nuwayhid et al. appear to support this concept because they show a greater vasodilating effect of estrogens in hypertensive ewes in which, presumably, the uterine vasculature is partially constricted. However, the observations include only one hypertensive pregnant animal and therefore need to be confirmed. In addition, it would be important to measure placental blood flow when the effect of estrogens on the hypertensive state is studied because of the experimental evidence showing that placental, endometrial, and myometrial vasculature may respond differently to various pharmacologic agents. Finally, it should be noted that the stress of surgery nearly abolishes the vasodilating effect of estrogens on the nonpregnant uterus. Hence there is at least one clear example of a situation in which estrogens, even in massive amounts, cannot release uterine vasoconstriction. For all these reasons, the effectiveness of estrogens in improving placental blood flow remains to be defined.

Placental transfer of free fatty acids

■ Elphick, M. C., Hudson, D. G., and Hull, D.: Transfer of fatty acids across the rabbit placenta, J. Physiol. **252:**29-42, 1975.

The transfer of fatty acids across the placenta was studied in anesthetized rabbits at 28 days' gestation by measuring umbilical arteriovenous differences, injecting 1-¹⁴C-palmitate into the mother and observing its appearance in the fetus, injecting 1-¹⁴C-palmitate into the fetus and observing its appearance in the mother, and measuring the fetal clearance rate. The effect of noradrenaline on the release of fatty acids and glycerol by fetal tissues was measured in vitro and in vivo. The results show that the concentration of free fatty acids (FFAs) in the maternal blood of anesthetized rabbits is relatively high and that there is a detectable uptake of fatty acids by the umbilical circulation. A significant, positive correlation is found between maternal concentration and umbilical arteriovenous difference of FFAs. Labeled palmitate injected in either maternal or fetal blood has a half-life of 30 to 60 seconds. Fetal white adipose tissue incubated in vitro releases FFAs and glycerol into the medium, and the rate of release increases fourfold or fivefold after addition of noradrenaline. Infusion of noradrenaline in the fetus leads to a rise in glucose and glycerol concentrations, but the change in FFA concentration is not significant.

On the basis of these observations, the authors conclude that (1) fatty acids can cross the rabbit placenta in amounts sufficient to provide the fatty acid components of the triglyceride and structural lipids accumulated by the growing fetus, (2) placental transport of fatty acids depends in part on maternal blood concentration, and (3) fetal circulating fatty acids are continually exchanging with fatty acid pools in the placenta and with maternal circulating FFAs.

■ Edson, J. L., Hudson, D. G., and Hull, D.: Evidence for increased fatty acid transfer across the placenta during a maternal fast in rabbits, Biol. Neonate **27:**50-55, 1975.

Organ weights and fat content, blood glucose, free fatty acids, and glycerol were measured at the twenty-eighth day of pregnancy and at term. The mothers had been fasted for 2 days prior to measurement. In the 28-day group, maternal and fetal blood levels of FFAs and glycerol were doubled in comparison to nonfasted controls. The fetuses from fasted does had increased fat stores both in the liver and adipose tissue. The overall increase in fat stores was 80% to 100%. It is suggested that during maternal fasting, increased amounts of maternal FFA cross the placenta into the fetal circulation and are incorporated into the fetal fat stores.

COMMENT: There are substantial quantitative differences among species in the placental transfer of nonessential FFAs from mother to fetus. The experiments by Elphick et al. and by Edson et al. show that in rabbits the fetus may acquire a large quantity of FFA from the mother when the FFA concentration in maternal plasma is elevated by fasting. This phenomenon has the paradoxical effect of increasing the amount of fat stored in the fetus when the mother is deprived of food. In other species (e.g., sheep), no metabolically significant transfer of FFA from mother to fetus is detectable, either normally or under conditions of maternal fasting (James et al.: A-V differences of free fatty acids and glycerol in the ovine umbilical circulation, Proc. Soc. Exp. Biol. Med. 138:823-826, 1971).

It should be noted that the fetal rabbit is born with a large content of fat, whereas the fetal lamb body contains only 2% to 3% lipids at term. Because of these differences among species, the extrapolation of conclusions from animal research to humans is difficult. In man the newborn infant is similar to the rabbit fetus in that it is born with a considerable amount of stored lipids. However, fetal growth rate is comparatively slow in man so that the daily rate of fat accumulation by the human body, expressed as mg/24 hr/kg of body weight, is much smaller than that in the rabbit and closer to that observed in fetal lambs.

Measurements of FFA uptake by the human fetus at delivery (Sabata et al.: The role of free fatty acids, glycerol, ketone bodies and glucose in the energy metabolism of the mother and fetus during delivery, Biol. Neonate 13:7-17, 1968) indicate that significant amounts of FFA are transferred to the fetus only when their concentration in maternal blood is elevated. In addition, at comparable maternal levels the rate of transfer is much less in humans than in the rabbit. Unfortunately, observations at the time of delivery do not represent normal in utero conditions. Therefore the contribution of maternal FFA to lipid storage by the human fetus remains uncertain. We do not know whether an increased level of FFA in maternal plasma, because of low caloric intake or other reasons, leads to a substantially increased fetal uptake and, if so, whether the FFA of maternal origin are oxidized or stored.

Atheromatous lesions of uterine arteries

■ Sheppard, B. L., and Bonnar, J.: The ultrastructure of the arterial supply of the human placenta in pregnancy complicated by fetal growth retardation, Br. J. Obstet. Gynaecol. 83:948-959, 1976.

The ultrastructure of the arterial supply of the human placenta was studied in fifteen pregnancies with severe fetal growth retardation. The group consisted of five patients with essential hypertension and superimposed preeclamsia, five patients with preeclampsia, and five with no hypertension. The patients were delivered by elective cesarean section between 29 and 37 weeks' gestation. Biopsies of the placental bed were taken under direct vision. Extensive placental infarction was invariably present, and the degree of infarction reflected the extent of pathologic changes in the spiral arteries. In both hypertensive and normotensive patients, the spiral and basal arteries of the decidua showed occlusive atheromatous lesions, with considerable fibrin deposition and accumulation of lipid-laden cells in both the intima and media of the vessel walls.

COMMENT: It is generally recognized that fetal growth retardation is an entity due to multiple etiologic factors. The article by Sheppard and Bonnar delineates what may be a type of growth retardation secondary to vascular lesions of the placenta. Of particular interest is the fact that these lesions can be found in normotensive as well as hypertensive patients and that they are localized in the decidual segments of the spiral and basal arteries. Therefore it would appear that they are the expression of an abnormal reaction of the uterine arteries to placentation, rather than the expression of a general circulatory disease of the mother. As to the cause of this abnormal reaction, Sheppard and Bonnar favor the theory of an immunologic response to the foreign trophoblastic antigens. Although this is a plausible theory, it should be kept in mind that experiments in animals thus far have failed to demonstrate an adverse effect on the placenta of antigenic differences between mother and fetus. To the contrary, the existence of these differences seems to favor placental growth.

CHAPTER 6

Biochemical maturation

Biochemical maturation of the developing embryo, fetus, and newborn is frequently assessed by measurement of enzyme activities in various tissues and organs of the maturing animal. In general terms, appearance, disappearance, increase, and decrease of specific enzymes as a function of time under these circumstances are seemingly controlled by one of two mechanisms. In some instances, regulation is imposed by changes in the external environment, such as change in oxygen concentration associated with birth. In other instances the developmental changes are programed to occur at some specified time interval after fertilization, regardless of specific environmental changes. In the former case, the mechanisms involved may be direct repression or depression by some environmental agent or closely related substance. In the latter case, the primary mechanism is not yet clear, although it may ultimately be expressed through repression or depression controlled by some metabolic intermediate.

Brain maturation

■ Sessa, G., and Perez, M. M.: Biochemical changes in rat brain associated with the development of the blood-brain barrier, J. Neurochem. 25:779-782, 1975.

A cell membrane fraction was prepared from whole rat brains of varying postmature ages (5 to 30 days) and from adults. This preparation was assayed for γ-glutamyl transpeptidase, 5'-nucleotidase, monoamine oxidase, and alkaline phosphatase activity. The first three of these enzymes increased as the animals matured, but the alkaline phosphatase decreased from day 15 onward. The transpeptidase is believed to be involved in amino acid transport, and therefore its increase in this capillary membrane–enriched brain fraction may reflect development of the blood-brain barrier.

COMMENT: Previous work from the authors' and other laboratories may be interpreted as showing the functional role of the transpeptidase in brain. The present article is an attempt to define the developmental aspects of the enzyme in maturation of the barrier.

Liver glucose metabolism maturation

■ Smith, R. W.: The effects of pregnancy and lactation on the activities in rat liver of some enzymes associated with glucose metabolism, Biochim. Biophys. Acta 411:22-29, 1975.

Various glycolytic and gluconeogenic enzymes in liver were measured in rats during pregnancy and at the height of lactation. Hexokinase and glucokinase increased relative to glucose-6-phosphatase, a metabolic change that favors glycolysis. Phosphofructokinase did not change relative to frutose diphosphatase, which should have had no effect on the direction of carbon flow through the glycolytic and gluconeogenic pathways. Pyruvate kinase increased relative to phosphoenolpyruvate carboxylase and pyruvate carboxylase, which should favor glycolysis. These changes in enzyme activity ratios may reflect the important metabolic role of glycolysis (carbohydrate breakdown) in pregnancy and in lactation.

COMMENT: Presumably, these changes result from hormonal stimuli. The changes may be a response to increased dietary intake of carbohydrate by the animals.

Liver enzyme maturation

- Herzfeld, A., Rosenoer, V. M., and Raper, S. M.: Glutamate dehydrogenase, alanine aminotransferase, thymidine kinase, and arginase in fetal and adult human and rat liver, Pediatr. Res. 10:960-964, 1976.

The enzymes listed in the title were analyzed by standard methods in specimens of rat and human liver at various periods in gestation, in the newborn, and in the adult. Thymidine kinase falls steadily from the fifteenth day of gestation (rat) until it reaches the adult level at about 1 week of age. The other enzymes rise during late fetal life and during the first 3 or 4 weeks after birth in rats, at which time they have reached the adult level. A similar pattern was found in a smaller number of human liver specimens.

COMMENT: These developmental patterns of enzyme activity are in accord with the metabolic requirements of the animal at the times studied. DNA synthesis is extremely active early in fetal life and falls steadily thereafter so that thymidine kinase, which catalyzes an essential reaction early in the biosynthetic pathway that eventually provides nucleotides for DNA synthesis, would be expected to parallel the rate of synthesis.

Liver mitochondria maturation

- Pollak, J. K.: The maturation of the inner membrane of foetal rat liver mitochondria, Biochem. J. 150:477-488, 1975.

Using very carefully prepared fetal, neonatal, and adult rat liver mitochondria, it was shown that there is a distinct biochemical maturation of the functional enzymes of liver mitochondria that occurs at about the time of birth. For example, the ratio of activities of the mitochondrial enzymes cytochrome oxidase/succinate–cytochrome c reductase changes from three just prior to birth to six in the adult rat. At the same time, the inner mitochondrial membrane changes from a permeable state to the relatively impermeable state found in the adult. Fetal rat liver mitochondria are not tightly coupled (closely controlled) to oxygen consumption, but after birth normal respiratory control, calcium uptake, and oxidative phosphorylation take place. When rat liver mitochondria from fetuses just prior to birth are incubated in oxygen, after preparation they appear to mature in vitro, developing some of the characteristics of the normal adult state. The mechanism of these changes is not clear but may involve uptake and/or metabolism of adenine nucleotides.

COMMENT: Presumably, these changes enable the newborn to utilize efficiently the oxygen available once the confines of intrauterine existence have been broached. Exactly why the fetal mitochondria should permit uncoupled respiration is not clear. No obvious advantage to the fetus exists.

Development of enzyme activity

- Telang, N. T., and Kothari, R. M.: Aspartate aminotransferase activity during early development of chicken embryo, Differentiation 4:61-64, 1975.

Aspartate aminotransferase (glutamic oxaloacetic transaminase) is a pyridoxal-dependent enzyme of importance in the metabolism of amino acids. Whole chicken embryos at various stages of development were assayed in crude homogenates by classic methods, and it was shown that the enzyme activity increases dramatically and suddenly at the time of differentiation of the definitive primitive streak in the embryo. The enzyme activity was virtually completely inhibited by isoniazid or iproniazid phosphate, as expected for a vitamin B_6-dependent enzyme. The increase in enzyme activity is associated with an increase in the rate of cell division in the embryo.

COMMENT: The increased activity of this enzyme at a specific time in development may reflect a need for increased interconvertibility of amino acids at this time so that the needs of growing tissues can be precisely met.

Liver enzyme induction

■ Alvares, A. P., and Kappas, A.: Induction of aryl hydrocarbon hydroxylase by polychlorinated biphenyls in the foetoplacental unit and neonatal livers during lactation, FEBS Lett. 50:172-174, 1975.

Polychlorinated biphenyls (PCBs) are known to induce nonspecific hydroxylases in the liver of many species. Pregnant rats were injected with a PCB mixture, and the placenta and fetal livers of the pregnant animals, newborns, and control animals were analyzed for benzo(a)pyrene hydroxylase activity as well as ethylmorphine N-demethylase activity and cytochrome P-450 content. The PCBs caused a tenfold induction in the hydroxylase activity of the placenta and a threefold increase in the fetal liver. This is a smaller response than that induced by 3-methylcholanthrene and is similar, in the livers, to that caused by phenobarbital. Liver enzymes in neonatal animals (exposed to the chemicals by way of the mother's milk) were also induced by the toxins.

COMMENT: These observations are interesting in that they show how the fetus as well as the adult can protect itself from possible toxicity of unnatural organic compounds. More important, the results suggest that the organism has encountered this same problem many times before in evolutionary history. Perhaps these "detoxification" mechanisms were important formerly in protection against unusual compounds in exotic plants or decaying foods, long before the profession of organic chemist or drug companies had even been created.

Placental enzyme maturation

■ Dean, J. C., and Gusseck, D. J.: Changing patterns of placental hexokinase isozymes during the course of gestation, Arch. Biochem. Biophys. 172:130-134, 1976.

The isozymes of hexokinase in rabbit and human placenta at various stages of gestation were separated by ion-exchange chromatography on DEAE-cellulose. In both the rabbit and the human, hexokinase I, a low-K_m enzyme, increases in concentration as gestation proceeds, until at term in the human it comprises almost all the glucose phosphorylating activity present. The concentration of hexokinase IV, the high-K_m enzyme, remains more or less constant throughout gestation in both species. These changes in isozyme concentration are correlated with a decreasing insulin sensitivity as the placenta develops.

COMMENT: It would be interesting to know why these changes in enzyme concentration take place. It is difficult to rationalize a requirement for insulin regulation of placental carbohydrate metabolism early in gestation that becomes less important later. Perhaps glucose becomes less readily available as gestation proceeds. This is yet another characteristic

of placental metabolism that appears to bridge species differences. (See Chapter 1 on aerobic production of lactic acid.)

Origin of dermoid cysts

■ Linder, D., McCaw, K. K., and Hecht, F.: Parthenogenic origin of benign ovarian teratomas, N. Engl. J. Med. **292:**63-66, 1975.

Benign ovarian teratomas are known to possess a normal 46,XX karyotype. Biopsies of teratomas from five patients were studied for chromosome analysis by cell culture, subsequent treatment with colchicine, and staining by the banding technique. Control tissues from the same patients were treated in the same way. The normal tissues were heterozygous for seventeen different chromosome polymorphisms examined, but the teratomas were uniformly homozygous at these loci. Similar cultures were also examined for electrophoretic polymorphism of 6-phosphogluconic dehydrogenase, phosphoglucomutase, adenylate kinase, adenosine deaminase, nucleoside phosphorylase, and lactic dehydrogenase. There were fewer instances of heterozygosity in the electrophoretic analyses of the tumors than in the corresponding normals.

These results are most consistent with a parthenogenic origin of the teratomas, which presumably arise from a single germ cell after the first meiotic division.

COMMENT: These observations are interesting as an example of one of the large number of ways in which chromosomal aberrations can occur in development.

Steroids and placental development

■ Pijnenborg, R., Robertson, W. B., and Brosens, I.: The role of ovarian steroids in placental development and endovascular trophoblast migration in the golden hamster, J. Reprod. Fertil. **44:**43-51, 1975.

The hamster is dependent on a source of ovarian steroids for maintenance of pregnancy because ovariectomy at any time during gestation causes death of the fetuses. The experiments reported here were designed to determine whether progesterone or progesterone plus estrogen could prevent this result of ovariectomy and to determine which effects were due to which hormone. It was shown that both progesterone and estradiol were required for maintenance of pregnancy in ovariectomized animals and that the principal effect of the hormones was to stimulate the formation of maternal vascular spaces beneath the haemochorial placenta, which permitted trophoblast migration to the maternal spiral arteries. Failure of the blood supply in the absence of the hormones presumably resulted in death of the fetuses.

COMMENT: Estrogen and progestin have been thought to be essential for maintenance of pregnancy because of their effect on the uterus, not its contents—which are usually considered to be autonomous. These results are one of the few examples of a direct effect of the steroid hormones on the placenta as such.

CHAPTER 7

Endocrinology

The long-term investment in basic research by endocrinologists who have studied endocrine changes during pregnancy is now beginning to yield substantial practical rewards. Knowledge of ranges of normal values, together with new, rapid and relatively simple but nevertheless accurate and precise methods, is making possible advances in fetal diagnosis and prognosis that were only dreamed of a few years ago. Effective treatment schemes are appearing close on the heels of the new diagnoses.

Hormone assays as diagnostic aids

- Buster, J. E., and Abraham, G. E.: The applications of steroid hormone radioimmunoassays to clinical obstetrics, Obstet. Gynecol. **46:**489-499, 1975.

- Mikhail, G.: Hormone assay and the gynecologist, Fertil. Steril. **27:**229-237, 1976.

These two articles provide an excellent review of the theory, technical principles, methods of application, and interpretation of results of the modern methods of hormone analysis as they can be used in caring for patients. The articles will reward thoughtful reading by all gynecologists, obstetricians, perinatologists, and pediatricians who must learn what tests to request, when and how often to obtain them, and how to interpret the results. It is essential that the conscientious physician obtain all the data needed for accurate diagnosis and therapy and also take care not to unnecessarily squander any limited resources.

Radioimmunoassay of steroids

- Barnard, G. J. R., Henman, J. F., and Collins, W. P.: Further studies on radioimmunoassay systems for plasma oestradiol, J. Steroid Biochem. **6:**107-116, 1975.

A variety of different techniques for the performance of radioimmunoassay of plasma estradiol are evaluated in this article. Comparisons of different radionuclides, antisera, separation techniques, measurements of radioactivity, and so forth were evaluated. The article includes many technical details of interest to laboratory directors and operators. Estradiol-6--carboxymethyl oxime linked to bovine serum albumin was shown to give an antiserum that led to the most accurate values even without chromatographic purification of the steroid. The radioisotope or specific chemical form of the radioactivity did not seem to affect the assays, and double antibody separation of free from bound steroid was found to be most satisfactory. The results are not necessarily applicable to all laboratories at all times in all circumstances, but they do indicate how variation in technique may affect results.

COMMENT (Barnard et al.): **An understanding and appreciation of the desirable and undesirable features of laboratory tests, and of their pitfalls, is best achieved by actual experience with them in the laboratory. Most clinicians do not have the time or opportunity** for laboratory experience, but they could get a better "feel" for the tests that they use by careful study of a summary methods article such as this one.

Radioimmunoassay of estriol

■ Goebelsmann, U., Katagiri, H., Stanczyk, F. Z., Cetrulo, C. L., and Freeman, R. K.: Estriol assays in obstetrics, J. Steroid Biochem. **6:**703-709, 1975.

The authors of this report describe the preparation of rabbit antibodies to estriol-6-carboxymethyl oxime linked to bovine serum albumin. The antigen was injected intradermally to give antibodies that are suitable for use in routine estriol assays. The methodology of the assay and its validation in terms of accuracy, sensitivity, precision, and specificity are provided in detail. Normal plasma estriol values at various stages of gestation are reported, and comparisons are provided of free and total estriol in plasma.

COMMENT: This reference provides basic information for the operation of a modern obstetrics and gynecology clinical endocrinology laboratory.

Urinary estriol in the diagnosis of complicated pregnancies

■ Aubry, R. H., Rourke, J. E., Cuenca, V. G., and Marshall, L. D.: The random urine estrogen-creatinine ratio; a practical and reliable index of fetal welfare, Obstet. Gynecol. **46:**64-68, 1975.

The investigators claim that analysis of random urine samples for total estrogen content and creatinine content, with calculation of an estriol/creatinine ratio, gives a valid index of fetal welfare. Twenty subjects were investigated in detail. As already described by others, there is a high correlation between the amount of estriol and the total estrogen in 24-hour urine collections. On the average, the creatinine excretion measured in 24-hour urine samples is relatively constant, particularly in individual subjects compared to themselves. In a population of different subjects, the expected biologic standard deviation is found for creatinine excretion. There is a high correlation between the total estrogen excretion and the estrogen/creatinine ratio in total urine samples when a population is considered in toto. Similarly, the estrogen/creatinine ratios in 24-hour urine collections are highly correlated with those determined in "random samples" collected in the morning following completion of the 24-hour collection from the same subjects. The authors do not present any specific numerical data on the correlation coefficient for the critical comparison of estrogen/creatinine ratio in truly random urine samples (i.e., nonserially correlated) and total estrogen content of the 24-hour urine samples in the *same* patient, but they claim that their method gives satisfactory clinical results.

COMMENT: Scientific "proof" that measurement of estriol in pregnant women improves the quality of the delivered infant may never become available, but most obstetricians believe that the analysis sometimes may be helpful. Analyses of urinary estriol will probably disappear except in special circumstances because the blood methods are more convenient. Attempts to make the urine analysis more convenient, such as the one described here, have not gained wide acceptance: sound statistical evidence has not been provided to support the concept that additional sources of variation are acceptable in the method because its biologic variability is already so large. These authors have made a beginning toward establishing the facts. Unfortunately, they use an estrogen method in which only 75% to 85%

of the total value determined is actually due to the specific fetal product estriol, and their statistical design is not optimal for deciding the question they pose.

Serum estriol

■ Hay, D. M., and Lorscheider, F. L.: Serum oestriol in normal pregnancy, Br. J. Obstet. Gynaec. **83:**118-123, 1976.

Total serum estriol determinations in pregnant women at various stages of gestation were measured, using a radio receptor rather than a radioimmunoassay. The overall pattern of increase in serum estrogens as pregnancy proceeded was similar to that found by other methods and other authors, with a more rapid increase in concentration after week 34 in normal pregnancy (Fig. 7-1). The authors found a statistically significant positive correlation between the infant birth weight and the last estriol value determined prior to delivery (r = .34).

COMMENT: The values shown are typical of many results for *total* (free plus conjugated) serum or plasma estriol. They are ten to twenty times greater than the values for free (that is, unconjugated) estriol, as shown in the following article. The marked change in

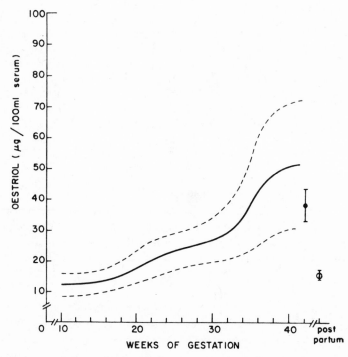

FIG. 7-1

Normal range of estriol values according to gestation. The curves of the mean and ± 1 SD have been smoothed. Average number of patients each week: eleven from 10 to 30 weeks; thirty-seven from 31 to 40 weeks; thirteen at 41 weeks; four at 42 weeks (●); and forty-six at 2 to 3 days postpartum (○). (From Hay, D. M., and Lorscheider, F. L.: Serum oestriol in normal pregnancy, Br. J. Obstet. Gynaecol. **83:**118-123, 1976.)

slopes in the third trimester is also typical. Although the correlation with birth weight is significant, the r is so small as to make prediction of weight from estriol extremely imprecise.

■ Buster, J. E., Sakakini, J., Killam, A. P., and Scragg, W. H.: Serum unconjugated estriol levels in third trimester and their relationship to gestational age, Am. J. Obstet. Gynecol. **125:**672-676, 1976.

Unconjugated serum estriol concentration was determined in a group of randomly selected subjects between 28 and 41 weeks' gestation and in a group of nine subjects who provided serial samples. Concentration values were converted to logarithms and studied as a function of gestational age (Fig. 7-2). Statistical analysis showed a transitory decline from the average upward trend at gestational age 34 to 36 weeks, with a subsequent increase to the original slope. Later there was a secondary decrease in slope at 41 weeks. The authors suggest that the results could be of value in predicting gestational age.

COMMENT: These normal values for unconjugated serum estriol should be compared to those for total serum estriol in the preceding article. If further studies confirm that this pattern of slope changes occurs in all pregnancies at the same time as found by these authors, it may become possible to add another valuable predictor of fetal age to those already available.

Use of plasma estrogen measurements in management of complicated pregnancies

■ Duenhoelter, J. H., Whalley, P. J., and MacDonald, P. C.: An analysis of the utility of plasma immunoreactive estrogen measurements in determining delivery time of gravidas with a fetus considered at high risk, Am. J. Obstet. Gynecol. **125:**889-898, 1976.

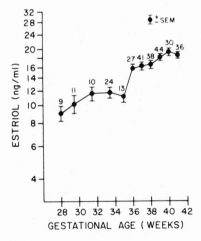

FIG. 7-2
The means and standard errors for the means from 285 unconjugated estriol determinations between weeks 28 and 41 of gestational age on a semilogarithmic plot. Figures indicate the numbers of samples for each point. (From Buster, J. E., Sakakini, J., Killam, A. P., and Scragg, W. H.: Serum unconjugated estriol levels in third trimester and their relationship to gestational age, Am. J. Obstet. Gynecol. **125:**672-676, 1976.)

A population of 622 pregnant women diagnosed as being at high risk (patients attending the obstetric complication clinic or hospitalized in the high-risk obstetric unit) were randomly divided into two groups, and plasma estrogens were repeatedly measured by a relatively nonspecific radioimmunoassay method. In one of the groups of patients the results were immediately reported to the responsible clinicians; in the other half they were not. The perinatal death rate was identical in both groups. In the group in which the results were not reported, there were ten infants who ultimately did well whom the authors state "would have been delivered 28 days or more prematurely if management had been based solely on the basis of abnormal immunoreactive estrogen levels." The authors conclude that the measurements were of little value and might even be hazardous.

COMMENT: These results contradict the opinion of many thoughtful physicians. No serious defects are evident in the prospective study except for the assumption that the results of estrogen measurements should dictate patient management. Thus the authors state that for the patients in the reported group, "Special notice was given to a physician if the plasma estrogen levels were consistently low or suddenly decreased. Prompt delivery was advised if a fall in concentration of plasma estrogens of more than 40 percent from previous values occurred and was confirmed in a subsequent sample. Delivery was also urged in the gravida in whom multiple plasma samples contained less than 20 ng. per milliliter after 34 weeks' gestation." These authors also used a method that includes estrogens other than estriol, which may have further impaired the clinical utility of the analyses.

Many clinicians would suggest that a report of a *normal* plasma estriol is reassuring information about the status of the fetus and that the criteria quoted from the article should lead to reevaluation of the progress of the gestation. They would *not* urge delivery on the basis of the laboratory results alone.

Estriol excretion

■ Young, B. K., Jirku, H., Kadner, S., and Levitz, M.: Renal clearances of estriol conjugates in normal human pregnancy at term, Am. J. Obstet. Gynecol. 126:38-42, 1976.

Estriol conjugates were measured in plasma and in urine by a complex separation method utilizing chromatography, followed by determination of the quantity of the various conjugates by radioimmunoassay. Five volunteers were studied and clearances of the various conjugates were measured in the customary way. The subjects were studied late in pregnancy and it was shown that more than 90% of the total estriol consisted of four conjugates: estriol-3-sulfate, estriol-16-glucosiduronate, estriol-3-glucosiduronate, and estriol-3-sulfate-16-glucosiduronate. The estriol-16-glucosiduronate was preferentially excreted, followed closely by the 3-glucosiduronate. The sulfoconjugates were excreted at a far smaller rate, perhaps because they are more tightly bound to the plasma proteins. The calculated renal clearance of the predominant 16-glucosiduronate approached the clearance of para-aminohippurate.

COMMENT: Since the kidney treats different steroid conjugates differently, the relative preponderance of the several compounds is different in blood and urine. It would appear that the predominant urinary constituent (estriol-16-glucosiduronate) is almost completely cleared from the renal plasma in one pass.

Estetrol in pregnancy

■ Tulchinsky, D., Frigoletto, F. D., Jr., Ryan, K. J., and Fishman, J.: Plasma estetrol as an index of fetal well-being, J. Clin. Endocrinol. Metab. 40:560-567, 1975.

Estetrol (15-α-hydroxyestriol, or E_4) is a recently described steroid hormone metabolite that is probably synthesized almost exclusively in the fetal liver. It has been suggested that measurement of this hormone in the maternal blood might be a good indicator of fetal well-being. As is the case with estriol, plasma estetrol concentration increases rapidly during the second half of gestation, although the hormone is frequently undetectable prior to the eighteenth week of pregnancy by the radioimmunoassay used by these authors. At term the plasma concentration was sevenfold that at 24 weeks of gestation. The careful clinical studies of these investigators demonstrate that measurement of plasma estetrol values in Rh-isoimmunization was not useful in evaluating fetal well-being, but in patients with hypertension or preeclampsia, subnormal plasma estetrol concentrations always preceded intrauterine fetal death.

COMMENT: Measurement of estetrol has certain theoretical advantages over estriol measurement for pregnancy monitoring, but these results suggest that in practice the measurements are of similar value.

Dehydroepiandrosterone sulfate loading test

■ Tulchinsky, D., Osathanondh, R., Finn, A.: Dehydroepiandrosterone sulfate loading test in the diagnosis of complicated pregnancies, N. Engl. J. Med. 294:517-522, 1976.

This article describes another investigation of dehydroepiandrosterone sulfate (DHA-S) infusions in pregnant women as an assessment of the status of pregnancy. Fifty milligrams of the conjugate were administered, and both estradiol and estetrol were measured in the blood at intervals thereafter. The infused steroid disappeared rapidly from the circulating blood with a half-life of about 30 minutes. The peak concentration of estradiol, a direct metabolic product made by the placenta from DHA-S, occurred 30 minutes after beginning the infusion. The mean preinfusion level in the normal subjects was 16 ng/ml, which increased to a mean of 44 ng/ml after infusion. The biosynthesized estetrol reached a maximum concentration at 4 hours after beginning the infusion. In those patients with low urinary estriol excretion who also showed evidence of chronic fetal distress (birth weight small for gestational age), there was a less than normal increase in estradiol and estetrol following the DHA-S infusion. Another group of patients with low urinary estriol excretion who ultimately delivered normal infants were found in nine out of ten cases to show a normal increase in plasma estradiol and estetrol as a result of the conjugate administration. The authors consider this test to be more accurate in assessing fetal well-being than measurements of estradiol, estriol, estetrol, or human placental lactogen.

■ Fraser, I. S., Leask, R., Drife, J., Bacon, L., and Michie, E.: Plasma estrogen response to dehydroepiandrosterone sulphate injection in normal and complicated late pregnancy, Obstet. Gynecol. **47:**152-158, 1976.

DHA-S (100 mg) was infused intravenously in subjects with either normal or complicated pregnancy. Unconjugated estradiol, estrone, and estriol concentrations were measured in blood at intervals after the infusion. The infusion resulted in a marked increase in estradiol in all patients, 174% to 478% above basal levels. Estrone increases were smaller and more variable, and estriol changes were not significant. No differences were observed between normal subjects and patients with preeclampsia, essential hypertension, retarded intrauterine growth, diabetes, or twin pregnancies. The authors believe that this procedure has no advantages over existing methods of assessing the endocrine function of the placenta except in the diagnosis of placental sulfatase deficiency.

COMMENT: These two contradictory articles demonstrate that no consensus has been reached about the value of this function test.

Placental sulfatase deficiency

■ Tabei, T., and Heinrichs, W. L.: Diagnosis of placental sulfatase deficiency, Am. J. Obstet. Gynecol. **124:**409-414, 1976.

Low concentrations of serum estriol or excretion of urinary estriol in pregnant women may be caused by the absence of sulfatase from the placenta. This enzyme hydrolyzes 16-α-hydroxydehydroepiandrosterone sulfate and other estrogen precursors, which normally must be hydrolyzed so that the free steroids can be aromatized. Four cases of placental sulfatase deficiency are described in which the lack of the enzyme was demonstrated by standard biochemical techniques and in which normal aromatase activity was also demonstrable in the placenta. The enzyme deficiency can be diagnosed by a laboratory test prenatally. DHA-S infused into either the amniotic fluid or the maternal peripheral circulation is converted to estradiol and estrone, which can be measured in blood or urine. If increases in these two hormones do not appear following the infusion, placental sulfatase deficiency is strongly suggested. The enzyme deficiency does not appear to affect the developing fetus that in the cases reported thus far has always been male.

■ Beastall, G. H., Kelly, A. M., England, P., Rao, L. G. S., MacGregor, M. W., and Paterson, M. L.: Urinary oestrogen and plasma human placental lactogen as initial screening tests for a placental sulphatase deficiency, Scott. Med. J. **21:**106-108, 1976.

This brief case report presents the essentials of management and diagnosis in a suspected case of placental sulfatase deficiency, complete with enzymic confirmation of the diagnosis by biochemical study of the placenta after delivery. The essential features were low urinary estriol excretions throughout the latter portion of pregnancy in the presence of normal serum prolactin values. The results show that DHA-S loading tests are not necessary for the diagnosis of this rare, presumably mutational, abnormality of gestation.

COMMENT: This rare metabolic abnormality is clinically important because of its potential for causing error in interpretation of estriol analyses in pregnancy. The outcome of pregnancy in the cases so far reported suggests that high blood concentrations of estriol are not important in the maintenance of normal pregnancy. The loading test described in the article by Tabei and Heinrichs involves saturation of the placental enzymes, which hydrolyzes steroid sulfates (sulfatase) and converts C-19 steroids into estrogens (aromatase). The high concentrations of steroid used in the test approximately measure the total activity of the enzymes in the placenta. The activity of these enzymes in other tissues is small compared to that in the placenta. A different application of metabolic measurements of DHA-S at normal concentrations is reviewed in Chapter 5.

High-risk pregnancy

■ Edwards, R. P., Diver, M. J., Davis, J. C., and Hipkin, L. J.: Plasma oestriol and human placental lactogen measurements in patients with high risk pregnancies, Br. J. Obstet. Gynaec. **83:**229-237, 1976.

Total plasma estriol was measured by a fluorometric technique, and plasma human placental lactogen (HPL) was measured by a commercial kit in 383 high-risk pregnancies. Eighty-five infants in these pregnancies were growth retarded, and 122 developed fetal distress or neonatal asphyxia. Of the infants whose mothers had either abnormal plasma estriol or HPL levels about two thirds were either growth retarded or showed fetal distress. The determinations clearly are of value in identifying in the total population of high-risk pregnancies a subpopulation in whom the hazards of delivery of a poor infant are increased.

COMMENT: These results are typical of those reported by a number of authors and show that the two tests studied are valuable diagnostic and prognostic aids when intelligently applied. The report is a calm appraisal of the clinical value of the tests and can be strongly recommended for detailed study. Estriol measurements may be slightly more precise, but HPL analyses are still somewhat easier to perform.

Human placental lactogen

■ Spellacy, W. N., Buhi, W. C., and Birk, S. A.: The effectiveness of human placental lactogen measurements as an adjunct in decreasing perinatal deaths; results of a retrospective and a randomized controlled prospective study, Am. J. Obstet. Gynecol. **121**:835-844, 1975.

In this investigation weekly serum HPL measurements were performed in a high-risk group of pregnancies. In confirmation of previous results, it was shown that identification of patients in whom this placental product was significantly decreased, effectively identified a group of subjects with fetuses at risk. When these patients were treated, the perinatal mortality was substantially reduced.

■ Stroobants, W. L. A., Van Zanten, A. K., de Bruijn, H. W. A., Van Doorm, J. M., and Husisjes, H. J.: Serial human placental lactogen estimations in serum and placental weight-for-dates, Br. J. Obstet. Gynaecol. **82**:899-902, 1975.

Serial HPL determinations were done with the aid of a commercial kit in 100 randomly selected pregnant women. The individual progress curves were examined for abnormality according to a variety of criteria, including consistent low values, defined decreasing concentration with time, transitory depressed value, and failure to increase. After delivery the abnormal values were compared with the outcome of pregnancy, and it was found that patients who showed a fall to a value more than 2 SD below the mean at a specified time and failed to recover frequently had small-for-dates placentas. The prediction was not uniform, however, giving a substantial number of false negatives. The single fetal death that occurred in this series was predicted.

■ Spellacy, W. N., Buhi, W. C., and Birk, S. A.: Human placental lactogen and intrauterine growth retardation, Obstet. Gynecol. **47**:446-448, 1976.

The authors reiterate their belief that a low serum HPL value during the last month of pregnancy is a substantial warning to the physician of the possibility of intrauterine growth retardation. Sixty percent of the women with intrauterine growth retardation had placental lactogen values less than 6 μg/ml.

■ Harrigan, J. T., Langer, A., Hung, C. T., Pelosi, M. A., and Washington, E.: Predictive value of human placental lactogen determinations in pregnancy, Obstet. Gynecol. **47**:443-445, 1976.

HPL determinations were made on blood of ninety-four patients late in the third trimester, using a commercial kit for analysis. As described by others, there was a correlation between birth weight and HPL concentration when all the patients were considered together, with an overall r of .6. In all but 2% of the patients a low birth weight was associated with low HPL in the blood but 5% of the subjects with normal weight infants also had low lactogen values in the circulation. The authors consider the determination to be valuable in the prediction of low birth weight.

COMMENT: Currently it would appear that measurements of serum HPL, estriol, or both, are valuable in identifying a group of pregnant women who may require special attention during gestation. The cost-effectiveness of the procedures has not been evaluated. One might envision a mass-screening approach in which the unit cost of each analysis became negligible with respect to the total cost of care during gestation. Under such circumstances the predictive value of the analyses might be quite substantial.

■ Schneider, A. B., Kowalski, K., and Sherwood, L. M.: Identification of "big" human placental lactogen in placenta and serum, Endocrinology **97:**1364-1372, 1975.

Recent investigations of the physical chemistry of a variety of polypeptide hormones have shown that many of them exist in a variety of physical forms in vivo with many instances of the existence of high molecular weights of the hormone. In this article it is shown that placental lactogen possesses this property also. The "big" form of HPL appeared to be identical in activity with the low molecular weight material.

Biosynthesis of human placental lactogen

■ Szczesna, E., Boime, I.: mRNA-dependent synthesis of authentic precursor to human placental lactogen: conversion to its mature hormone form in ascites cell-free extracts, Proc. Natl. Acad. Sci. USA **73:**1179-1183, 1976.

mRNA containing the information necessary for the biosynthesis of HPL was isolated from human placenta and was translated in an enzyme-ribosome preparation prepared from ascites tumor cells. The product was characterized by the usual methods, and it was found that unpurified ascites cell preparations gave a product identical to that secreted by the placenta (molecular weight, 22,200). When the protein-synthesizing machinery was purified, a higher molecular weight product was produced. Investigation of this material showed that it was an HPL precursor that is cleaved in the intact animal prior to secretion of the hormone.

COMMENT: It would now appear that the majority of secreted proteins are synthesized in a precursor form that must then be modified. The necessity for the processing is not well-understood but may involve intracellular transport from the site of synthesis to the sites of storage or secretion, or may be related to the secretory process itself.

Placental hormones

■ Beas, F., Salinas, A., Gonzalez, F., Teran, C., and Szendro, P.: A human placental hormone (UTPH) with uterine growth and DNA promoting effects, Horm. Metab. Res. **7:** 515-520, 1975.

Further investigations of a protein from human placenta are described in this article. The material was extracted with 0.1 N acetic acid and gel filtration in a column of Sephadex G-75. The protein extract was injected into prepubertal mice where it exerted a growth-promoting effect on the weight of the uterus. A substantial amount of the protein was required to stimulate the growth, which was quite dramatic. Hydrolysis of the extract with acid abolished its biologic activity. The activity was also abolished when antiserum to the protein was administered simultaneously with the extract, but the effects were not inhibited by estradiol, progesterone, or HCG. The uterotrophic effect of the placental extract may be due to its stimulation of incorporation of precursors into RNA and DNA. The authors have previously reported results that suggest that the protein is not identical with any other placental or pituitary protein hormone.

COMMENT: Evidence is gradually accumulating for the existence of a variety of polypeptides with growth-regulating properties. The material studied here may be another example, and hopefully studies of this kind will eventually greatly clarify our understanding of organ growth and differentiation.

Placental weight and maternal hormone concentrations

■ Spellacy, W. N., Conly, P. W., Cleveland, W. W., and Buhi, W. C.: Effects of fetal sex and weight and placental weight on maternal serum progesterone and chorionic gonadotropin concentrations, Am. J. Obstet. Gynecol. **122:**278-282, 1975.

A large series of pregnant women was investigated to determine possible relationships between hormone concentration and other parameters. Neither HCG nor progesterone concentrations in the serum correlated with infant weight or infant sex. There was no correlation between the HCG concentration and the serum progesterone concentration. The only significant correlation found was between the serum progesterone level and the weight of the placenta, but the correlation is so small as to have no predictive value.

COMMENT: Prediction of fetal and placental weight or functional capacity by some simple prenatal test remains an elusive goal, probably because the biologic correlation contains more inherent variability than most investigators will readily accept. An interesting relationship between hormone concentrations, organ size, and nutrition is reviewed in Chapter 2.

Placental progesterone metabolism

■ Tabei, T., and Troen, P.: Formation of 6-hydroxylated progesterone in the human placenta and response to HCG, J. Clin. Endocrinol. Metab. **40:**697-704, 1975.

Minced human placenta preparations were incubated in buffer with radioactive steroid substrates, chiefly 5-pregnenolone. No coenzymes were added, but HCG or human prolactin were added to some vessels. The major radioactive product of the incubation in every case was progesterone (40% to 60% conversion). 6-β-Hydroxyprogesterone was a minor product (2% to 4% conversion). An even smaller amount of 6-α-hydroxyprogesterone was also found. In some, but not all, experiments the HCG increased the amount of 6-β-hydroxylation, whereas HPL had no effect. The physiologic importance of these observations is not known.

COMMENT: Although the major features of placental steroid metabolism are now known, it is obvious that many quantitatively less important pathways remain to be investigated and evaluated for biologic and clinical significance. One of the objectives of this kind of investigation is to find some unique metabolic reaction in the placenta in which there is no large metabolic "reserve." Such a reaction might then serve as a functional test of the placenta and might be diagnostically or prognostically useful.

Placental ACTH

■ Rees, L. H., Chard, T., Evans, S. W., and Letchworth, A. T.: Possible placental origin of ACTH in normal human pregnancy, Nature (Lond.) **254:**620-622, 1975.

Plasma and placental extract concentrations of ACTH were measured with highly specific antibodies in a radioimmunoassay. The maternal plasma concentration rose steadily from the sixteenth to the fortieth week of gestation, approximately doubling during that period of time. Extracts of placentas also contained large amounts of ACTH activity measurable by radioimmunoassay, which was far in excess of the amount that might be accounted for by sequestered blood. Dexamethasone suppression tests in which urinary free cortisol was measured showed that in late pregnancy the adrenals were less readily suppressed than in the nonpregnant state.

COMMENT: Many reports of placental production of ACTH have been published, but few have been as convincing as this one. Perhaps the tropin is secreted to make certain that gestation is not interferred with by pituitary inadequacy.

Placental content of chorionic gonadotropin

- Hobson, B., and Wide, L.: Relationship of the sex of the foetus to the amount of human chorionic gonadotrophin in placentae; single and dizygotic twin placentae compared, J. Endocrinol. **64:**117-123, 1975.

HCG was assayed by both biologic and radioimmunologic methods in human placentas. It had previously been shown that the amount of HCG in the term placenta was higher when the fetus was a female singleton, and the present studies were made to further examine this differentiation. In the case of dizygotic twins of unlike sex, it was found that there was no sex differentiation of HCG content. The values for the twin placentas are midway between those previously found for male and female singleton placentas.

COMMENT: The results support the previous postulate that the fetal gonads regulate placental HCG production by an unknown mechanism.

Placental growth hormone action

- Croskerry, P. G., and Smith, G. K.: Prolongation of gestation by growth hormone: a confounding factor in the assessment of its prenatal action, Science **189:**648-650, 1975.

It was previously reported (see *Perinatal Medicine,* volume one, p. 7) that growth hormone administered to pregnant rats had a selective stimulatory action on brain growth. The present report describes further investigation of the phenomenon. The effect of purified bovine growth hormone on length of gestation in the rat was measured, and it was found that the treated animals delivered 1 day later than the controls (22 days after conception instead of 21). This difference could account for the previously reported difference in brain size.

COMMENT: These investigations emphasize the complexity of interactions between hormone effects, nutrition, and other factors in intact animals. Only multiple, carefully controlled experiments of many different kinds by different investigators can unravel these complexities. Here it would now appear that growth hormone improves nutrient utilization in malnourished animals and in addition prolongs gestation. Both these effects can increase brain size.

Newborn steroids

- Schindler, A. E., and Wuchter, J.: Studies on steroids in urine of the male newborn, Biol. Neonate **27:**192-207, 1975.

The steroids present in urine of newborn males during the first 5 days of life were analyzed in detail by a variety of careful analytical techniques. The amount of steroid present was determined by gas-liquid chromatography. The qualitative and quantitative patterns of steroids present in the newborn urine are more similar to those of amniotic fluid than to those of fetal and newborn blood. Of particular interest is the high concentration of 16-hydroxylated and 16-dehydro steroids. The 16-hydroxylated compounds are typically produced by the hydroxylases present in the fetus, particularly the fetal liver. A portion of the 16-dehydro compounds may be produced enzymically, although these substances can also be produced from the 16-hydroxysteroids during the analytical procedure.

COMMENT: No similar analyses seem to be available for female newborns. The comparison between the sexes might be interesting. The available data are convincing evidence that the amniotic fluid is mainly a product of the fetal kidney.

Menstrual cycle of the baboon

■ Goncharov, N., Aso, T., Cekan, Z., Pachalia, N., and Diczfalusy, E.: Hormonal changes during the menstrual cycle of the baboon *(Papio hamadryas)*, Acta Endocrinol. (Kbh.) **82:** 396-405, 1976.

A variety of steroid hormones and luteinizing hormones were measured in the peripheral plasma in normally cycling female baboons. The changes seen were similar to those found in the human except in the luteal phase, when progesterone was much lower and the ratios of progesterone to 20-α-dihydroprogesterone, pregnenolone, androstenedione, estradiol, and estrone were not as high during the luteal phase in the baboon as in humans. Details of the results may be found in many figures in the original article. Thus the pattern of steroid secretion is similar but the quantitative aspects are different in these two species.

COMMENT: These data emphasize the potential usefulness of this large primate in studies of reproduction when the objective is to obtain data directly transferable to the human.

Molecular mechanism of steroid hormone action

■ Eide, A., Hoisaeter, P. A., and Kvinnsland, S.: Estradiol receptor in uterine tissue from neonatal mice. Influence by cyclic AMP, J. Steroid Biochem. **6:**1121-1125, 1975.

The estradiol receptor was studied by standard techniques in the uteri of newborn mice less than 5 days old. The receptor was found to be present in cytosol, and high concentrations of dibutyryl-cyclic AMP caused a decrease in the receptor with a sedimentation coefficient of 8 and an increase in the receptor.

■ Kang, Y., Anderson, W. A., and DeSombre, E. R.: Modulation of uterine morphology and growth by estradiol-17β and an estrogen antagonist, J. Cell Biol. **64:**682-691, 1975.

The effect of an estrogen antagonist, CI628, and of estrogen on the uterus of virgin female rats was studied. CI628 caused a marked hypertrophy of the uterine epithelium, a change greater in magnitude than that induced by estrogen. However, estrogen produced a marked hyperplasia of the uterine epithelium over 48 hours, and CI628 or CI628 plus estrogen did not.

■ Martinez-Vargas, M. C., Gibson, D. B., Sar, M., and Stumpf, W. E.: Estrogen target sites in the brain of the chick embryo, Science **190:**1307-1308, 1975.

Specific autoradiograms of high specific activity tritium-labeled estradiol showed that the hormone was concentrated in brain cells of the medial preoptic and ventral hypothalamic regions as early as day 10 in the incubated chick embryo. Hormone appeared in other sites of the brain later in embryonic development. In other target organs, demonstration of concentration of the hormone in cells has been correlated with action of the hormone.

■ Anderson, J. N., Peck, E. J., Jr., and Clark, J. H.: Estrogen-induced uterine responses and growth: relationship to receptor estrogen binding by uterine nuclei, Endocrinology **96:**160-167, 1975.

The effects of estradiol and estriol injections into immature rats were measured in uterus. Accumulation and retention of the estrogen receptor in the nucleus of the cells was measured, and a variety of biochemical events induced by estrogen were also measured. The two hormones were of equal potency when the accumulation by the nucleus was measured, but estradiol disappeared from the nucleus more rapidly than estriol. The two hormones were of equal potency in stimulating glucose utilization, water imbibition, and incorporation of ^{14}C-glucose into lipid, protein, and RNA in the uterine cells. Moreover, the activity of RNA polymerase was equally stimulated by the two hormones. By contrast, estriol failed to stimulate true uterine growth unless it was administered repetitively. Thus the responses to the hormone are similar but are modulated by the degree to which the receptor hormone complex is retained in the nucleus.

■ Spelsberg, T. C., Pikler, G. M., and Webster, R. A.: Progesterone binding to hen oviduct genome: specific versus nonspecific binding, Science **194:**197-198, 1976.

Radioactive progesterone receptor complex from chick oviduct cytosol was allowed to bind to oviduct or spleen nuclei at various salt concentrations, as well as to isolated chromatin from oviduct or spleen and purified DNA. At low ionic strength, binding to nuclei and chromatin in both tissues is nonsaturable and nonspecific. Purified DNA binding of the progesterone receptor complex is nonspecific at all salt concentrations. At high ionic strength, binding of the hormone receptor complex is saturable and tissue specific, the binding being high with the target organ oviduct and low with the spleen. These results correlate well with the observed hormone-induced increases in RNA polymerase, which are an essential part of the response to the hormone. The investigation emphasizes that in this complex field the experimental conditions are crucial to an understanding of the results.

■ Means, A. R., Woo, S., Harris, S. E., and O'Malley, B. W.: Estrogen induction of ovalbumin mRNA: evidence for transcription control, Mol. Cell. Biochem. **7:**33-42, 1975.

Studies of estrogen and progesterone action in the chick oviduct have greatly advanced knowledge in this area. It has been shown that both of these steroid hormones, which stimulate the production of the specific proteins ovalbumin and avidin, exert their effects by the derepression of the genes responsible for the information required for the synthesis of the proteins. The mRNA produced as a result of the derepression can be purified on a preparative scale to apparent homogeneity. This mRNA can then be used to synthesize (with the aid of a reverse transcriptase) a radioactive complementary DNA copy. The complementary DNA can then be used for further genetic analysis, and in the case of ovalbumin it was shown that the gene which coats for the ovalbumin mRNA is represented only once in each haploid genome.

Careful studies of the quantitative aspects of estrogen action in this system suggests that the hormone acts by pure translational control of the synthesis of the tissue-specific protein.

COMMENT: This group of articles is included to indicate the status of fundamental re-

search in this exciting area. A detailed summary may be found in a three-part review by O'Malley (N. Engl. J. Med. 294:1322-1328, 1372-1381, 1430-1437, 1976).

As now understood, the active hormone enters the target cell, which contain a specific cytosol hormone-binding protein called a receptor (R_C). The hormone combines with the receptor ($H \cdot R_C$), which is then transformed and moves with the attached hormone into the nucleus ($H \cdot R_N$). There it finds a specific site or sites on the DNA, guided by an acidic protein in the chromatin that specifically binds to a site on the receptor. The nuclear receptor hormone complex then somehow facilitates the transcription of specific genes in the DNA. The protein or proteins whose structure is specified by this messenger RNA transcript is the hormone "effect." After a number of false starts, it is satisfying to seemingly understand in large part these complex molecular actions of the steroid hormones as they direct the activities of their target cells. Knowledge of receptor concentration and activity may permit clinical modulation of target cell sensitivity in situations such as fertility control, endocrine sensitive tumors, and so on. Synthetic hormones and antagonists may be designed on the basis of receptor specificity. Knowledge of regulation of DNA function might someday permit direct treatment of genetic disease.

Control of prostaglandin synthesis by angiotensin

■ Gimbrone, M. A., Jr., and Alexander, R. W.: Angiotensin II stimulation of prostaglandin production in cultured human vascular endothelium, Science **189**:219-220, 1975.

Human endothelial cells were obtained by collagenase treatment of term umbilical cord veins. The cells derived from the luminal surface of the vessels were grown in tissue culture, and PGE-like material was assayed in the tissue culture medium or on samples of fractured cells by a specific radioimmunoassay. The cells produced substantial amounts of immunoreactive PGE, and the synthesis was inhibited by indomethacin (50% inhibition at 6×10^{-9} gm/ml). In this system, addition of angiotensin II to the serum-free, chemically defined medium that was used to feed the cells gave a maximal prostaglandin response approximately a hundred times greater than that in the unstimulated cells at a concentration of 5×10^{-7} M hormone. The phenomenon described may be important in the local control of vascular permeability and tone in small vessels and of platelet-dependent thrombotic phenomena.

COMMENT: See Comment following the review of Ham et al.

Uterine prostaglandins

■ Ham, E. A., Cirillo, V. J., Zanetti, M. E., and Kuehl, F. A., Jr.: Estrogen-directed synthesis of specific prostaglandins in uterus, Proc. Natl. Acad. Sci. USA **72**:1420-1424, 1975.

Rat uterine prostaglandins and cyclic nucleotides were measured by radioimmunoassay procedures, and it was found that prostaglandin F (PGF) concentration in the uterus varied with the stage of the estrus cycle, being highest at proestrus. Estradiol administration to oophorectomized animals caused a substantial increase in PGF, and the response was abolished by simultaneous treatment with indomethacin. Cyclic GMP was increased by estradiol, whereas cyclic AMP was reduced. Similar changes were seen in the rate of synthesis of PGF as a function of stage of the menstrual cycle. Presumably, the observed effects are related to the estrogenic environment of the tissue.

COMMENT: The observations in these two reports support the concept that prostaglandins may serve as endocrine-regulated "second messengers."

■ Keirse, M. J., Williamson, J. G., and Turnbull, A. C.: Metabolism of prostaglandin $F_{2\alpha}$ within the human uterus in early pregnancy, Br. J. Obstet. Gynaecol. **82:**142-145, 1975.

Human uterine tissues were obtained from hysterectomies for abortion done between the seventh and sixteenth weeks of gestation. Tissues obtained from different parts of the uterus were homogenized, and the homogenates were then incubated with tritiated $PGF_{2\alpha}$ and nicotinamide adenine dinucleotide (NAD). $PGF_{2\alpha}$ was rapidly metabolized in two tissues—placental villous tissue and membranes. Most of the radioactivity was recovered in a metabolite tentatively identified as 15-oxo-$PGF_{2\,alpha}$. Since the enzyme 15-hydroxyprostaglandin dehydrogenase would have oxidized both PGE_2 and $PGF_{2\,alpha}$, these data suggest that both prostaglandins would be rapidly metabolized by the placenta and placental membranes.

COMMENT: **Prostaglandin-metabolizing enzymes may be important in the maintenance of pregnancy and avoidance of spontaneous abortion. The higher metabolic activity in fetal tissues supports a fetal role in regulating the onset of labor. These observations may help explain the high dosage required for therapeutic abortions when prostaglandins are given intra-amniotically.**

Placental prostaglandins

■ Schlegel, W., and Greep, R. O.: Prostaglandin 15-hydroxydehydrogenase from human placenta, Eur. J. Biochem. **56:**245-252, 1975.

An NAD-linked prostaglandin 15-hydroxyprostaglandin dehydrogenase was purified more than 12,000-fold from human placental soluble cell sap by standard enzymic methods. This enzyme inactivates the biologically active compounds. Kinetic analyses of the purified enzyme were made, and numerical values for the kinetic constants are reported.

COMMENT: **The enzyme may be important in inactivation of the biologically potent prostaglandins. Preparation of the highly purified enzyme will permit studies of its specificity and so forth, which are prerequisite to understanding its biologic function.**

Prostaglandins in preeclampsia

■ Keirse, M. J. N. C., Hicks, B. R., and Turnbull, A. C.: Prostaglandin dehydrogenase in the placenta before and after the onset of labour, Br. J. Obstet. Gynaecol. **83:**152-155, 1976.

15-Hydroxyprostaglandin dehydrogenase determinations were done in the placentas of forty-four normal patients. The placentas were obtained before or after spontaneous labor or after oxytocin-induced labor. The enzymic activities were the same before and after labor, and oxytocin induction had no effect on the enzyme content of the tissue.

COMMENT: **This experiment would appear to rule out changes in catabolism of prostaglandins by the placenta as an explanation for the increase in amniotic fluid prostaglandins that occurs during labor.**

■ Demers, L. M., and Gabbe, S. G.: Placental prostaglandin levels in pre-eclampsia, Am. J. Obstet. Gynecol. **126:**137-139, 1976.

Prostaglandin analyses were done by radioimmunoassay on placenta obtained immediately after delivery. Specific antisera against PGE and PGF were used. Results in twenty normal patients were compared to those in twenty-two subjects with preeclampsia. PGE concentra-

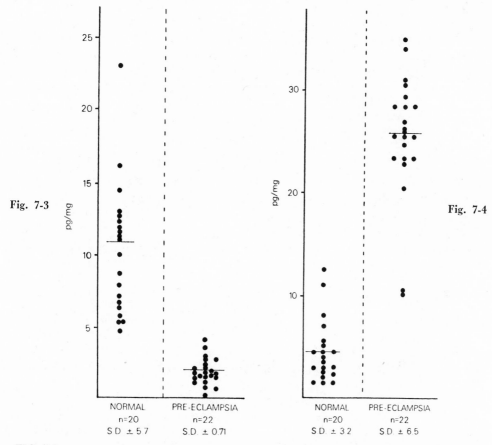

FIG. 7-3
PGE levels in placental tissue from twenty control patients and twenty-two patients with preeclampsia. Results are expressed as picograms per milligram of wet tissue weight. The solid line across the data points indicates the mean value. Standard deviations are listed at the bottom of the figure. (From Demers, L. M., and Gabbe, S. G.: Placental prostaglandin levels in pre-eclampsia, Am. J. Obstet. Gynecol. **126:**137-139, 1976.)

FIG. 7-4
PGF levels in placental tissue taken from the same patients as in Fig. 7-3. Results are expressed as picograms per milligram of wet tissue weight. (From Demers, L. M., and Gabbe, S. G.: Placental prostaglandin levels in pre-eclampsia, Am. J. Obstet. Gynecol. **126:**137-139, 1976.)

tions in preeclampsia were significantly lower than those in normal subjects (Fig. 7-3), whereas PGF concentrations were significantly increased (Fig. 7-4). No correlation between the concentration of prostaglandin in the placenta and severity of the preeclampsia was found.

COMMENT: These striking changes demonstrate that it will be necessary to study specific compounds (and enzymes) before the role of the prostaglandins in health and disease can be understood. PGF is a potent vasoconstrictor, and the results suggest that it may be an etiologic factor in the disease.

Neonatal ovary regulation

■ Kolena, J.: Ontogenic development of the responsiveness in cAMP synthesis to LH and PGE$_1$ and gonadotropin receptors in the rat ovary, Biol. Neonate **29**:96-103, 1976.

Responsiveness of the neonatal ovaries to luteinizing hormone (LH) and PGE$_1$ were measured at various ages by assessing the cyclic AMP formation response to added hormones. Whereas the ovary responded to prostaglandin at all ages from 2 to 20 days, the response to luteinizing hormone did not appear until 9 days of age. Measurement of gonadotropin receptors in similar tissues showed that the receptors were present from the time of birth.

COMMENT: This experiment suggests that luteinizing hormone effects on the ovary are not mediated by PGE$_1$.

Placental hydroxylases

■ Juchau, M. R., and Zachariah, P. K.: Displacement of carbon monoxide from placental cytochrome P-450 by steroids: antagonistic effects of androstenedione and 19-norandrostenedione, Biochem. Biophys. Res. Commun. **65**:1026-1032, 1975.

Binding of carbon monoxide to placental microsomes was measured spectrophotometrically under a variety of conditions and with various added reagents, including steroids and reducing agents. Addition of androstenedione to the enzyme preparation caused the disappearance of the P-450 carbon monoxide complex adsorption spectrum. Presumably, carbon monoxide was released from the enzyme. The effect of androstenedione was reversed by 19-*nor*androstenedione or 19-*nor*testosterone. The known effect of the 19-*nor*steroids in augmenting carbon monoxide binding was similarly reversed by androstenedione. The effects observed were independent of the sequence of the addition of substrate, cofactor, and so forth. The androstenedione binding spectra are of the type I classification, which suggests that the steroid binds to a site other than the heme site so that the effect on carbon monoxide binding must be of an allosteric nature.

■ Zachariah, P. K., and Juchau, M. R.: Interactions of steroids with human placental cytochrome P-450 in the presence of carbon monoxide, Life Sci. **16**:1689-1692, 1975.

Placental microsomes were prepared in a conventional manner and were examined spectrally for formation of the complex between cytochrome P-450 and carbon monoxide. It was found that after reduction of the pigment with NADPH, addition of normal aromatization substrates such as androstenedione, 19-hydroxyandrostenedione, 19-oxoandrostenedione, and testosterone eliminated or prevented the absorbance maximum normally induced by carbon monoxide. By contrast, 19-*nor*androstenedione, 19-*nor*testosterone, pregnenolone and benzo(a)pyrene did not eliminate the peak. The results are interpreted to mean that in the presence of steroid substrates for hydroxylation, carbon monoxide is either displaced from the pigment or cannot form the heme complex. Reduction with dithionite, on the other hand, consistently permitted the appearance of the specific carbon monoxide–dependent absorption maximum. Presumably, binding of the steroids to the active site of the pigment is sufficiently tight to prevent complex formation with carbon monoxide.

COMMENT: The complex experimental results reported in these two articles appear to resolve several vexing questions about the mechanism of placental steroid hydroxylation.

They permit the enzymic reaction to be considered as very similar in mechanism to other P-450–dependent hydroxylases.

Pregnancy proteins

- Lin, T., Halbert, S. P., and Kiefer, D.: Quantitative analysis of pregnancy-associated plasma proteins in human placenta, J. Clin. Invest. **57:**466-472, 1976.

This study determined the concentration of four pregnancy-associated plasma proteins (PAPPs) in human placenta. The gestational ages of the pregnancies from which placental tissue was obtained are not given. Immunochemical methods were used to identify four PAPPs, one of which was shown to be human placental lactogen (HPL). In addition, measurements of albumin, transferrin, IgA, and IgM were also made on the placental extracts. The results demonstrated that the four proteins PAPP-A, PAPP-C, PAPP-B, and HPL were all at much higher concentrations in placental tissue than could be accounted for by their concentrations in maternal blood. This contrasted to the determinations of pregnancy zone protein (PZP) whose concentration in placental tissue never exceeded that which could be accounted for by its concentration in maternal blood, a finding similar to those for IgM and IgA in the placenta. The data are consistent with placental synthesis of the four PAPPs and with the conclusion that pregnancy zone protein is synthesized elsewhere in the mother. From the concentrations of proteins in maternal and fetal blood and their concentrations in placental tissue, calculations of the placental blood volume derived from the mother and the fetus were made. The calculations estimated that in a 400 gm placenta approximately 25% of the blood in the placenta would be derived from the mother and 75% from the fetus with a blood volume of approximately 140 ml.

COMMENT: In contrast to HPL, whose biologic activity was studied in parallel with its original purification, the other three PAPPs have no known biologic role.

- Damber, M. G., Von Schoultz, B., Stigbrand, T., and Tärnvik, A.: Inhibition of the mixed lymphocyte reaction by the pregnancy zone protein, FEBS Lett. **58:**29-32, 1975.

This study tested the effect of PZP, a protein that has been shown not to be produced in the placenta but elsewhere in the mother, on mixed lymphocyte cultures. PZP was purified by adsorption on staphylococci coated with rabbit anti-**PZ** antiserum. The incorporation of ^{14}C-thymidine into DNA in mixed lymphocyte cultures was reduced by approximately 50% in the presence of high concentrations of pregnancy zone protein (160 to 170 μg/ml). There was no significant effect at PZP concentrations of 35 to 40 μg/ml.

COMMENT: The high concentration of PZP required to produce the effects reported renders their in vivo significance questionable.

Rat alpha-fetoprotein

- Benassayag, C., Vallette, G., Cittanova, N., Nunez, E., and Jayle, M. F.: Isolation of two forms of rat alpha-fetoprotein and comparison of their binding parameters with estradiol-17β, Biochim. Biophys. Acta **412:**295-305, 1975.

Rat alpha$_1$-fetoprotein, which is present in blood for only a few days after birth in the rat, has been shown to bind estradiol very strongly. The protein was highly purified by affinity chromatography, and its binding properties were examined. Under appropriate conditions the purified protein gave two distinct bands on polyacrylamide gel electrophoresis.

The binding was studied by electrophoresis and by equilibrium dialysis. The purified alpha-fetoprotein which migrated less rapidly on electrophoresis contained approximately one binding site for estradiol per molecule, whereas the other fraction consistently gave a smaller number of available sites for binding. The binding constant is approximately 0.2×10^8 M for the slow form and is greater for the more rapidly migrating protein, which has the lower number of binding sites. The isolated alpha-fetoprotein is therefore heterogenous.

COMMENT: The reappearance of this transitory fetal antigen in hepatic neoplasia has aroused great interest. The fact that it binds estradiol avidly makes it even more mysterious. The human alpha$_1$-fetoprotein does *not* bind estradiol appreciably.

Pregnancy sex hormone–binding globulin

■ De Hertogh, R., Thomas, K., and Vanderheyden, I.: Quantitative determination of sex hormone–binding globulin capacity in the plasma of normal and diabetic pregnancies, J. Clin. Endocrinol. Metab. **42:**773-777, 1976.

A plasma protein, sex hormone–binding globulin, increases in concentration during pregnancy, probably as a result of the increased estrogen present. It can be measured by its capability of binding dihydrotestosterone, which is not present in large amounts in normal pregnancy. The amount of the globulin increased about sevenfold in the first half of pregnancy and by another 30% in the second half, plateauing late in gestation. The increase was somewhat greater in diabetic pregnancy, and in diabetics the increased binding globulin was paralleled by increased unconjugated estradiol concentrations in the blood.

COMMENT: The biologic role of this protein is unknown, but its behavior in pregnancy, which is similar to that of corticosteroid- and thyroxin-binding globulins, must be understood for proper interpretation of hormone assays done during gestation.

Specificity of steroid-binding protein

■ Laurent, C., De Lauzon, S., Cittanova, N., Nunez, E., and Jayle, M.-F.: The comparative specificity of three oestradiol-binding proteins, Biochem. J. **151:**513-518, 1975.

Binding of a variety of steroids, particularly estradiol, to three proteins was studied. The proteins were rat alpha-fetoprotein, rat liver microsomal 17β-hydroxysteroid dehydrogenase, and a model protein, rabbit anti-**estradiol** gamma globulin. Binding was measured either with the aid of radioactivity, fluorescence, or enzyme activity. In a detailed study of the binding capacity of these three proteins for a great variety of steroids with differing structural features, it was shown that the two naturally occurring proteins (alpha-fetoprotein and 17β-hydroxysteroid dehydrogenase) recognize by some kind of a template mechanism the edge of the steroid defined by C-4, C-6, C-8, and C-15. By contrast, the antibody gamma globulin, which was conjugated through position 6 to bovine serum albumin (for use as an antigen), recognized the opposite edge of the steroid molecule—that defined by C-2, C-11, C-10, and C-17.

COMMENT: The geometric relationships shown here are illustrative of the mechanisms by which specific steroids are recognized by cells.

Fetal thyroid

■ Chopra, I. J., and Crandall, B. F.: Thyroid hormones and thyrotropin in amniotic fluid, N. Engl. J. Med. **293:**740-743, 1975.

A sensitive and precise radioimmunoassay was used to measure thyroxin, 3,3′,5-triiodothyronine (T_3), 3,3′-5′-triiodothyronine (reverse T_3), and thyrotropin in amniotic fluid at various stages in gestation. Thyroxin concentration does not vary greatly as gestation advances but reverse triiodothyronine falls steadily from week 15 to term. Triiodothyronine (3,3′,5-triiodothyronine) was undetectable, as was thyrotropin. Reverse triiodothyronine in amniotic fluid was much higher than the corresponding value in maternal serum, and the authors suggest that this measurement may aid in the diagnosis of both fetal thyroid function and the identification of pregnancies of more than 30 weeks' gestation.

COMMENT: Although reverse triiodothyronine has little calorigenic activity, it may be an important intermediate in thyroxin-thyronine interconversions. This article should be studied carefully by physicians responsible for management of maternal thyroid disorders during pregnancy or in the fetus and newborn.

Fetal status in hypothyroidism

■ Porterfield, S. P., Whittle, E., and Hendrich, C. E.: Hypoglycemia and glycogen deficits in fetuses of hypothyroid pregnant rats, Proc. Soc. Exp. Biol. Med. **149:**748-753, 1975.

Female rats were thyroidectomized just after mating and were used for experimentation on the last day of pregnancy (day 22). It was found that the weight gain of the hypothyroid animals was less than normal, and the total weight of the fetuses was much less than the weight of those from pair-fed, nonthyroidectomized controls. Likewise, the livers of the hypothyroid mothers were smaller than normal. Glycogen in liver and muscle was decreased by thyroidectomy in both the mothers and offspring. The total glycogen content of these organs was therefore much reduced from normal, being affected both by the size of the organ and the concentration of the carbohydrate polymer.

COMMENT: Maternal thyroidectomy early in pregnancy prevents the normal and essential accumulation of glycogen stores that occurs late in pregnancy. Because glucose is an important metabolic substrate in pregnancy, this metabolic failure of carbohydrate storage probably accounts for the small size of the animal. The most important immediate result to the fetus is a marked hypoglycemia.

Normal prolactin concentrations

■ Schenker, J. G., Ben-David, M., and Polishuk, W. Z.: Prolactin in normal pregnancy: relationship of maternal, fetal and amniotic fluid levels, Am. J. Obstet. Gynecol. **123:**834-838, 1975.

Prolactin was measured by a radioimmunoassay method in normally cycling women and normal men and in serum of pregnant women as well as cord blood serum and amniotic fluid. Normal male and female serum contained 4 to 30 ng/ml of prolactin, which rose at term in uncomplicated pregnancy to 208 ± 8 ng/ml. Cord blood contained a higher concentration, and amniotic fluid contained concentrations much higher than those found in the mother's serum (Fig. 7-5). These results are similar to those already reported in a smaller group of samples by the same authors.

COMMENT: More data are needed to establish the normal limits of variation of this hormone in pregnancy with precision, but the general patterns of increase are established in this careful investigation. In addition to its role in lactation, the polypeptide probably

126 *Perinatal medicine: review and comments*

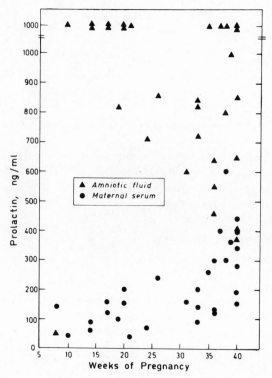

FIG. 7-5
Prolactin levels in maternal serum and in amniotic fluid during various stages of pregnancy.
(From Schenker, J. G., Ben-David, M., and Polishuk, W. Z.: Prolactin in normal pregnancy:
relationship of maternal, fetal and amniotic fluid levels, Am. J. Obstet. Gynecol. **123:**834-838,
1975.)

has effects on salt and water-balance regulation. The latter function is probably related
to the presence of the hormone in amniotic fluid.

Postpartum amenorrhea

■ Delvoye, P., Delogne-Desnoeck, J., and Robyn, C.: Serum-prolactin in long-lasting lactation
amenorrhoea, Lancet **2:**288-289, 1976.

Serum prolactin, LH, and follicle-stimulating hormone (FSH) were measured by
radioimmunoassay in postpartum women living in Central Africa. In this area where
breast feeding is often prolonged up to 24 months, the basal serum prolactin concentrations
were high until 15 months after giving birth. Three months postpartum the suckling stimulus
to circulating prolactin concentration disappears, as already reported elsewhere. The results
suggest that prolactin is involved in the etiology of prolonged postpartum amenorrhea and
birth spacing.

Prolactin in pituitary-ovarian function

■ Bonnar, J., Franklin, M., Nott, P. N., and McNeilly, A. S.: Effect of breast-feeding on
pituitary-ovarian function after childbirth, Br. Med. J. **4:**82-84, 1975.

Radioimmunoassay measurements of plasma LH and FSH, total estrogens and progesterone, prolactin, and HCG beta-subunit are reported for a group of women who consistently breast-fed their infants from the time of delivery onward. The values were compared to women who did not breast-feed their infants. As described previously by others, the main difference between the groups was the persistently higher concentration of prolactin in the lactating women. As a result, and in the presence of normal FSH concentrations, ovarian function was inhibited in these women, and plasma estrogens remained low without evidence of ovulation.

COMMENT: These results should convince the remaining doubters of the relationship between prolactin, lactation, and relative infertility.

Relaxin in humans

■ Weiss, G., O'Byrne, E. M., and Steinetz, B. G.: Relaxin: a product of the human corpus luteum of pregnancy, Science **194:**948-949, 1976.

By means of a radioimmunoassay using antibody to porcine relaxin, it was shown that the blood draining human ovaries having a corpus luteum contains a higher control concentration of material that interacts with the antibody used. The secretion of this immunologically determined material correlates well with secretion of progesterone by the corpus luteum.

COMMENT: Perhaps radioimmunoassay will finally permit clarification of the biologic role of this old hormone.

Fetal pancreatic development

■ Freie, H. M. P., Pasma, A., and Bouman, P. R.: Quantitative analysis of pancreatic islet development and insulin storage in the foetal and newborn rat, Acta Endocrinol. **80:**657-666, 1975.

Histologic and insulin concentration studies of fetal rat pancreas were made. Insulin concentration rose from low levels beginning about day 19 to adult levels on day 22 and remained stable after birth. During the same time, the percentage of islet tissue rose slowly from 0.7% at day 19 to 1.5% on day 22 with a more rapid postnatal increase to 3.6% at the fifth day. No measurements were made prior to day 19.

■ Asplund, K., Andersson, A., Jarrousse, C., and Hellerstrom, C.: Function of the fetal endocrine pancreas, Isr. J. Med. Sci. **11:**581-590, 1975.

The authors review earlier work from their own laboratory and that of other investigators. In the rat, immunoreactive glucagon and insulin in the fetal pancreas are present prior to visibility of the specific cells that synthesize these hormones, which appear at about day 11 and the cells appearing at about day 15. The fetal pancreas does not readily release insulin on glucose stimulation, and this response is not well established in the rat until 2 days following delivery. On the other hand, glucose does stimulate insulin synthesis during fetal life. There is thus a dissociation between insulin synthesis and insulin release in the fetus. Treatment with glucose does not induce sensitivity of the fetal pancreas to glucose as a releasing agent. It is clear that regulation of fetal pancreatic function requires further study.

COMMENT: These two studies provide more facts about the initiation of regulation of carbohydrate metabolism in the fetus, but a clear overall scheme is still not available.

Fetal carbohydrate metabolism

■ Schwartz, A. L., and Rall, T. W.: Hormonal regulation of incorporation of alanine-U-^{14}C into glucose in human fetal liver explants, Diabetes **24:**650-657, 1975.

In a continuation of previous studies of human fetal liver carbohydrate metabolism, experiments were done with fetal liver explants in organ culture. Glucagon and dibutyryl cyclic AMP were added to the cultures and were shown to produce a twofold to tenfold increase in conversion of alanine into glucose and/or glycogen. Insulin additions reversed the effects of the nucleotide or glucagon, while the synthetic corticosteroid triamcinolone stimulated gluconeogenesis from alanine. This striking stimulation of gluconeogenesis may account for a substantial fraction of the glucose needs of the developing fetus. The mechanism of the effect is not known with certainty but apparently does not require increased uptake of amino acid by the tissue or induction of specific enzymes.

COMMENT: **The varied kinds and amounts of nutrients required by the developing fetus are provided by the maternal organism, but the composition of the maternal blood must also be suitable for the continuing metabolic needs of the mother as well as the fetus. As a result, some metabolic interconversions of foodstuffs are required in the fetus from early in gestation. Gluconeogenesis permits the fetus to utilize excess amino acids for synthesis of carbohydrate skeletons.**

Insulin effects on placenta

■ Podskalny, J. M., Chou, J. Y., and Rechler, M. M.: Insulin receptors in a new human placenta cell line: demonstration of negative cooperativity, Arch. Biochem. Biophys. **170:** 504-513, 1975.

Experiments were done in a newly established culture of normal human trophoblasts derived from a term placenta (JHC-1 cells). This cell line has been cloned once. Iodinated insulin–binding studies were done in the usual way, separating bound from free hormone by centrifugation. The labeled hormone bound rapidly and specifically, and it was shown by dilution experiments that the binding sites exhibited negative cooperatively. That is, dissociation was accelerated when a greater fraction of the insulin receptors was occupied. The Scatchard plots for binding were nonlinear, but the hormone had an apparent association constant of 4.8×10^8 M.

COMMENT: **After considerable disagreement, it would now appear to be established that the placenta is an insulin-sensitive organ. It follows that some of the pathology of the fetoplacental unit in the pregnant diabetic may be the result of inadequate maternal insulin for regulation of placental metabolism. Alternatively, inadequate control of the pregnant diabetic may stimulate fetal hyperinsulinism with other undesirable consequences such as macrosomia and placental hypertrophy.**

Insulin effects on muscle

■ Asplund, K.: Protein synthesis and amino acid accumulation during development in the rat: dissociation of diaphragm and heart muscle sensitivity to insulin, Horm. Res. **6:**12-19, 1975.

This study compared the effect of insulin in vitro on hemidiaphragms and heart muscle obtained from rat fetuses from shortly before the end of gestation, fetal age 21.5 days, through the forty-first postnatal day. The study demonstrated an effect of insulin in stimulating the uptake of alpha-aminoisobutyric acid (AIB) in both diaphragm muscle and heart muscle from fetal life throughout the postnatal period. In contrast, insulin stimulated the incorporation of tritiated leucine only into heart muscle and into hemidiaphragms. An effect of insulin on protein synthesis could be demonstrated in hemidiaphragms beginning on the third postnatal day. The authors speculate that this study may have demonstrated a different effect of insulin on two separate muscle tissues, skeletal muscle and heart muscle.

COMMENT: These experimental results reemphasize the fact that insulin is not simply a hormone that regulates glucose uptake by certain cells. Instead, it is a general regulator of cell nutrition and growth, with different effects on different cells and metabolites. Glycogen deposition is also different in heart and diaphragm.

Hypoglycemia in the young calf

- Bloom, S. R., Edwards, A. V., Hardy, R. N., Malinowska, K. W., and Silver, M.: Endocrine responses to insulin hypoglycaemia in the young calf, J. Physiol. **244**:783-803, 1975.

The young calf is remarkably sensitive to hypoglycemia induced either by adrenalectomy or insulin. The mechanisms of protection of the blood sugar concentration were studied in detail. Hypoglycemia was induced with insulin, and it was found that there was first an increase in adrenocorticosteroids, followed by significant increases in epinephrine and plasma glucagon concentrations. These responses were transient and were related to changes in adrenal blood flow. With large doses of insulin, glucocorticoid output was not maintained during prolonged hypoglycemia, and it was necessary to treat these animals with glucose infusions if they were to be saved. The results are surprising in that the adrenocorticoid response in young calves insulted by hypoglycemia occurs prior to that of the adrenal medulla.

COMMENT: These results emphasize again the importance of the adrenal cortex in protecting against hypoglycemia.

Mechanism of glucagon action

- Vinicor, R., Higdon, G., Clark, J. F., and Clark, C. M., Jr.: Development of glucagon sensitivity in neonatal rat liver, J. Clin. Invest. **58**:571-578, 1976.

Before birth the fetal hepatic glycogenolytic and gluconeogenic enzyme systems are relatively insensitive to glucagon but not dibutyrl cyclic AMP. Shortly after birth the liver becomes sensitive to glucagon and responds in the usual way by releasing cyclic nucleotide. Measurements of sensitivity to glucagon were made in fetal and neonatal liver at various times in development. Fig. 7-6 shows the response found. It is clear that the sensitivity of the cyclase increases with increasing age of the animal, and the response appears to be an increase in the maximal capacity of the enzyme. The latter may be related to the number of glucagon receptor sites for this membrane-bound enzyme. The early lack of sensitivity to glucagon may in part explain fetal and neonatal hypoglycemia, since the tissue cannot respond in the usual way to stressful situations.

COMMENT: The alterations in responsiveness to carbohydrate-regulating hormones at birth are outstanding examples of changes triggered by a change in environment of the developing organism.

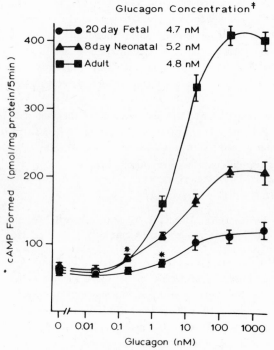

FIG. 7-6

Effects of glucagon concentration on adenylate cyclase activity. Partially purified liver membranes (20-40 µg of protein per tube) were incubated for 5 minutes at 30° C for determination of cyclic AMP formation. Points are means ‡ SEM of triplicate determinations in three experiments on three different membranes for each age. *, Concentration of glucagon giving initial significant stimulation of hepatic adenylate cyclase over basal activity; ‡, concentration of glucagon giving half-maximal stimulation of hepatic adenylate cyclase. (From Vinicor, R., Higdon, G., Clark, J. F., and Clark, C. M., Jr.: Development of glucagon sensitivity in neonatal rat liver, J. Clin. Invest. **58**:571-578, 1976.)

Hormone effects

■ Walters, M. R., Lawrence, A. L., and Hazelwood, R. L.: Amino acid transport by the rat uterus during the estrous cycle and pregnancy, Biol. Reprod. **12**:383-388, 1975.

Uterine tissue was obtained from rats at different stages of the estrus cycle and at days 2, 7, 14, and 20 of gestation. Tissue from pregnant animals was cleaned and did not include fetal and associated placental tissue. The uterine tissue was cut into small segments and incubated in vitro with glucose and tritiated aminoisobutyric acid, and ^{14}C-labeled mannitol was added as a reference marker for extracellular fluid volume within the uterine tissue. Fig. 7-7 taken from their report shows that the AIB uptake corrected for the changes in extracellular fluid volume occurring in the uterus at different stages of estrous cycle was altered, and the direction of change in AIB uptake parallels changes in uterine size. Similarly the AIB uptake corrected for mannitol uptake changed during gestation, with the highest levels of alpha-aminobutyric acid minus mannitol uptake per gram of uterus found in late gestation between 14th and 20th days. Thus the changes in AIB uptake during the

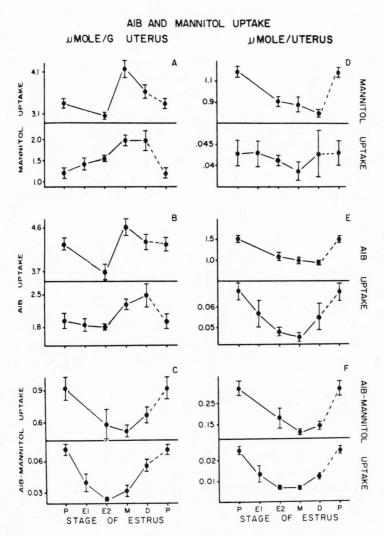

AIB AND MANNITOL UPTAKE

ɥMOLE/G UTERUS   ɥMOLE/UTERUS

STAGE OF ESTRUS

FIG. 7-7

Changes in uterine absorption of D-mannitol and AIB during the estrus cycle. In each doublet of curves **A** to **F**, the upper represents data from 10 mmolar initial ambient concentration and the lower, 0.5 mmolar. These concentrations were selected to allow evaluation of uterine uptake phenomena (1) at a concentration (0.5 mmolar) near amino acid plasma levels at which the rate of uptake by way of active components may be affected by either changing K_m or V_m and (2) at a concentration (10 mmolar) much greater than plasma levels when V_m is probably the rate-limiting factor. However, concentrations used in the medium external to the tissue may measure intracellular rates of uptake characteristic of much lower plasma amino acid concentrations (see text). Points and bars, respectively, represent mean ± SEM (n = 4.6). Broken line indicates a return to the first stage presented. Abbreviations for cycle stages are *P,* proestrus; *E1,* early estrus; *E2,* late estrus; *M,* metestrus; and *D,* diestrus. (From Walters, M. R., Lawrence, A. L., and Hazelwood, R. L.: Amino acid transport by the rat uterus during the estrus cycle and pregnancy, Biol. Reprod. **12:**383-388, 1975.)

estrous cycle and gestation correlated with changes in uterine weight, suggesting some mechanism that synchronizes amino acid transport to nutritional requirements in the uterus.

COMMENT: The observed changes are probably steroid hormone effects, but this hypothesis needs investigation.

Placental permeability

■ Ganazzani, A. R., Fraioli, F., Fioretti, P., and Felber, J. P.: Placental impermeability to maternal ACTH in the rabbit, Experientia **31:**245-246, 1975.

Synthetic human ACTH was labeled with radioactive ^{125}I and purified. The radioactively labeled hormone was injected peripherally in pregnant rabbits, and fetal blood and placental samples were taken for counting. The radioactivity disappeared rapidly from the maternal circulation, and virtually none was found in the fetal blood or organs. These results are similar to those found for ACTH and other protein hormones in humans.

COMMENT: This result can probably now be accepted as established for most species.

Implantation

■ Bergstrom, S., and Nilsson, O.: Embryo-endometrial relationship in the mouse during activation of the blastocyst by oestradiol, J. Reprod. Fertil. **44:**117-120, 1975.

Implantation may be studied in rats by delaying the process with progesterone and subsequently "reactivating" the blastocyst by estrogen injection. Investigation of this process by transmission and scanning electron microscopy showed that estrogen causes swelling of the trophoblast and an apparent separation of the developing embryo from the uterine surface by the development of a layer of secretion. Thereafter the process of implantation proceeds by erosion and so forth as usual. The authors of this article interpret these changes as indicating that arrest of implantation is caused by reduction of metabolic activity in the trophoblast by means of a reduced supply of nutrients. Estrogen administration reverses this process and permits implantation to proceed.

COMMENT: The mechanism of hormonally delayed implantation is imperfectly understood. The ultrastructural changes involved in one species are carefully described in this article, but the authors' suggestions regarding mechanism must be considered speculation until direct evidence for their hypothesis is presented.

Lecithin metabolism in the fetus

■ Hallman, M., and Raivio, K. I.: Formation of disaturated lecithin through the lysolecithin pathway in the lung of the developing rabbit, Biol. Neonate **27:**329-338, 1975.

Fetal rabbit lung preparations were incubated with radioactive precursors for the biosynthesis of phospholipids. The precursors included labeled choline, labeled S-adenosylmethionine, and doubly labeled lecithin, lysolecithin, and phosphatidylethanolamine. Detailed consideration of the labeling patterns resulting from these experiments suggested that the mature pattern of disaturated lecithin is achieved by biosynthesis by way of cytidine phosphate choline in association with a lysolecithin loop pathway in which previously synthesized unsaturated lecithin is deacylated and subsequently reacylated with a saturated fatty acid. The methylation pathway appears to be less important under all circumstances.

COMMENT: See Comment following the review of Ekelund et al.

Fetal lung phospholipids

■ Ekelund, L., Arvidson, G., Astedt, B.: Cortisol-induced accumulation of phospholipids in organ culture of human fetal lung, Scand. J. Clin. Lab. Invest. **35**:419-423, 1975.

Human fetal lung at various gestational ages was incubated with or without cortisol in organ culture. The phospholipid content of the cultures was measured, as was the incorporation of radioactively labeled choline into lecithin. The steroid treatment increased the phospholipid content in the cultured tissue, particularly the lecithin fraction. Likewise steroid increased the incorporation of radioactivity into lecithin.

COMMENT: The articles by Ekelund et al. and Hallman and Raivio are included as a sample of the available material on the biochemistry of lung phospholipid. No consensus has been reached about the mechanisms of maturation of lung composition, although the empirical facts about phospholipid composition and surfactant activity appear to be established. (See Chapter 11.)

Sexual differentiation

■ Resko, J. A.: Fetal hormones and their effect on the differentiation of the central nervous system in primates, Fed. Proc. **34**:1650-1655, 1975.

In the rhesus monkey the major hormonal differences between male and female fetuses are found in the testosterone/progesterone ratio, which is high in the male because of the biosynthesis of testosterone in the fetal testis. The author proposes that the anti-androgen effect of progesterone is of vital importance in the differentiation of the hypothalamic centers into those with responsiveness typical of male or female in the adult. These results are in accord with those obtained by administration of the steroid hormones to pregnant rhesus monkeys. In both the normal and experimental situation, typical masculine or feminine behavior results from corresponding high or low testosterone/progesterone ratios.

COMMENT: These speculations illustrate the primitive state of research in this area.

CHAPTER 8

Immunology

Substantial advances in understanding of the molecular features of the immunologic response have been achieved in recent years. This new information has not yet been helpful in understanding clinical mysteries such as the failure to reject the fetal "graft."

Effect of immunologic status on reproductive capability

■ Beer, A. E., Scott, J. R., and Billingham, R. E.: Histoincompatibility and maternal immunological status as determinants of fetoplacental weight and litter size in rodents, J. Exp. Med. **142:**180-196, 1975.

Various sublines of defined strains of mice, hamsters, or rats were mated within or outside of their own genetic line, and at specified times in gestation the resulting pregnant females were examined. The number of viable fetuses present and the weights of the individual fetoplacental units, fetuses, and placentas were measured. Weights of the spleens and the para-aortic lymph nodes were also measured. In some experiments sensitized tolerant females were used.

In general, histoincompatibility between the mother and the fetuses caused hypertrophy and increased cellularity of the lymph nodes in the mother and a somewhat increased size of placentas or fetoplacental units. Likewise, sensitized animals showed increased placental weights, whereas tolerant mothers had normal or decreased fetoplacental unit size in most instances.

The result of this partial immunologic response is to yield larger and perhaps more vigorous offspring, which may be a selective advantage in evolution.

COMMENT: In these experiments there was not only a failure to reject the fetal graft, but also the apparent immune response in the maternal organism seemingly gave rise to *more* vigorous offspring. The results may be related to a form of heterosis (hybrid vigor), in addition to the immunologic circumstances of the matings.

Placental proteins and the response to the fetal graft

■ Strelkauskas, J. J., Wilson, B. S., Dray, S., and Dodson, M.: Inversion of levels of human T and B cells in early pregnancy, Nature (Lond.) **258:**331-332, 1975.

In this study the proportion of T and B lymphocytes was determined in women during different stages of pregnancy. The percentage of B cells was determined by direct rosette techniques, using mixtures of human erythrocytes coated with anti–**human** kappa or anti–**human** lambda light-chain antibodies. The percentage of T cells was determined by indirect rosette techniques, using human erythrocytes coated with anti-**rabbit** light-chain antibodies. The lymphocytes were first sensitized with specific rabbit anti–**human** T cells antiserum. From the twenty-second week of gestation until term the proportion of T and B cells was identical to that found in four nonpregnant women serving as controls; however, from the seventh to the twentieth week of pregnancy the percentage of T cells was very low and the percentage of B cells much higher than both later in pregnancy and in the nonpregnant women. The biphasic lymphocyte response during pregnancy, consisting of an early inversion phase and a later stable phase, parallels changes in serum chorionic gonadotropin (HCG) levels. The authors speculate that HCG may possibly have an immunoregulatory role in pregnancy.

COMMENT: These results suggest that in early pregnancy a part of the foreign cell recognition system (suppressor T cells) is depleted so that the fetal "graft" is not rejected. The mechanism of the suppression is not clear, but it occurs at about the same time that placental HCG production is maximal. Perhaps the two phenomena are related.

■ Gusdon, J. P., Jr., and Witherow, C. C.: The effects of active immunity against placental proteins on pregnancy in monkeys, Am. J. Obstet. Gynecol. **126**:308-312, 1976.

Female squirrel monkeys were actively immunized against human placental lactogen (HPL), or soluble human or squirrel monkey placenta extract. The titers obtained were low and irregular among the immunized animals, but the incidence of pregnancy in the injected animals was significantly reduced. Crude HPL extract was a more potent antigen than purified HPL.

COMMENT: These experiments confirm the belief that failure to reject the fetal graft is not the result of a failure or attenuation of the maternal immune response.

■ Werthamer, S., Govindaraj, S., and Amaral, L.: Placenta, transcortin, and localized immune response, J. Clin. Invest. **57**:1000-1008, 1976.

In this study the authors isolated from human placental tissue a cytoplasmic protein similar to, but not identical with, human plasma transcortin. The placental protein exhibited antigenic and biochemical similarity to plasma transcortin; however, it had a smaller sedimentation coefficient and bound cortisol less strongly than did plasma transcortin. The placental protein was shown to be localized within the cytoplasm of syncytiotrophoblastic cells of frozen placental tissues sectioned at 5 μm. The placental protein was shown to inhibit the incorporation of tritiated thymidine into phytohemagglutinin-stimulated lymphocytes by 78%. The researchers speculate that this placental protein may be an additional factor helping to block maternal cellular immune responses in late pregnancy.

COMMENT: Placentas contain a number of proteins whose function is unknown. The effect of this one on lymphocytes is tantalizing, but obviously the substance requires additional investigation.

Human chorionic gonadotropin-like protein in tumor cells

■ Naughton, M. A., Merrill, D. A., McManus, L. M., Fink, L. M., Berman, E., White, M. J., and Martinez-Hernandez, A.: Localization of the β-chain of human chorionic gonadotropin on tumor cells and placental cells, Cancer Res. **35**:1887-1890, 1975.

■ McManus, L. M., Naughton, M. A., and Martinez-Hernandez, A.: Human chorionic gonadotropin in human neoplastic cells, Cancer Res. **36**:3476-3481, 1975.

Peroxidase labeled antibody to the beta chain of HCG was used to stain various tissues for putative human chorionic gonadotropin. Human placenta and the BeWo line of human trophoblast in tissue culture were used as positive controls and normal tissues as negative controls (presence and absence of stain in cell cytoplasm). Twenty-eight different human tumors of various kinds were stained, and of these, twenty-five showed evidence for the presence of the antigen. These results are probably related to the T cell–inhibiting properties of a closely related protein that is present in commercial HCG preparations and that may account for maternal tolerance of the fetal graft. (Personal communication: Naughton, M. A., 1977.)

COMMENT: Three aspects of these experiments are striking. First is the possibility that a substance chemically similar to HCG may in fact be the immunosuppressor that permits growth of the eutherian mammals in utero. Second is the recognition of another example of phenotypic expression of embryonic genes in cancerous cells. Third is the difficulty of assigning potent biologic activities to specific protein molecules.

Pregnancy proteins from placenta

■ Boss, J. H., Dishon, T., and Rosenmann, E.: Placental antigens and fetoproteins in the urine of rats, indicators of resorption of conceptuses, Gynecol. Invest. **6**:285-290, 1975.

Specific antisera to rat placental antigens, alpha-fetoprotein (AFP) and alpha-M-fetoprotein (AMFP) were prepared in rabbits. Rats were mated and serum and urine were tested with the antisera during and after normal pregnancy and after attempts to interfere with pregnancy by injections of nephrotoxic serum or *E. coli* endotoxin. AFP and AMFP were found in the serum during pregnancy and to the fifth postpartum day. AFP, but not AMFP, also appeared in urine during pregnancy. By contrast, the placental antigens usually did not appear in the urine during pregnancy, but were frequently found following interruption and resorption of the conceptus.

COMMENT: These experiments show that in rats, at least, placental proteins can enter the maternal circulation and theoretically could induce antibody formation. (See also the comment on the review by Lin and Halbert.)

■ Lin, T.-M., and Halbert, S. P.: Placental localization of pregnancy-associated plasma proteins, Science **193**:1249-1252, 1976.

Monospecific antisera to PAPP-A and PAPP-C, HPL (HCS), and pregnancy zone protein (PZP) were prepared by absorption of rabbit antisera with plasma from nonpregnant women. The purified antisera were then used for the immunofluorescence technique of localization of the proteins in term human placentas. PAPP-A, PAPP-C, and HPL were localized in the syncytiotrophoblast, whereas PZP was detected in both trophoblast and blood vessel walls.

COMMENT: These experiments are in a sense the inverse of those in the previous article. Here, immunologic techniques were used to show that certain proteins which appear in serum during pregnancy likely arise from the placenta.

Transmission of maternal immunologic tolerance to the fetus

■ Auerbach, R., and Clark, S.: Immunologic tolerance: transmission from mother to offspring, Science **189**:811-813, 1975.

Soluble material from heterologous erythrocytes injected into mice produces tolerance (immunologic nonresponsiveness) to subsequent injections of similar intact erythrocytes into the treated mice. The tolerance produced is "systemic in nature, presumably dependent on serum-mediated blocking of the immune response." Treatment of pregnant mice or conception in treated females consistently gave litters that were immunologically tolerant. Rearing experiments with foster mothers showed that the factor(s) responsible for production of tolerance were transmitted to the offspring mainly by suckling.

COMMENT: Passive transmission of immunologic tolerance, perhaps by transfer of antigen-antibody complexes from mother to fetus through suckling, is an example of maternal modification of the immunologic responsiveness of the offspring, not unlike the well-known transmission of passive immunity from mother to child. Perhaps these phenomena, coupled with the delayed development of active immune responsiveness in the newborn, evolved to permit him to fit immediately into his new environment.

Human placental alkaline phosphatase

- Lehmann, F.-G.: Immunologic relationship between human placental and intestinal alkaline phosphatase, Clin. Chim. Acta **65:**257-269, 1975.

Highly purified, crystalline human placental and human intestinal alkaline phosphatase were prepared. Rabbit antisera to these proteins showed reactions of partial identity to each other but not to human alkaline phosphatases from other organs when analyzed by double diffusion immunoassay. Similar results were obtained by quantitative precipitation analysis.

- Lehmann, F.-G.: Immunological methods for human placental alkaline phosphatase (Regan isoenzyme), Clin. Chim. Acta **65:**271-282, 1975.

Using a highly specific antiserum to placental alkaline phosphatase, various immunoassay methods for determination of the enzyme in serum were evaluated. An absorption technique onto fixed antibody gave the most accurate and specific results. When the analysis was applied to serum from patients with a variety of malignant tumors, 26% of the patients showed an elevated activity of the isozyme compared to that found in healthy, nonpregnant blood donors.

COMMENT: These articles describe a highly specific method for the measurement of a placental protein that appears in maternal serum in large amounts and a demonstration that synthesis of this protein is derepressed in certain tumors.

Immunology of implantation

- Sacco, A. G., and Mintz, B.: Mouse uterine antigens in the implantation period of pregnancy, Biol. Reprod. **12:**498-503, 1975.

Mouse uterine tissue was obtained at about the time of implantation and was used as an antigen for the formation of antibodies in rabbits. The antibodies thus produced were used in the Ouchterlony technique in a search for specific antigens associated with implantation. Two uterine antigens, not found in any other tissue except the duodenum, were found with these techniques. One of them is identical to the duodenal protein and the other is probably related to a proteolytic implantation-initiating factor already described by these authors. This specific protein is a proteolytic eenzyme whose function is as yet unknown.

COMMENT: Both organ-specific antigens and antigens shared among several tissues, organs, animals, or species are theoretically possible because of the differences and similarities be-

tween and among cells. The physiologic significance of such observations are rarely deducible on purely immunologic evidence, but when proteins have already been discovered in an organ, immunologic investigations may simplify studies of the protein's distribution and so forth.

Immunosuppression in pregnancy

■ Tomoda, Y., Fuma, M., Miwa, T., Saiki, N., and Ishizuka, N.: Cell-mediated immunity in pregnant women, Gynecol. Invest. 7:280-292, 1976.

Lymphocytes and serum from normal pregnant women were used in the mixed lymphocyte culture test for transplantation antigenicity. Likewise, phytohemagglutinin was used to test the overall function of T cell lymphocytes. It was found that cell-mediated immunity as measured by phytohemagglutinin was much lower in the second trimester than in nonpregnant women. The suppression of lymphocyte stimulation appeared to be transmitted by the serum of pregnant women. This suppression might be due to alpha-fetoprotein. Similar effects of alpha-fetoprotein on the mixed lymphocyte culture test were obtained, which may demonstrate an effect on transplantation antigens as well as on cell-mediated immunity during pregnancy.

COMMENT: The results described in this article should be compared to those reported in the article by Strelkauskas et al.

CHAPTER 9

Parturition

Relatively little new information about fundamental aspects of parturition was published from 1975 to 1976. However, it would appear to be increasingly certain that a surge in fetal corticoid synthesis may be the elusive initiator of labor in many species, and that there is a distinct possibility that the steroid hormones act by means of prostaglandins. These compounds presumably activate the contraction process as local hormones or neuromuscular transmitters.

Length of gestation

■ McCarthy, T. G.: The relationship of a "short period" to conception, Br. J. Obstet. Gynaecol. **82**:158-161, 1976.

A retrospective analysis was done on the time interval between menstruation and delivery and on the birth weight of the infants from 918 patients delivered at a London hospital during 1963. The data were analyzed separately for fifty-two patients who had had bleeding interpreted as a "short period" following conception and the 155 randomly selected control patients. If one assumed that the bleeding episode in the fifty-two patients occurred after conception and truly represented minimal bleeding when menstruation would normally have occurred, then there was a high percentage of "postterm" pregnancies. This was not the case when the bleeding episode was not interpreted as a short period following conception, but rather as a menstrual period just prior to conception. The menstruation-delivery intervals were as follows: for the control group, 282.2 ± 18.8 days; for the study group, calculating from the last full period, 302.1 ± 21.6 days; and calculating from the short period, 271.8 ± 22.7 days.

COMMENT: **Women with some bleeding around the time of conception are probably a heterogenous group, including some in whom bleeding occurs following conception and others in whom bleeding occurs just prior to conception. Perhaps the proper interpretation of the results will await infant birth weight distribution studies compared with other indices of maturity or some other independent assessment of age.**

Diagnostic amniocentesis for gene defect

■ Henry, G., Wexler, P., and Robinson, A.: Rh-immune globulin after amniocentesis for genetic diagnosis, Obstet. Gynecol. **48**:557-559, 1976.

Theoretically, diagnostic amniocentesis could induce Rh-sensitization due to bleeding, and these investigators recommend the administration of Rh-immune globulin whenever the possibility of incompatibility exists. In their experience, fifty-six patients who received Rh-immune globulin showed no sensitization except one patient who underwent two amniocenteses, the second of which was not followed by administration of the immune globulin.

COMMENT: These case report data seem to make a clear case for the necessity of this simple addition to the routine procedure followed in amniocentesis.

Initiation of labor

■ Gustavi, B.: Release of lysosomal acid phosphatase into the cytoplasma of decidual cells before the onset of labor in humans, Br. J. Obstet. Gynaecol. **82:**177-181, 1975.

The author obtained decidual cells from twelve women in elective caesarean section at term and from ten women at midpregnancy hysterotomy. The cells were assayed cytochemically for the lysosomal marker enzyme, acid phosphatase. Decidual cells from midpregnancy were well preserved and showed a good distribution of the enzyme throughout the cytoplasm in a granular form, presumably in the lysosomes. The term decidual cells were varied in their appearance. Some were well preserved, whereas others showed degenerative changes such as cytoplasmic vacuoles, nuclear pyknosis, and cellular shrinkage. These cells also showed diffuse staining of the cytoplasm with the marker enzyme, indicating lysosomal release of the enzyme.

Prostaglandin synthesis

■ Keirse, M. J. N., and Turnbull, A. C.: The fetal membranes as a possible source of amniotic fluid prostaglandins, Br. J. Obstet. Gynaecol. **83:**146-151, 1976.

Amniotic and chorionic membranes at term from primigravidas who had a normal pregnancy and labor were studied. The membranes were freed of decidual and placental tissue, and prostaglandin synthesis was studied by an isotope dilution technique. Homogenates were incubated with labeled arachidonic acid in the presence of an excess of $PGF_{2\alpha}$ and PGF_2 was added to trap newly formed prostaglandins. PGE_2 synthesis from labeled arachidonic acid was 4% in the chorion and 2% in the amnion, 5% in the combined membranes, and 2% in boiled membranes. The prostaglandins are rapidly metabolized as well.

COMMENT: Prostaglandin synthesis and metabolism occur in many tissues, but the relatively high rates of these processes in chorion suggest that these compounds may have a vital role in this tissue. It is tempting to speculate, as Keirse et al. do, that the chorion is the source of the large amounts of prostaglandins in the amniotic fluid. The histochemistry (Gustavi) is compatible with a steroid-triggered enzyme release of prostaglandin precursors that might be involved in the onset of labor.

■ Schultz, F. M., Schwarz, B. E., MacDonald, P. C., and Johnston, J. M.: Initiation of human parturition. II. Identification of phospholipase A_2 in fetal chorioamnion and uterine decidua, Am. J. Obstet. Gynecol. **123:**650-653, 1975.

These authors assume, as postulated by Karim, that prostaglandins occupy "a central role in the onset of human parturition." Therefore they have studied the biogenesis of prostaglandins in humans. Uterine decidua and chorion laeve were separated following vaginal delivery and were used after homogenization as enzyme preparation in incubation with labeled phosphatidylcholine and phosphatidylethanolamine. From the isolated products of the incubation mixture it was possible to establish that both the decidua and chorioamnion contained phospholipase A activity (which gives the 2-lysophosphatide). Taken with the previous demonstration of esterified arachidonic acid in amniotic fluid, these results suggest that the necessary precursor for prostaglandin synthesis, free arachidonic acid, can be produced in the uterus.

COMMENT: Although this kind of experimentation may not appear to be exciting, it forms an essential part of the chain of evidence required to show that a given tissue can synthesize a compound of interest, such as a prostaglandin.

Steroids and parturition

■ Baldwin, D. M., and Stabenfeldt, G. H.: Endocrine changes in the pig during late pregnancy, parturition and lactation, Biol. Reprod. **12**:508-515, 1975.

Plasma concentrations of progestins, corticosteroids, and estrogens were determined just before, during, and after parturition in pigs. Progestational steroids decreased slowly in late gestation and then showed a sharp drop just prior to parturition. Corticosteroids showed a marked increase in concentration just prior to farrowing. Estrogen concentrations increased until after parturition, whereupon a pronounced decline occurred. These changes are much like those seen in sheep.

■ Murphy, B. E. P., Patrick, J., and Denton, R. L.: Cortisol in amniotic fluid during human gestation, J. Clin. Endocrinol. Metab. **40**:164-167, 1975.

Cortisol in amniotic fluid at various stages of gestation in normal human subjects was measured by a specific binding protein assay method. Cortisol increased steadily in the amniotic fluid from week 10 of human gestation, with a slower rate of increase between 20 and 35 weeks, followed by a dramatic increase in the last few weeks before delivery. This increase is independent of any change in the maternal serum level. The results shown in Fig. 9-1 are in accord with the hypothesis that corticosteroid production by the fetus is somehow related to the onset of labor.

COMMENT: It is of interest that the sharpest increase in amniotic fluid cortisol occurs in humans at about week 35, which is also the time at which maternal estriol values begin to increase sharply. The data suggest strongly that corticoids are important in the initiation of labor in most species, including the human.

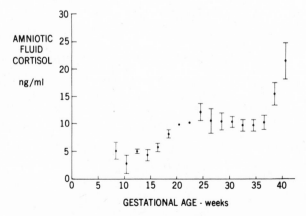

FIG. 9-1
Mean amniotic fluid cortisol at various gestational ages prior to the onset of labor. The bars show the SEM. (From Murphy, B. E. P., Patrick, J., and Denton, R. L.: Cortisol in amniotic fluid during human gestation, J. Clin. Endocrinol. Metab. **40**:164-167, 1975.)

■ Fencl, M. D., and Tulchinsky, D.: Total cortisol in amniotic fluid and fetal lung maturation, N. Engl. J. Med. **292:**133-136, 1975.

Cortisol was determined by radioimmunoassay in amniotic fluid obtained at various stages of gestation. There was a steady increase in the concentration of the hormone in the fluid as gestation advanced, and at 40 weeks the mean was two and a half times greater than that observed halfway through gestation. Further increase was found in postmature fetuses. The cortisol values were correlated with the L/S ratio (r = .83). No respiratory distress syndrome of the newborn occurred in subjects with an amniotic fluid cortisol greater than 60 ng/ml.

CHAPTER 10

Pathophysiology of pregnancy

■ Condie, R. G.: A serial study of coagulation factors XII, XI and X in plasma in normal pregnancy and in pregnancy complicated by pre-eclampsia, Br. J. Obstet. Gynaecol. **83:**636-639, 1976.

Sixty primigravidas were followed from 12 weeks of gestation through to the puerperium. Forty-eight remained normal and twelve developed preeclampsia. An additional ten non-pregnant women were used as controls. Assay of factors XII, X, and XI was carried out by the usual methods. Factor XII started to rise by 20 weeks of gestation and reached a peak at 135% above normal at 38 weeks of gestation. The patients with preeclampsia had a significantly higher level than that in normal pregnancy from 20 weeks of gestation onward. Factor XI level started to rise at 12 weeks of gestation and reached a peak at 139% of normal at 38 weeks. The level was lower than that in normal pregnancy in those patients with preeclampsia. The factor X rise started at 12 weeks and reached a peak at 30 weeks of gestation, the peak being 163% above normal. In patients with preeclampsia, factor X started to rise later at 20 weeks of gestation, but reached a similar peak at 38 weeks, that is, 165% of normal.

COMMENT: This study demonstrates that changes in the pregnant patient's physiology in preeclampsia precede symptomatology. It thus appears if one is going to look for the etiology of preeclampsia one must look quite early in pregnancy. The study of Brosens et al. (The role of the spiral arteries in the pathogenesis of preeclampsia, Obstet. Gynecol. Annu. 1:177-191, 1972) demonstrating the lack of trophoblastic invasion of the entire length of the spiral arteries in those patients developing preeclampsia would also indicate changes preceding symptomatology.

■ Cohen, W. R.: Influence of the duration of the second stage labor on perinatal outcome and puerperal morbidity, Obstet. Gynecol. **49:**266-269, 1977.

Forty thousand four hundred and three primigravidas were analyzed for the duration of their second stage of labor. No significant increase was observed in perinatal mortality with progressive lengthening of the second stage of labor, and many of the patients had a second stage longer than 180 minutes. There was a progressive increase in the frequency of low Apgar scores with a longer second stage; however, this phenomenon was not observed in patients who were managed using a fetal heart rate monitor. There was no significant difference in the frequency of low 5-minute Apgar scores for the various groupings of second stage duration. (See Table 10-1.)

COMMENT: This article would seem to question the long-held teaching that a prolonged second stage in labor is associated with an increased incidence of fetal difficulty. This study contradicts the conclusions drawn from the collaborative study, which showed a definite increase in the incidence of neurologic abnormalities in those babies born after greater than a 2-hour second stage (Women and their pregnancies, U.S. Department of Health, Education, and Welfare Pub. No. 73-379). It would seem somewhat hazardous to change the prac-

TABLE 10-1

Perinatal outcome and duration of second stage labor*

Duration (min)	Number of cases	Perinatal mortality (per 1000)	Neonatal mortality (per 1000)	Low 1-minute Apgar score† (%)	Low 5-minute Apgar score (%)
0–29	623	6.5	0.0	3.2 (4.4)	0.6
30–59	1257	4.8	2.4	3.1 (4.2)	0.7
60–89	1007	3.0	1.0	3.5 (2.7)	0.3
90–119	599	0.0	0.0	3.7 (4.3)	0.2
120–149	425	2.4	0.0	4.5 (5.9)	0.0
150–179	237	0.0	0.0	6.3 (3.3)	0.8
180+	255	3.9	0.0	7.1 (5.7)	1.6
Total	4403	3.4	1.8	3.8 (4.3)	0.5

*From Cohen, W. R.: Influence of the duration of the second stage labor on perinated outcome and puerperal morbidity, Obstet. Gynecol. 49:266-269, 1977.
†Distribution of data for total series is statistically significant ($\chi^2 = 15.6$, p $<$ .025), but the relative rates of depressed neonates among monitored patients (in parentheses) are not ($\chi^2 = 3.9$, p $>$ .5).

tice of a maximum 2-hour second stage, even in the monitored fetus, on the basis of a good 5-minute Apgar score, since 1% of babies with good 5-minute Apgar scores had neurologic damage diagnosed at 1 year of age (Pediatr. Clin. North Am. 13:635, 1966).

■ Harris, R. E., Thomas, V. L., and Shelokov, A.: Asymptomatic bacteriuria in pregnancy: antibody-coated bacteria, renal function, and intrauterine growth retardation, Am. J. Obstet. Gynecol. **126**:20-25, 1976.

The authors screened 1400 pregnant women without urinary tract symptoms for urinary tract infection. Those with greater than 10^5 bacteria in a clean voided urine were recultured. Seventy patients (5%) had confirmed asymptomatic bacteriuria. All patients with bacteriuria were given fluorescent antibody (FA) tests, and half (thirty-five) were FA positive. The bacteria found in the asymptomatic patients were predominantly *Escherichia coli* and *Klebsiella pneumoniae*. The 24-hour creatinine clearance test was lower in the patients who had FA-positive, asymptomatic bacilluria as compared to those who were negative. Of the patients with FA, 58% had a creatinine clearance of less than 90 ml/min, whereas only one of twenty-nine patients with a negative FA test had a clearance less than 90. Bacteriuria recurred in 29% of the patients with a positive FA test and 23% with a negative FA test.

COMMENT: The FA test would appear to offer significant advantages in the diagnosis of those patients having asymptomatic bacteriuria who may be more likely to have chronic pyelonephritis. However, as is demonstrated by this article, the presence of negative FA bacteria does not rule out the subsequent development of acute pyelonephritis.

■ Gabbe, S. G., Dizerega, G. S., and Mestman, J. H.: Remission of diabetes mellitus during pregnancy, Am. J. Obstet. Gynecol. **125**:264-265, 1976.

The authors discuss a patient 39 years of age, gravida 4, para 3, who was seen at approximately 24 weeks of gestation in her fourth pregnancy. At that time her fasting blood sugar was 226 mg/dl. She was placed on a 2000 calorie diet and 20 units of NPH insulin, which was gradually increased to 44 units. Her fasting blood sugar stabilized at 120 mg/dl. During the following month the patient's fasting blood sugar decreased and her insulin dose was tapered. At 33 weeks of gestation her blood pressure rose, and the patient was admitted for evaluation. At 34 weeks of gestation the insulin dose was reduced to 10 units, and by 35 weeks the insulin was discontinued. The patient's preeclampsia worsened at 37 weeks and labor was induced. Seven hours after the induction the patient delivered a 6 pound 2 ounce male infant with Apgar scores of 8 and 9.

COMMENT: Normally the dosage of insulin required by a diabetic increases progressively throughout pregnancy. This is believed to be due to the increase in HPL, rising progesterone as well as estrogen levels, and increased production of insulinase by the placenta. Clinically it has often been taught that a fall in insulin requirements in the third trimester is a signal that the placenta is failing. This patient demonstrates that such is not always the case. This patient was managed with estriol determinations and contraction stress tests. The fact that the contraction stress tests were normal stayed the hands of her physicians, even though the insulin requirement had fallen and the patient's estriol determinations were low. It would seem extremely important to make the maximum use of the tools that one has at hand and, if there is question of maturity of the fetus, *not* to induce or deliver the fetus unless more than one test would indicate fetal jeopardy.

- Bear, R. A.: Pregnancy in patients with renal disease. A study of 44 cases, Obstet. Gynecol. **48:**13-18, 1976.

The study reviews thirty-seven patients managed at the renal clinics of the New England Medical Center between the years 1955 and 1973. The author has divided the results into those patients with serum creatinine values of less than or greater than 1.5 mg/dl. There were thirty-six pregnancies observed in twenty-nine patients in the low-creatine group. Serum creatinines in this group ranged from 0.4 to 1.4 mg/dl. Diastolic hypertension was noted in eight of twenty-six pregnancies. Normal vaginal delivery of a healthy infant resulted in twenty-eight cases. There were eight pregnancies in eight patients with serum creatinines greater than 1.6 mg/dl. In four patients there was a significant rise in serum creatinine during pregnancy. Hypertension developed in seven of the eight cases. Only one normal delivery was recorded in this group of eight pregnancies.

COMMENT: Severe renal disease in pregnancy continues to present significant problems. It would appear from these data that there is certainly a marked difference in pregnancy outcome in those patients whose serum creatinine values are higher than 1.5 mg/dl. Even though the study is small, it is consistent with other studies indicating the seriousness of the outcome of pregnancy in this situation. The reason for such a poor outcome has always been blamed on a reduced uterine blood flow associated with pregnancy-associated renal disease; however, to the best of our knowledge, this has never been actually demonstrated. What has been demonstrated is a smaller-than-normal placenta in these cases and a higher incidence of intrauterine growth retardation. In a significant number of cases this might be associated with the vasospasm that is manifest generally by hypertension in the patient. However, in some patients no hypertension is present, and yet the prognosis for the fetus remains poor. The etiology of this type of fetal wastage in chronic renal disease at present is totally unexplained.

- Morrison, J. C., and Wiser, E. L.: The use of prophylactic partial exchange transfusion in pregnancies associated with sickle cell hemoglobinopathies, Obstet. Gynecol. **48:**516-520, 1976.

The article reports thirty-six pregnant patients with sickle cell anemia or one of its severe variants, sickle cell C or sickle cell thalassemia, who were treated by a partial exchange transfusion. Patients were treated in the following manner: They entered prenatal care between 12 and 16 weeks. The uncomplicated cases were seen every 2 weeks until the twentieth week and then they were seen weekly until delivery. At each clinic visit a reticulocyte count, hematocrit, and hemoglobin electrophoresis were obtained. If the patients had a crisis, they were hospitalized and treated with partial exchange transfusion prior to the twenty-eighth week. If no crisis occurred prior to the twenty-eighth week, they were admitted at 28 weeks and given partial exchange transfusion by doing a 500 ml phlebotomy from the patient and giving 2 (300 to 400 ml) units of buffy coat–poor, washed blood cells. That procedure was repeated until the hemoglobin A percentage was over 40 and the hematocrit was greater than 35. If the hemoglobin A level fell below 20% or the hematocrit decreased below 25, the exchange was repeated. Patients were allowed to go into spontaneous labor. These patients were compared with another group of twenty-nine gravidas treated from 1965 to 1970 in a similar manner except for exchange transfusion. In the partial exchange transfusion patients there was one maternal mortality. A patient who refused the second exchange transfusion went into labor at 39 weeks with a hemoglobin A of 5% and a hematocrit of 18. There was one patient with pneumonia and one with pyelonephritis. The perinatal mortality was very low with only one stillbirth and one neonatal death. In the twenty-nine patients who comprised the retrospective study, there were four maternal deaths, and the perinatal wastage was 48%.

COMMENT: Sickle cell anemia, sickle cell C disease, or sickle cell thalassemia are all conditions associated with a significant maternal mortality, in some studies up to 10%, and an extremely significant perinatal mortality, in some studies up to 50%. In the past the treatment has been predominantly symptomatic insofar as the mother is concerned, treating crises when they occur and only transfusing when very low levels of hematocrit, usually less than 20, had been reached. At least two groups, Morrison's in Memphis and Pritchard's in Dallas, are taking a good hard look at the possibility that many of the maternal and perinatal complications can be ameliorated by keeping the patient's hematocrit at a significantly higher level. This can be done either through partial exchange transfusion or through multiple transfusions to maintain the hematocrit above 35. The preliminary results are certainly encouraging; however, it must be kept in mind that this is not a prospective randomized study, and other forms of therapy may account for some of the benefits.

The principal problem, of course is going to be that these patients who have had multiple transfusions and are getting more transfusions with this type of therapy will develop more and more antibodies to donor blood. Thus it will be harder and harder to accomplish the desired goals.

■ Chesley, L. C.: Rheumatic cardiac disease in pregnancy: long-term follow up, Obstet. Gynecol. **46:**699-705, 1975.

Two hundred sixty women with cardiac disease seen during their pregnancy from 1937 through 1942 have been traced through the year 1974. Table 10-2 accurately depicts the survival over time in three functional cardiac classifications. Cardiac decompensation accounted for 60% of the deaths. The data indicate there is no adverse effect of subsequent pregnancies on maternal survival rates if one looks at each functional classification separately .

TABLE 10-2

Comparison of women with rheumatic cardiac disease with and without later pregnancy*

	Original number	Patient-years	Deaths	Dead (%)	Average annual death rate (per 1000)
Class I					
All women	168	4169.5	98	58.3	23.50
No later pregnancy	168(59)†	1564.5	40	67.8	25.55
Later pregnancies	109†	2605.0	58	53.2	22.25
Class II					
All women	61	1244.0	45	73.8	36.15
No later pregnancy	61(36)†	780	27	75.0	34.60
Later pregnancies	25†	464	18	72.0	38.80
Classes III or IV					
All women	57	782.5	52	91.3	66.5
No later pregnancy	57(43)†	526.0	41	95.5	78.0
Later pregnancies	14‡	256.5	11	78.7	42.9

*From Chesley, L. C.: Rheumatic cardiac disease in pregnancy: long-term follow up, Obstet. Gynecol. **46**:699-705, 1975.

†Interval from initial delivery to later conception credited to "No later pregnancy": the numbers in parentheses are the actual numbers of women who had no later pregnancy.

‡Follow-up begins at the conception of the first later pregnancy.

COMMENT: Although rheumatic cardiac disease is at a much lower incidence in the pregnant population than it was prior to the penicillin era, it still does occur from time to time. One of the significant questions that has always been posed has been whether such disease is accelerated by subsequent pregnancies. Only a meticulous study such as this one presented by Chesley carried out over a long time with very high rates of follow-up could provide a reasonable answer. From this study it seems clear that subsequent pregnancy does not affect the course of rheumatic cardiac disease adversely.

■ Selvin, S., and Garfinkel, J.: Paternal age, maternal age and birth order and the risk of a fetal loss, Hum. Biol. **48**:223-230, 1976.

This study includes a retrospective analysis of data obtained from 1.5 million birth certificates and fetal death certificates recorded during the period of 1959 through 1967 in New York State. The data excludes similar information from New York City for the same time period. Fetal deaths included all those deaths in utero after 20 weeks' estimated gestational age. Two groups of infants were excluded: (1) illegitimate births, since father's age was not recorded, and (2) infants with congenital malformations. The data were analyzed for the effects of paternal and maternal age and birth order on fetal mortality rate. A multiple logistic function was employed to separate the interdependent effects of parental age and birth order. The study demonstrated that all three factors—maternal and paternal age, as well as birth order—have separate and approximately equal effects on the risk of fetal death.

COMMENT: Table 10-3 from their report presents the data and illustrates the extremely low fetal death rate in the second-born infant, demonstrated in other studies as well. The

TABLE 10-3

The numbers of fetal deaths, total recorded pregnancies and fetal death rates for paternal age, maternal age and birth order—New York State, 1959-1967 (excluding New York City)*

	Fetal deaths	Pregnancies	Rate (per 1000 pregnancies)
Birth order			
1	4,450	368,790	12.1
2	3,268	367,045	8.9
3	3,496	300,392	11.6
4	2,792	196,460	14.2
5	1,934	111,384	17.4
6+	3,023	128,775	23.5
Total	18,963	1,472,846	12.9
Paternal age			
≤ 19	358	28,064	12.8
20-24	3,005	310,228	9.7
25-29	4,388	433,962	10.1
30-34	4,275	348,652	12.3
35-39	3,576	214,767	16.7
40-44	2,112	95,094	22.3
45-49	875	30,250	28.9
50-54	266	8,473	31.4
≥ 55	108	3,356	32.2
Total	18,963	1,472,846	12.9
Maternal age			
≤ 14	2	133	15.0
15-19	1,289	117,185	11.0
20-24	4,448	475,579	9.4
25-29	4,687	417,190	11.2
30-34	4,033	275,247	14.7
35-39	3,146	146,590	21.5
40-44	1,256	38,934	32.3
≤ 45	102	1,988	51.3
Total	18,963	1,472,846	12.9

*Reprinted from Selvin, S., and Garfinkel, J.: Paternal age, maternal age and birth order and the risk of a fetal loss, Hum. Biol. **48**:223-230, 1976; by permission of The Wayne State University Press.

data in Table 10-3 have been plotted graphically by us and are presented in Fig. 10-1, which shows the increasing rate of fetal death after age 30 in both parents.

■ Mujtaba, Q., and Barrow, G. N.: Treatment of hyperthyroidism in pregnancy with propylthiouracil and methimazole, Obstet. Gynecol. **46**:282-286, 1975.

The authors report twenty-six pregnancies in which the mother was hyperthyroid and treated during her pregnancy with antithyroid medication. Four pregnancies were lost, two being abortions and two stillbirths. Neonatal goiter was found in four infants, and five additional infants had congenital abnormalities, including developmental retardation, scalp defects, hypospadias, imperforate anus, and aortic atresia. Fourteen children were born without any goiters or other abnormalities. Cord blood protein-bound iodine or T_4 determinations were done on eleven newborns and in only one was there less than 4.5 μg of iodine per

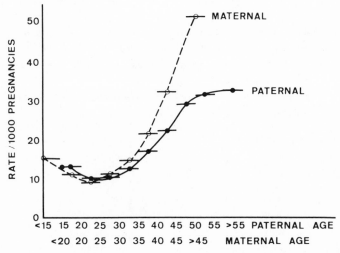

FIG. 10-1

Fetal mortality rate versus parental age. We plotted the data from Table I of the original. (Data from Selvin, S., and Garfinkel, J.: Paternal age, maternal age and birth order and the risk of a fetal loss, Hum. Biol. **48:**223-230, 1976.)

deciliter. Seven patients had long-acting, thyroid-stimulating hormone (LATS) assays. Of the four babies that developed neonatal thyrotoxicosis, two were from mothers whose LATS level was above 300%; however, three of the patients whose offspring developed neonatal thyrotoxicosis had an LATS level above 300%. These same three children also had goiters; in addition, one further child had a goiter, and in this child no LATS level had been obtained.

COMMENT: It was pointed out in the discussion portion of this original article that the fetal thyroid appears to be very sensitive to iodides. In a previous study (Barrow: Neonatal goiter after maternal propylthiouracil therapy, J. Clin. Endocrinol. 25:403-408, 1965) four of the five children who developed goiters had been born to women who received iodides in addition to their antithyroid therapy during pregnancy. Thus it is important that the problem of neonatal thyrotoxicosis be kept in mind. It has been suggested that all patients who are thyrotoxic during their pregnancy have LATS levels determined. Those patients whose levels are greater than 300% of normal appear to be at risk for having a thyrotoxic infant. That this is not always the case is pointed out by the patient in this series whose LATS level was greater than 500% above normal with a normal infant.

The treatment with propylthiouracil or methimazole is extremely effective in most cases. The patient should be kept slightly hyperthyroid; however, in some situations this cannot be accomplished and the patient becomes hypothyroid, thus needing thyroid hormone supplementation. The thyroid hormone of choice is triidothyronine because it does have the potential advantage of some placental transfer.

These researchers quote another article (Milham and Elledge: Maternal methimazole and congenital effects in children, Teratology 5:125, 1972) in which three cases of congenital scalp defects have been found in mothers treated with methimazole therapy. These authors reported one patient with scalp defects who delivered two infants. In both these pregnancies the mother was given methimazole. Our own experience has been that extensive use of methimazole has not been associated with an increased incidence of scalp lesions.

An attempt has been made at in utero treatment on one occasion (Ramsey: Attempted prevention of neonatal thyrotoxicosis, Br. Med. J. 2:1110, 1976). The mother, a treated hyperthyroid with high LATS levels and a previous child who died of neonatal thyrotoxism, was given carbimazol, 5 mg three times a day. The fetal heart rate remained normal throughout pregnancy; however, the day after delivery the child developed tachycardia. Treatment was again begun with carbimazol and the child did well.

- Stein, G., Milton, F., Bebbington, P., Wood, K., and Coppen, A.: Relationship between mood disturbances and free and total plasma tryptophan in postpartum women, Br. Med. J., p. 457, Aug. 21, 1976.

The investigators measured plasma 5-hydroxytryptamine in eighteen women postpartum. The women rated themselves each day in terms of depression. Daily 5-hydroxytryptamine levels were taken. The study demonstrated that those patients who appeared to have severe depression had free plasma tryptamine levels similar to those found in depressive illness.

COMMENT: These changes in 5-hydroxytryptamine levels may be the result of changes in steroids occurring in the postpartum period. Since depressive episodes may also occur when patients are taking contraceptive medication, the same type of levels would be worthy of measurement in this situation. If this compound is altered in terms of its brain metabolism by steroid compounds, it would be yet another effect of the steroid compounds on the central nervous system.

- Soffronoff, E. C., Kaufmann, B. M., and Connaughton, J. F.: Intravascular volume determinations and fetal outcome in hypertensive diseases of pregnancy, Am. J. Obstet. Gynecol. 127:4-9, 1977.

The authors studied fifty-one hypertensive nulliparous and parous patients, twenty-three normotensive nulliparous, and twelve normotensive multiparous patients who were followed in the prenatal clinic at Pennsylvania Hospital. Plasma volumes were determined using the Evans blue dye method. Table 10-4 indicates the results found in terms of plasma volume, red cell volume, and blood volume.

It is apparent that there is a significant decrease in blood volume in patients with the chronic hypertension, mild preeclampsia, and severe hypertensive disease and that with severe hypertension there is also a significant decrease in the blood cell mass.

COMMENT: Blekta et al. (Volume of whole blood and absolute amount of serum proteins in the early stage of late toxemia pregnancy, Am. J. Obstet. Gynecol. 106:10, 1970) demonstrated that the patients destined to develop preeclampsia had a significantly lower circulating plasma volume before the onset of symptoms. The question arises as to whether the decrease in plasma volume is an etiologic factor in causing the disease or a result of the disease. This would have profound implications for treatment. If it is one of the etiologic factors in the disease (Goodlin: Severe pre-eclampsia: another great imitator, Am. J. Obstet. Gynecol. 125:747, 1976), then obviously, expanding the plasma volume as suggested by Goodlin would be the correct way to approach the problem. If decrease in plasma volume is simply a result of the disease, this type of therapy would be an incorrect course to pursue. Proper control trials in a prospective fashion should be performed to determine if expanding plasma volume is correct or incorrect.

TABLE 10-4
Tabulation of groups studied*

Group	Plasma volume		Red cell volume		Blood volume	
	cc/M² of BSA	p†	cc/M² of BSA	p	cc/M² of BSA	p
Normotensive nullipara (control)	2,057‡ ± 183	—	1,031 ± 146	—	3,088 ± 274	—
Normotensive multipara	2,186 ± 273	0.05	1,105 ± 120	0.05	3,291 ± 348	0.02
Chronic hypertension	1,844 ± 154	0.001	1,011 ± 103	NS§	2,855 ± 222	0.01
Transient hypertension	1,921 ± 244	0.01	969 ± 163	NS	2,890 ± 359	0.01
Mild preeclampsia	1,776 ± 340	0.001	1,061 ± 130	NS	2,837 ± 443	0.05
Severe hypertensive disease	1,500 ± 183	0.001	891 ± 73	0.01	2,391 ± 219	0.001

*From Soffronoff, E. C., Kaufmann, B. M., and Connaughton, J. F.: Intravascular volume determinations and fetal outcome in hypertensive diseases of pregnancy, Am. J. Obstet. Gynecol. **127:**4-9, 1977.
†Two-tailed t test.
‡Mean ± SD.
§Not significant.

In addition to the significance in terms of the etiology, the blood volume may have significance in terms of prognosis. Arias (Expansion of intravascular volume and fetal outcome in patients with chronic hypertension and pregnancy, Am. J. Obstet. Gynecol. **123:**610-616, 1975) has demonstrated that failure to achieve a blood volume expansion of at least 60 ml/kg was associated with increased intrauterine growth retardation and fetal death.

■ Gibbs, C. P., and Noel, S. C.: Human uterine artery responses to lidocaine, Am. J. Obstet. Gynecol. **126:**313-315, 1976.

Six term uterine arterial segments were obtained from cesarean section hysterectomy specimens and seven segments from pregnant uteri specimens. These arteries were dissected free of surrounding fat and connective tissue and cut into tubular rings approximately 3 to 4 mm in length. The rings were allowed to stabilize in Krebs-Henseleit solution that was being perfused with 95% oxygen and 5% carbon dioxide. They were then attached to a tension balance that measured isometric contractions. A baseline tension of 500 mg was placed on the arterial segment, then 1000 µg/ml of lidocaine without preservative or epinephrine was added to the bath. When the drug was added, a significant increase in the tension of the vessels developed. The increase was greater in the pregnant specimens and there was a greater response—that is, all the pregnant specimens responded to the lidocaine—whereas only four out of the seven nonpregnant specimens contracted.

COMMENT: Morishima et al. (Transfer of lidocaine across the sheep placenta to the fetus, Am. J. Obstet. Gynecol. **122:**581, 1975) have demonstrated that intravenous administration of lidocaine to maternal sheep decreases uterine blood flow. This may explain the decrease in fetal heart rate that occasionally occurs with paracervical block and would place the decrease on a hypoxic basis. Such studies lend support to the admonition not to use paracervical block in the presence of late decelerations.

■ Gusdon, J. P., Jr., Anderson, S. G., and May, W. J.: A clinical evaluation of the "roll-over test" for pregnancy-induced hypertension, Am. J. Obstet. Gynecol. **127**:1-3, 1977.

The investigators studied sixty multigravida and sixty primigravida patients between the twenty-eighth and thirty-second week, using the "roll-over test." Twenty patients who had a positive test were primigravidas, and ten of these developed hypertension. Only three of forty patients who had negative tests developed hypertension. In multigravidas 25% with a positive test developed hypertension. In patients with a negative test, only three of forty-eight patients developed hypertension. Thus the test seemed to have a relatively high false positive rate, around 50%, and a relatively low false negative rate.

COMMENT: The roll-over test developed by Gant et al. (A clinical test useful for predicting the development of acute hypertension in pregnancy, Am. J. Obstet. Gynecol. 120:1, 1974) would seem to be most helpful in the prospective diagnosis of preeclampsia. Unfortunately, the tests may have a significantly higher false positive rate than originally described by Gant (around 10%) (A study of angiotensin II pressor response throughout primigravida pregnancy, J. Clin. Invest. 52:682, 1973) but according to Gibbs and Noel does have roughly the same false negative rate (around 7% to 10%) as that described by Gant. Thus the test is most helpful in eliminating a patient from the suspicious hypertensive category, rather than affirming the patient who will develop the disease.

■ Jekel, J. F., Harrison, J. T., Bancroft, D. R. E., Tyler, N. C., and Klerman, L. V.: A comparison of the health of index and subsequent babies born to school age mothers, Am. J. Public Health **65**:370-374, 1975.

This study reports data on the mortality rate and prematurity rate of babies subsequently born to young mothers who had been introduced to the young mothers program in New

TABLE 10-5
Obstetric outcomes among index and subsequent infants*

Outcome	Index (N = 180)		Subsequent (N = 103)	
	Number	*Percent*	*Number*	*Percent*
Survival				
Perinatal death	2	1.1	9	8.8
Living infants	178	98.9	94	91.3
Total	180	100.0	103	100.0

$$\chi_1^2 = 8.26, \; p < 0.01$$

Birth weight				
Less than 1000 gm	2	1.1	3	2.9
1000–2499 gm	19	10.6	25	24.3
2500+ gm	159	88.3	75	72.8
Total	180	100.0	103	100.0

$$\chi_1^2 = 11.04, \; p < 0.01$$

*From Jekel, J. F., Harrison, J. T., Bancroft, D. R. E., Tyler, N. C., and Klerman, L. V.: A comparison of the health of index and subsequent babies born to school age mothers, Am. J. Public Health **65**:370-374, 1975.

Haven, Conn. The comparison was made between these infants and subsequent pregnancies and the first-born index infant that brought the mother to the young mothers program initially. It was a 5-year prospective study and at the termination of the follow-up period on January 31, 1972, seventy-nine mothers had delivered a total of 103 babies. Table 10-5 taken from this study points out the striking increase in perinatal mortality among the subsequent-born children to the young mothers (8.8% versus 1.1%). In addition, there was a marked increase in low birth weight babies (27.2% versus 11.7%) for infants. This study demonstrated that subsequent pregnancies had terminated in less healthy babies than those from the first pregnancies, despite the fact that the mothers were now older. Second, it exposed the important role of preterm delivery in increasing perinatal mortality. All but two of the 103 infants were delivered to mothers who were still under 20 years of age. The women kept far fewer prenatal clinic visits during the subsequent pregnancies than during the first pregnancy. However, during subsequent pregnancies seven received no prenatal care and the average number of prenatal clinic appointments that were kept was five. (See Table 10-5.)

COMMENT: This article reemphasizes the importance of good prenatal care. These patients, according to traditional teaching, should have had a poorer pregnancy outcome when they were younger; however, they had intense team perinatal care then with excellent results. When older, without good prenatal care the results were poor. The lesson is that prenatal care had more impact than age on reproductive outcome. One cannot dismiss the possibility that early reproduction may have an adverse biologic effect on subsequent pregnancies, and this may be compounded by poor prenatal care.

- Scott, J. R., and Rose, N. B.: Effect of psychoprophylaxis (Lamaze preparation) on labor and delivery in primiparas, N. Engl. J. Med. **294:**1205-1207, 1976.

The authors studied 129 primiparous patients who had completed Lamaze classes. They chose an equal number of controls, the control being the next primiparous patient whose delivery was without prepared childbirth but who was of the same economic status; the same age, plus or minus 5 years; and at least 37 weeks' gestation at the time of delivery.

TABLE 10-6
Pharmacologic methods of pain relief used during labor and delivery*

Analgesia and anesthesia	Number of mothers		P value
	Lamaze group	Control group	
None during first stage of labor	36	9	< 0.001
Sedatives or tranquilizers	28	39	NS†
Narcotics	84	109	< 0.001
Paracervical	13	15	NS
Epidural or caudal	18	52	< 0.001
Saddle	6	8	NS
General anesthesia	4	5	NS
Pudendal	83	59	< 0.001
Local infiltration only	13	5	NS

*From Scott, J. R., and Rose, N. B.: Effect of psychoprophylaxis (Lamaze preparation) on labor and delivery in primiparas, reprinted by permission from The New England Journal of Medicine **294:**1205-1207, 1976.
†Not significant.

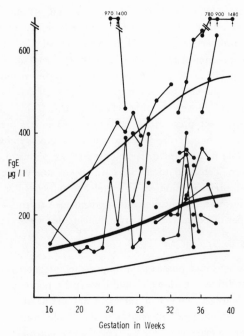

FIG. 10-2
Circulating levels of FgE (●—●) in 20 patients with severe preeclampsia. The normal range (mean ±2 SD after logarithmic transformation of the data) is also shown. (From Gordon, Y. B., Ratsky, S. M., Baker, L. R. I., Letchworth, A. T., Leithton, P. C., and Chard, T.: Circulating levels of fibrin/fibrinogen degradation fragment E measured by radioimmunoassay in pre-eclampsia, Br. J. Obstet. Gynaecol. **83**:287-291, 1976.)

The results showed a higher percentage of patients taking Lamaze training had spontaneous deliveries and, in addition, significantly less use of narcotics and sedatives in the patients who had undergone Lamaze training. (See Table 10-6.)

COMMENT: There is little doubt that proper preparation for childbirth and proper Lamaze training are good education and can lead to a reduced narcotic intake during labor. Reasonably, this should be better for both the mother and the baby. The problem arises when the patient is persuaded that any narcotic would be dangerous for her or the baby. Thus, if she requires some narcotic during her pregnancy, she feels that she is damaging the baby, and therefore the entire procedure is a failure for her. This is a great tragedy and can be avoided by proper instruction during the preparation classes. It should be emphasized that pain thresholds vary widely and that for relief during labor, some individuals will need narcotics that in the vast majority of instances will have little or no effect on the child.

■ Gordon, Y. B., Ratky, S. M., Baker, L. R. I., Letchworth, A. T., Leithton, P. C., and Chard, T.: Circulating levels of fibrin/fibrinogen degradation fragment E measured by radioimmunoassay in pre-eclampsia, Br. J. Obstet. Gynaecol. **83**:287-291, 1976.

Fibrinogen E was determined in normal pregnancy based on 1300 estimates from 200 normal women. There were forty patients with mild or moderate preeclampsia, defined as

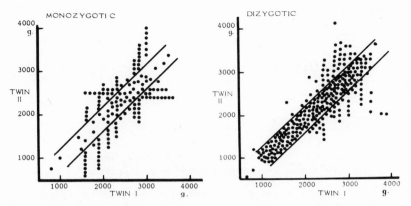

FIG. 10-3

Variations in twin pregnancy birthweights. Area between solid lines represents weight difference of 440 g. (From Daw, E., and Walker, J.: Biologic aspects of twin pregnancy in Dundee, Br. J. Obstet. Gynaecol. 82:29-34, 1975.)

a diastolic blood pressure of 90 to 100 mm Hg with no proteinuria. Twenty patients had severe preeclampsia, defined as a diastolic blood pressure greater than 110 mm Hg and proteinuria in a sterile urine specimen. Ten patients had essential hypertension. In the normal subjects the levels of fibrinogen E rose progressively from the sixteenth week of pregnancy to reach a plateau by the thirty-sixth week. Of the forty patients with mild or moderate preeclampsia, only one showed consistently elevated levels. Six of the twenty patients with severe preeclampsia had consistently elevated levels of fibrinogen E. (See Fig. 10-2.)

COMMENT: There seems to be little doubt that preeclampsia is associated with excess fibrin deposition (McKay et al.: Am. J. Obstet. Gynecol. 66:507, 1953), and there may also be a microangiopathic hemolytic anemia (Seftel and Metz: Haemolytic anaemia, thrombocytopenia and uraemia in eclampsia, S. Afr. Med. J. 31:1037-1041, 1957). From this article it is apparent that high levels of degradation products of fibrinogen are present in significant amounts only in severe preeclampsia and only after the onset of symptomatology: thus fibrin deposition may be a result rather than a cause of the preeclampsia.

■ Daw, E., and Walker, J.: Biological aspects of twin pregnancy in Dundee, Br. J. Obstet. Gynecol. **82:**29-34, 1975.

This study presents a retrospective review of 712 twin pregnancies that occurred in Dundee, Scotland, between 1956 and 1971. Maternal age, parity, and maternal size were compared with the incidence of both monozygotic and dizygotic twinning. The study confirmed previous reports that the incidence of twinning in relation to maternal age is shifting from a previous peak in the 35- to 39-year-old age group. Monozygotic twinning had a maximum incidence in the youngest age group (19 years old and younger). Fig. 10-3 taken from this report demonstrated that there was a much higher incidence of discrepant birth weight between the twins with monozygosity compared with dizgotic twinning.

COMMENT: An obvious limitation of an analysis such as this is the absence of description of placental arrangement and its weight. The large discrepancy in weight of monozygotic twins emphasized the importance of environment on fetal weight.

CHAPTER 11

Fetal monitoring

■ Grennert, L., Gennser, G., Persson, P. H., and Kullander, S.: Ultrasound and human-placental-lactogen screening for early detection of twin pregnancies, Lancet **1:**4-6, 1976.

The investigators examined about 4900 women using ultrasonic screening for twin gestation. Ninety-five percent of the twins were diagnosed by this method. The investigators noted that in the past 5 years the average gestational age for the detection of multiple pregnancies has fallen from 33 weeks to 25 weeks, and they attribute this to the use of ultrasound. In addition, they have found that 95% of the twin gestations have HPL that is greater than 1 SD above the normal for the gestational age. Thus they postulate that this could be used as a less expensive screening method of determining which patients should use ultrasound for the ultimate diagnosis of twin pregnancies.

COMMENT: **The problem of detection of the twin pregnancy remains with us. About 50% of twin pregnancies will be diagnosed before the thirty-fourth week. In this study the authors have lowered their diagnostic age from 33 to 25 weeks, which they attribute to ultrasound, and believe that this can be further lowered perhaps with the use of HPL. It is important that the diagnosis be made prior to the twenty-eighth week so that those patients can have bedrest between the twenty-eighth and thirty-fourth week. Only with this type of therapy is there the possibility of increase in fetal survival in twin pregnancies.**

■ Chik, L., Sokol, R. J., Rosen, M. G., and Borgstedt, A. D.: Computer interpreted fetal electroencephalogram. II. Patterns in infants who were neurologically abnormal at 1 year of age, Am. J. Obstet. Gynecol. **125:**541-544, 1976.

From a group of twenty-five fetal electroencephalographic tapes of infants known to be neurologically abnormal at 1 year of age, nine were known to have been monitored during labor for at least 1½ hours. In addition, there was 30 minutes during which the program detected more than 70% artifact-free data. Seven thousand one hundred and twenty-five 10-second epochs were available for analysis. Low-voltage irregular accounted for 17.85% of these epochs, MIX accounted for 30.5%, high-voltage slow accounted for 18%, and trace alternans, 33.2%; less than 0.2% of the epochs showed depression or isoelectricity. There was a significant increase in low-voltage irregular in these nine abnormal infants when compared to the eleven normal infants in whom the percentage of low-voltage irregular was 4.41%.

COMMENT: **In this article by Chik et al. the work of Rosen and his group on fetal electroencephalogram does seem to demonstrate the correlation of a low voltage electroencephalogram pattern and subsequent neurologic abnormalities.**

This type of study, that is, long-term follow-up, needs to be conducted in evaluation of all current methods of fetal monitoring. Unfortunately, seldom is this done, and it is heartening to see it being done in the studies on fetal electroencephalography; however, one must

ask what was the electroencephalogram pattern of the sixteen patients who were damaged but did not meet the criteria of 1½ hours of monitoring of which at least 70% was artifact-free. The clinical value of a technique with a less than 50% yield of usable information must also be questioned.

- Milunsky, A., and Alpert, E.: Prenatal diagnosis of neural tube defects. I. Problems and pitfalls: analysis of 2495 cases using the alpha-fetoprotein assay, Obstet. Gynecol. 48:1-5, 1976.

- Milunsky, A., and Alpert, E.: Prenatal diagnosis of neural tube defects. II. Analysis of false positive and false negative alpha-fetoprotein results, Obstet. Gynecol. 48:6-12, 1976.

All patients had amniotic fluid analyzed during the second trimester. Of women who had had a previous child with neural tube defect, 1.4% were found to be carrying a second affected child. Of women who had borne two previously affected children, 12% were found to be carrying a third affected fetus. The frequency of neural tube defects in patients not at risk was 1 in 310. Other disorders giving an elevated alpha-fetoprotein (AFP) level included fetal death, spontaneous abortion, and stillbirth. False positive elevations of AFP in the amniotic fluid were observed in 122 cases. There was only one false negative AFP value, and this was found in a patient who subsequently delivered a child with a myelomeningocele and multiple congenital abnormalities.

COMMENT: These articles point out the occurrence of neural tube defects and the pitfalls of using simply previous history and polyhydramnios to diagnose neural tube defects. Despite the importance of the use of AFP, there is a relatively high incidence of false positives associated with AFP according to the data presented. Thus one must utilize not only alpha-fetoprotein but also ultrasound or amniography in arriving at a positive diagnosis of neural tube defect. Elevated levels of AFP may also be found in a variety of other conditions, including the congenital nephrotic syndrome (Wiggelinkhuizen et al.: Alpha fetoprotein in the antenatal diagnosis of the congenital nephrotic syndrome, J. Pediatr. 89:452-455, 1976).

- Wald, N., Barker, S., Peto, R., Brock, D. J. H., and Bonnar, J.: Maternal serum alpha-fetoprotein and previous neural tube defects, Br. J. Obstet. Gynaecol. 83:213-216, 1976.

The authors examined twenty-one women who in the past had pregnancies associated with a neural tube defect and matched these with women who did not have such a history. Maternal serum AFP was done by radioimmunoassay. In only three instances was the maternal serum AFP higher in the index pregnancies than in the control pregnancies, whereas in nine it was lower. Thus there is no evidence that patients with a normal pregnancy who have a previous history of neural tube defect would have an elevated AFP in the maternal serum.

- Rodeck, C. H., Campbell, S., and Biswas, S.: Maternal plasma alpha-fetoprotein in normal and complicated pregnancies, Br. J. Obstet. Gynaecol. 83:24-32, 1976.

The authors measured plasma AFP in thirty-six normal women and fourteen normal men who had no past history of liver disease and were taking drugs. They had 543 samples obtained from 480 normally pregnant women. There were 110 complicated pregnancies, which included preeclampsia, 38; hypertension, 28; small-for dates babies, 44; low urinary estrogen excretion, 38; retarded ultrasonic cephalometry growth rates, 32; and fetal distress in labor, 37. AFP were determined by radioimmunoassay. There was a demonstrated marked rise starting at 8 weeks of pregnancy, and it reached its maximum at 32 weeks. From 32 weeks onward there was a gradual drop to term. The vast majority of the estimates of AFP

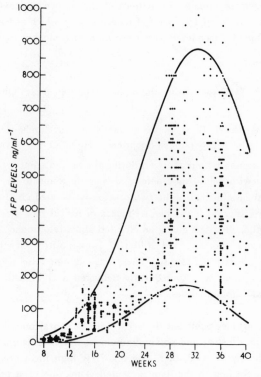

FIG. 11-1
Maternal plasma AFP levels in normal pregnancies (543 samples) showing the 90% range.
(From Rodeck, C. H., Campbell, S., and Biswas, S.: Maternal plasma alpha-fetoprotein in
normal and complicated pregnancies, Br. J. Obstet. Gynaecol. **83:**24-32, 1976.)

fell within the 90% normal range. Two patients above the 95th percentile at 38 weeks'
gestation had infants with large cutaneous hemangiomas. (See Fig. 11-1.)

- Cowchock, F. S., and Jackson, L. G.: Diagnostic use of maternal serum alpha-fetoprotein
  levels, Obstet. Gynecol. **47:**63-68, 1976.

These investigators examined 150 amniotic fluid specimens from patients undergoing
amniocentesis for conditions unassociated with pregnancy complication and whose infants
were normal at delivery. This group formed the normal controls of AFP levels. They also
studied AFP levels in maternal serum from the same patients. They found that the values
began to rise in maternal serum at about 12 to 14 weeks postconception and reached a peak
at about the twenty-fourth to twenty-sixth week. Amniotic fluid concentrations, on the other
hand, are high early in gestation and begin to drop steadily so that about the nineteenth to
twentieth week they are at low levels and remain low throughout the remainder of the pregnancy. There was no correlation between AFP levels in maternal serum and amniotic fluid. In
the same article the authors report fourteen patients studied over a 2-year period who had elevated serum levels of amniotic fluid AFP. In each case there was a fetal abnormality or a
fetomaternal transfusion. The amniotic fluid was also elevated when tested in these patients.

■ Hay, D. M., Forrester, P. I., Hancock, R. L., and Lorscheider, F. L.: Maternal serum alpha-fetoprotein in normal pregnancy, Br. J. Obstet. Gynaecol. **83:**534-538, 1976.

The authors have done consecutive maternal serum determinations of AFP on sixty-three patients throughout their pregnancy. These patients all delivered a singleton fetus that was healthy. The gestational age of the newborn was calculated from the date of the last menstrual period as well as examination of the newborn. Elevated levels of AFP could be detected at 10 weeks' gestation. The levels peaked at 32 weeks and then fell by about 50% by term. The average day-to-day coefficient of variation for blood specimens was 3.6%. The hour-to-hour coefficient of variation for specimens taken between 8 A.M. and 12 noon was 6.4%.

■ Weiss, R., Macri, J. N., Elligers, K., Princler, G. L., McIntire, K. R., and Waldman, T. A.: Amniotic fluid α-fetoprotein as a marker in prenatal diagnosis of neural tube defects, Obstet. Gynecol. **47:**148-151, 1976.

Amniotic fluid levels of AFP were obtained from 237 patients. The normals were between 7 and 13 weeks of gestation. They were obtained during suction curettage for elective legal abortion. A large number of samples were obtained from pregnancies culminating in the delivery of newborns with a variety of neural tube defects. It was found that the highest concentration of AFP is, in early gestation, from 7 to 9 weeks; then there is a gradual decrease until the twenty-sixth week of gestation. In the patients with neural tube deformity, high levels of AFP were found in the amniotic fluid in thirteen of fourteen patients prior to the twenty-sixth week of gestation. After the twenty-sixth week, twenty-one fluids were analyzed. Of these, one case of spina bifida and two cases of anencephaly gave no detectable levels of AFP.

■ Edwards, R. P., and Balfour, R. P.: The clinical diagnosis of major congenital abnormalities of the fetal central nervous system, Br. J. Obstet. Gynaecol. **83:**422-424, 1976.

These investigators report on 207 major congenital malformations of the central nervous system out of 30,388 pregnancies in the Mill Road Maternity Hospital, Liverpool. Open neural tube defects were found in 190 patients, 100 of whom had an anencephalic infant. Polyhydramnios was present in 93% of the anencephalic group. Fetal malpresentation or clinical suspicion of a cephalic abnormality was present in 26%. Clinical suspicion was responsible for the diagnosis of malformations of the central nervous system in only 51% of cases. The majority of the diagnoses were made in the last 4 to 6 weeks of gestation.

■ Norgaard-Pedersen, B., Jorgensen, P. I., and Trolle, D.: Alpha-fetoprotein concentration in amniotic fluid during the last trimester in normal pregnancies and in pregnancies with severe fetal abnormalities, Acta Obstet. Gynecol. Scand. **55:**59-62, 1976.

The authors examined the amniotic fluid in the last trimester of pregnancy in a group of ninety-four normally pregnant women and seven women with abnormal pregnancies. One hundred twenty-nine amniotic fluid samples were obtained from normal patients and twelve amniotic fluid samples from affected patients. A standard curve was established from the normal values. It demonstrated a gradual decrease in AFP levels as term approached. In the ten cases of anencephaly, two fell within the normal range and the remainder were elevated. (See Fig. 11-2.)

■ Chard, T., Kitau, M. J., Ledward, R., Coltart, T., Embury, S., and Seller, M. J.: Elevated levels of maternal plasma alpha-fetoprotein after amniocentesis, Br. J. Obstet. Gynaecol. **83:**33-34, 1976.

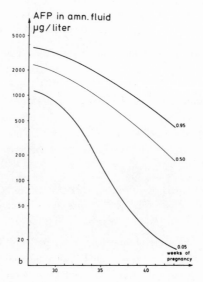

FIG. 11-2
Smoothed curve for amniotic fluid AFP in the last trimester of pregnancy. (From Norgaard-Pedersen, B., Jorgensen, P. I., and Trolle, D.: Alpha-fetoprotein concentration in amniotic fluid during the last trimester in normal pregnancies and in pregnancies with severe fetal abnormalities, Acta Obstet. Gynecol. Scand. **55:**59-62, 1976.)

The investigators collected maternal blood samples before and after amniocentesis in sixty-five women. Gestational ages ranged from 14 to 40 weeks. Maternal plasma AFP was done by radioimmunoassay. The results demonstrated a significant rise in maternal blood AFP after amniocentesis had been performed (150% above the preamniocentesis level) in eleven of the sixty-five patients. (See Fig. 11-3.)

COMMENT (Chard et al.)**: This is an important study that needs confirmation. The etiology of this marked increase following amniocentesis is not readily apparent. To implicate AFP transfer is difficult, considering the magnitude of the increase in maternal blood.**

■ Dow, T. G. B., Rooney, P. J., and Spence, M.: Does anaemia increase the risks to the fetus caused by smoking in pregnancy? Br. Med. J. **4:**253-254, 1975.

The patients selected were ten normal women late in the second trimester of pregnancy with hemoglobin levels of 11 gm/dl or greater, the second group was ten women late in the second trimester of pregnancy whose hemoglobin was less than 10 gm/dl, and the third group was ten normal nonpregnant women with hemoglobin levels over 11 gm/dl. All women were regular cigarette smokers. Change in carboxyhemoglobin concentration was estimated spectrophotometrically. In the nonpregnant group the rise in carboxyhemoglobin concentration with a cigarette was 2.1%. A significantly greater increase was found in the normal pregnant group, 3.9%, and this effect was more pronounced in the pregnant anemic woman, 5%.

COMMENT: The fact that the carboxyhemoglobin content rises more significantly after cigarette smoking in the pregnant woman who is anemic would lead one to speculate that there may be a correlation between hemoglobin levels, cigarette smoking, and birth weight.

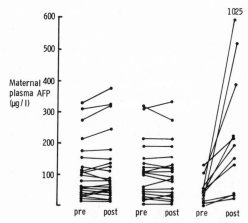

FIG. 11-3
Maternal plasma AFP levels before and after amniocentesis. The right-hand panel shows subjects in which there was a significant rise in levels (more than 150%) and the remaining panels, subjects in which there was no significant rise. The first two panels are separate to avoid the confusion of too many overlapping lines. (From Chard, T., Kitau, M. J., Ledward, R., Coltart, T., Embury, S., and Seller, M. J.: Elevated levels of maternal plasma alpha-fetoprotein after amniocentesis, Br. J. Obstet. Gynaecol. **83:**33-34, 1976.)

To the best of our knowledge, this has not been tested and should be investigated. Although cigarette smoking is to be discouraged in pregnant women, it certainly should be pointed out as a more significant hazard to the patient who is anemic during pregnancy.

- Redman, C. W. G., Beilin, L. J., Bonnar, J., and Wilkinson, R. H.: Plasma-urate measurements in predicting fetal death in hypertensive pregnancy, Lancet **2:**1370-1373, 1976.

This study consisted of 332 patients with hypertension. Of these, 238 patients were in a trial of antihypertensive treatment in pregnancy, of which 117 were randomly assigned to active treatment with methyldopa. The results indicate that plasma urate values exceeding 0.36 mmol/L were associated with a significant perinatal mortality. After 28 weeks of pregnancy, low maternal plasma urate concentrations were associated with a low perinatal mortality even in infants of hypertensive mothers. There was a better correlation between plasma urate concentrations and perinatal mortality than between the degree of diastolic elevation and perinatal mortality. (See Table 11-1.)

COMMENT: This simply confirms an older observation that hyperuricemia correlates with the severity of preeclampsia and perinatal mortality. The hyperuricemia is probably due to a reduced glomerular filtration rate. It may also be associated with a marked decrease in renal plasma flow. Thus the marked increase in perinatal mortality and hyperuricemia may both be a reflection of the increase in vascular reactivity in the vessels both in the placenta and the kidney.

- Lee, C. Y., Di Loreto, P. C., and Logrand, B.: Fetal activity acceleration determination for the evaluation of fetal reserve, Obstet. Gynecol. **48:**19-26, 1976.

The study was done over a 20-month period during which fetal activity determination was performed 462 times on 410 patients. The determination was obtained by placing an

TABLE 11-1

Eventual perinatal mortality by plasma-urate*†

Gestation	≤0.23 mmol/L (3.9 mg/dl)	0.24-0.35 mmol/L (4.0-5.9 mg/dl)	0.36-0.41 mmol/L (6.0-6.9 mg/dl)	≥0.42 mmol/L (7.0 mg/dl)	Number of pregnancies ending with each period
126–153 days (20 wk)					
Stillbirths	5 (4.7%)	2 (4.4%)	3 (50%)		0
Neonatal deaths	0	0	0		0
Livebirths	101	44			0
154-181 days (24 wk)					
Stillbirths	2 (1.4%)	2 (2.9%)	2 (40%)	3 (50%)	3
Neonatal deaths	2 (1.4%)	0	0	1 (17%)	0
Livebirths	140	68	3	2	0
182–209 days (28 wk)					
Stillbirths	2 (1.3%)	1 (0.9%)	1 (11%)	4 (40%)	8
Neonatal deaths	0	2 (1.8%)	2 (22%)	3 (30%)	1
Livebirths	158	107	6	3	2
210–230 days (32 wk)					
Stillbirths	0	2 (1.4%)	1 (6%)	7 (39%)	6
Neonatal deaths	0	1 (0.7%)	2 (12%)	5 (28%)	4
Livebirths	124	139	14	6	9
231–244 days (34 wk)					
Stillbirths	0	1 (0.7%)	1 (6%)	2 (15%)	2
Neonatal deaths	0	1 (0.7%)	1 (6%)	2 (15%)	2
Livebirths	100	146	18	9	10
245–258 days (36 wk)					
Stillbirths	1 (1.3%)	0	0	1 (6%)	2
Neonatal deaths	0	1 (0.6%)	1 (4%)	0	2
Livebirths	78	162	22	15	30
6 wk postpartum (all patients)					
Stillbirths	0	17 (7.9%)	3 (6%)	3 (9%)	32/332‡
Neonatal deaths	0	7 (3.2%)	1 (2%)	1 (3%)	(9.9%)
Livebirths	32	190	49	29	

*From Redman, C. W. G., Beilin, L. J., Bonnar, J., and Wilkinson, R. H.: Plasma-urate measurements in predicting fetal death in hypertensive pregnancy, Lancet 2:1370-1373, 1976.
†All stillbirths and neonatal deaths after 24 weeks.
‡Total perinatal mortality summarized includes 2 deaths occurring at 38 weeks.

ultrasonic transducer on the mother's abdomen to record continuously the fetal heart rate and placing an externally recording tocodynamometer, also on the mother's abdomen, to record uterine activity and fetal activity. The mother was also asked to record her own fetal activity using a marker on the oscillograph. A positive fetal activity determination test was acceleration of the fetal heart rate with fetal activity. Baseline fluctuations of the heart rate were studied, and simultaneous oxytocin challenge tests (OCTs) were done on 298 patients. In those patients in whom the fetal activity test was positive and the OCT was negative, there was one fetal death due to abruptio placentae. Late decelerations were not observed during labor in the remainder of the infants. In twelve cases the fetal activity test was positive, the OCT was questionable but probably negative, and in seven cases with a positive fetal activity the simultaneous OCT was unsatisfactory. In all these instances the infant was delivered in excellent condition. In 137 instances there was a positive fetal activity test, but no OCT was performed; all these fetuses were delivered in good condition. Two fetuses had negative fetal activity and positive OCTs and were delivered in good condition.

■ Buster, J. E., Sakakini, J., Jr., Killam, A. P., and Scragg, W. H.: Serum unconjugated estriol levels in the third trimester and their relationship to gestational age, Am. J. Obstet. Gynecol. **125:**672-676, 1976.

The authors measured serum unconjugated estriol using a specific radioimmunoassay. There were two groups of subjects. The first group were randomly selected subjects in whom samples were obtained (1 to 9 samples between 28 and 41 weeks' gestation). The second group consisted of 9 subjects who provided serial samples. The investigators demonstrated a decrease in estriol between the thirty-third and thirty-fourth week, with a surge of estriol between the thirty-fifth and thirty-sixth week that was remarkably consisent in the patients studied.

COMMENT (Buster et al.): **This, too, may provide another means of attempting to date pregnancies, particularly in the third trimester; however, the series provided by the authors is relatively small and studies would need to be done to confirm the surge in patients having various diseases such as diabetes and hypertensive vascular disease in pregnancy. It would also be important to look at this surge in relationship to patients having premature delivery between the thirty-fourth and thirty-sixth week of pregnancy. It is conceivable that the surge is a prelabor phenomenon and may occur regardless of when labor does occur.**

■ Odendaal, H. J., Neves Dos Santos, L. M., Henry, M. J., and Crawford, J. W.: Experiments in the measurement of intrauterine pressure, Br. J. Obstet. Gynaecol. **83:**221-224, 1976.

The investigators attempted to determine the validity of the recording of intrauterine pressures. Ten patients had one catheter adjusted to independent transducers, and it was found that these recordings were essentially similar. Twenty patients had two catheters. One had the tip cut off and the other was used as a control. There was no difference in the number of contaminated catheters whether or not the tip had been cut off. In ten patients one of two catheters was not flushed throughout the labor. In four of the ten patients the catheter not being flushed was blocked, whereas the blockage occurred in only one of the flushed catheters. In ten patients one catheter was flushed during insertion and the other was not, but both were flushed every 30 to 60 minutes while catheters remained open. In two patients suspected of having attenuated signals from a catheter blockage, a peristaltic pump was attached so that it caused a flow of liquid from the transducer to the catheter tip, and the flow rate was increased until no further effect was noted. In both these patients the intensity of the contractions increased to a value consistent with clinical observation.

COMMENT: These authors have found that there may be significant signal attenuation in the recordings that we see in our intrauterine pressure tracings. This is particularly important and stresses the significance of flushing frequently if one is to obtain anywhere near accurate representation of intrauterine pressure.

■ Farahani, G., Vasudeva, K., Petrie, R., and Fenton, A. N.: Oxytocin challenge test in high-risk pregnancy, Obstet. Gynecol. **47:**159-168, 1976.

The authors examined 333 high-risk patients with 767 oxytocin challenge tests. Two hundred eighty-eight patients had a total of 689 negative OCTs. Of these, only one patient who had a negative OCT within a week prior to labor had any evidence of late deceleration during labor. All these patients had normal fetal heart rate tracings during labor and delivered healthy infants. All but two of the infants with negative oxytocin challenge tests had Apgar scores of 7 or more at 5 minutes. These two had Apgar scores of 6 at 5 minutes. Of these patients, there was one false-negative test, and that was a fetus that died within 1 week of the negative OCT. There were twenty-six positive oxytocin challenge tests on twenty-four patients, twenty-two of whom were delivered by cesarean section.

■ Freeman, R. K., Goebelsmann, U. T., Nochimson, D., and Cetrulo, C.: An evaluation of the significance of a positive oxytocin challenge test, Obstet. Gynecol. **47:**8-13, 1976.

In the antepartum period 810 OCTs were done in 390 high-risk pregnancies. Seventy-nine tests were interpreted as positive in sixty-six patients. The patients with positive tests had a higher incidence of hypertension. Perinatal mortality among sixty-six patients with positive OCTs was 15% compared to 4% among the 324 patients who had no positive OCT. In a group with positive OCT, thirteen of sixty patients with live births had babies with Apgar scores of less than 7 at 5 minutes. Among the 324 with a negative OCT, 5.2% had low 5-minute Apgar scores. Intrauterine growth retardation was present in 37% of the patients with a positive OCT versus only 10% in those with a negative OCT. Of the sixty-six patients with positive OCTs, 57 were monitored with 24-hour urinary estriol determinations. Of these 46% had 24-hour urinary estriols that averaged less than 2 SD below the mean for gestation. Fifteen (26%) had estriols that fell by over 35%. In only four patients the estriol was both low and falling. All the perinatal deaths and all but one of the low Apgar score babies occurring in singleton births were from patients with low or falling 24-hour urinary estriol excretions.

■ Odendall, H.: Fetal heart rate patterns in patients with intrauterine growth retardation, Obstet. Gynecol. **48:**187-190, 1976.

The author examined 953 patients, 324 of which were said to be totally uncomplicated. He looked at the incidence of tachycardia and bradycardia in the groups with growth retardation as compared to the normal patients, growth retardation being defined as babies below the 10th percentile of weight for gestational age. They found no difference in the incidences of tachycardia and bradycardia. There was, however, a significant difference in the incidences of variable and late decelerations. Variable decelerations were seen in 8% of the uncomplicated labors and in 26% of the labors associated with growth retardation of the infant. Late deceleration was seen in 16% of the patients with uncomplicated labors and in 27% of those in labor with growth retarded infants. There was no difference in the beat-to-beat variability, but a significant difference was found in the incidence of low Apgar scores, being defined as an Apgar score of less than 7 at 5 minutes. This occurred in 16% of the infants with growth retardation and 8% of the normal infants.

COMMENT: The studies by Farahani et al. and Freeman et al. have demonstrated the value of the contraction stress test in the management of high-risk pregnant patients. The important point is the extremely low false negative rate in this test. Exactly what the incidence of false positives was could not be demonstrated in this article, since the vast majority

of patients with positive OCTs were delivered by cesarean section. Freeman's study showing an increase in positive OCTs in the intrauterine growth-retarded fetus confirms previous observations (Lowe et al.: Fetal asphyxia during the intrapartum period in intrauterine growth-retarded infants, Am. J. Obstet. Gynecol. 113:351-357, 1972), which showed an increased incidence of metabolic acidosis in these infants with intrauterine growth retardation (IUGR) at the time of delivery:

	Mild acid	*Severe acid*
IUGR	52%	48%
Borderline	78%	22%

These reports suggest that estriol measurements are useful adjuncts to the OCTs. For further discussion of the use of estriol in high-risk pregnancy, see Chapter 7.

Odendall's article confirms the high incidence of variable and late decelerations associated with intrauterine growth retardation.

■ Spellacy, W. N., Buhi, W. C., and Burke, S. A.: The effectiveness of human placental lactogen measurements as an adjunct in decreasing perinatal deaths. Results of a retrospective and a randomized controlled prospective study, Am. J. Obstet. Gynecol. 121:835-844, 1975.

These researchers studied the results of all the patients who had serum HPL levels measured during a 6-year period. Those pregnancies in which a perinatal death occurred after the thirtieth week were studied. There were seventy-one fetal deaths occurring in women having HPL determinations done during the 6-year period. In thirty-six of the seventy-one deaths there was a low HPL value, less than 4 μg/ml. The highest results were seen in severe toxemia: eighteen of twenty-one fetal deaths were predicted by a low HPL value. In the prospective study 230 women were enrolled. The women were assigned to two groups, depending on whether their hospital numbers were odd or even. Both groups were fundamentally high-risk pregnancies and both groups had HPLs done at each visit. In one group the HPL data were given to the physician to help manage the pregnancy, and in the other group they were not. The fetal death rate was 14.2% in the controlled group and 2.6% in the HPL-managed group, which would seem to point toward benefit from the use of the HPL in high-risk pregnancy.

COMMENT: In all probability, measurements of HPL levels are of use in high-risk pregnancy, particularly in the patient with hypertensive vascular disease; however, their use in pregnancies complicated by diabetes as well as erythroblastosis is certainly questionable. This test is an easy one to do and thus should be considered in the armamentarium of the physician managing the patient with toxemia of pregnancy.

■ Edwards, R. P., Diver, M. J., Davis, J. C., and Hipkin, L. J.: Plasma oestriol and human placental lactogen measurements in patients with high risk pregnancies, Br. J. Obstet. Gynaecol. 83:229-237, 1976.

Three hundred eighty-three patients with an at risk pregnancy were investigated. Fetal distress was diagnosed if there was meconium in the amniotic fluid, if the Apgar score was 6 or less at 1 minute and/or 10 minutes, or if the fetal heart rate was abnormal. Abnormal fetal heart rate consisted of decelerations related to uterine contractions. Total plasma estriol levels were considered abnormal if they were less than 10 μg/dl or if they were more than 1 SD below the normal mean value on more than one occasion after 35 weeks. Of 129 patients, a suspicion of fetal growth retardation was correct in seventy-one cases, a 55%

correct suspicion on the basis of estriol data. Of the 254 patients with normal estriols levels, the incidence of fetal growth retardation was 5.5%. Thus fetal growth retardation was five times as common with an abnormal plasma estriol.

HPL measurements were also done, and it was found that with abnormal HPL levels, fetal growth retardation was eight times more common.

When both estriol & HPL levels were abnormal, fetal growth retardation was twenty times more common.

COMMENT: One of the more difficult diagnoses to make is intrauterine growth retardation. It would appear from some preliminary reports that putting patients with such a diagnosis at bedrest may result in some benefit. The diagnosis of this condition by ultrasound alone may be inaccurate in as high as 25% to 50% of cases. Therefore it is somewhat encouraging to know that the use of both estriol and HPL data can assist in making this diagnosis. Both are relatively easy to obtain. Used both as a screening tool and then in conjunction with serial studies of biparietal diameter, estriol and HPL measurements should enable the clinician to be more accurate in a significantly higher percentage of cases.

■ Rochard, F., Schifrin, B. S., Goupil, F., Legrand, H., Blottiere, J., and Sureau, C.: Nonstressed fetal heart rate monitoring in the antepartum period, Am. J. Obstet. Gynecol. **126:**699-706, 1976.

The heart rate patterns were classified into reactive, nonreactive, and sinusoidal patterns. A reactive pattern had a stable baseline rate between 120 and 160 beats per minute, the range of baseline variability is 6 beats per minute, and accelerations accompanied fetal movement. The nonreactive pattern had a stable baseline rate, the variability was consistently less than 6 beats per minute, and there were no accelerations with fetal movement. Sinusoidal patterns were periodic oscillations in the fetal heart rate superimposed on a nonreactive pattern. The results showed that of nineteen fetuses demonstrating a persistent nonreactive pattern, five, or 26%, died in utero or in the neonatal period; eleven, or 58%, required prolonged neonatal care; and only three of the nineteen were mildly affected. In those infants with persistently reactive patterns, forty-one, or 80%, tolerated labor without distress and were delivered in good condition; six babies developed fetal distress during labor; and four were affected with intrauterine growth retardation, the respiratory distress syndrome, or anemia. Sinusoidal heart patterns were observed only in infants with severe isoimmunization. Of the twenty babies having this type pattern, 50% either died in utero or in the neonatal period, and an additional 40% required prolonged hospitalization.

COMMENT: This article presents preliminary results on a potentially useful method for assessing antepartum fetal status. The fact that the normal fetus is capable of reacting to an external stimulus was demonstrated many years ago by Sontag and Wallace (Changes in rate of human fetal heart in response to vibratory stimuli, Am. J. Dis. Child. 51:583-589, 1936), when he found that the normal fetus reacted with movement to a sound source placed on the mother's abdomen. Subsequently it has been found that the normal fetus reacts to fetal movement with a tachycardia, whereas the fetus that is abnormal, that is, distressed, does not. Unfortunately there are other situations in which the fetus does not react with cardiac acceleration, such as a deep sleep state. It appears that the incidence of false negatives utilizing this test is relatively low, as is the case with the contraction stress test. On the other hand, it is also apparent from the preliminary results that the incidence with false positive tests, that is, seemingly abnormal tests in what is otherwise a normal fetus, is

quite high (about 40% to 50%). This is also true for the contraction stress test. Thus both these tests give the obstetrician a sense of confidence in permitting the fetus to stay in its environment for a longer period. They should not be used singly as indications to remove the fetus from its environment unless the fetus has demonstrated that it is mature and that there would be no problems associated with delivery at that point.

■ Ron, M., and Polishuk, W. Z.: The response of the fetal heart rate to amniocentesis, Br. J. Obstet. Gynaecol. **43:**468-770, 1976.

The authors recorded the fetal heart rate for 10 minutes prior to amniocentesis and up to 90 minutes afterward. Fetal heart rate acceleration was defined as an increase of at least 20 beats per minute that was sustained for 2 minutes. Eighty-eight amniocenteses were done for medical indications. Of these, 82% showed fetal heart acceleration within 30 seconds of puncture of the amniotic sac. In ten patients there was a delay of 5 minutes between puncture of the abdominal and uterine walls. In ten patients acceleration of the fetal heart rate occurred after penetration of the uterine wall only without entering the amniotic cavity. Of the eighty-eight patients in whom the fetal heart rate acceleration occurred, 97.7% delivered healthy babies with a good Apgar score. In 2.3% there were evidences of fetal distress before or during labor. In nineteen amniocenteses there was no fetal heart rate acceleration response. In this group eight or 42.2%, delivered infants with a low Apgar score and there were two perinatal deaths.

COMMENT: These investigators have found an acceleration of the fetal heart rate in the vast majority of patients with either puncture of the amniotic sac or simply penetration of the uterine wall. The obvious question is why would there be an acceleration of the fetal heart rate with penetration of the uterine wall only. It would have been of interest in this study to have recorded uterine activity to investigate the most likely explanation: that uterine wall penetration may stimulate uterine contractions, which would alter uterine blood flow. A decrease in uterine blood flow would be associated with a slight decrease in fetal oxygen tension, which could trigger the tachycardia.

■ Sabbagha, R. E., Barton, F. B., and Barton, B. A.: Sonar biparietal diameter. I. Analysis of percentile growth differences in two normal populations using same methodology, Am. J. Obstet. Gynecol. **126:**479-484, 1976.

The authors have examined 198 patients with similar socioeconomic status from the sixteenth week of pregnancy through term. There were 107 white patients and 91 black patients in the group. Pregnancies were uncomplicated. The dates were established by a known last menstrual period and a spontaneous delivery ±2 weeks of the estimated date of confinement, calculated from that last known menstrual period and the delivery of the normal term neonate. Slight differences were found between the black and white population, particularly beyond 36 weeks (the blacks were about 2 mm larger in biparietal diameter than the whites), but they were not significant from a clinical standpoint. An excellent growth curve was established with percentile limits which shows a significant increase in biparietal diameter from 16 weeks through term. (See Fig. 11-4.)

COMMENT: In a subsequent article these investigators used the normal growth patterns of the biparietal diameter as established to demonstrate the progressive growth of fetuses and the fact that in general the normally growing fetus does tend to fall within certain percentile limits of the fetal growth curve and to stay in that limit through pregnancy (Sab-

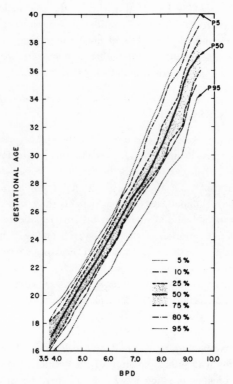

FIG. 11-4
Note the variation in gestational age for different BPDs (black and white fetuses). (From
Sabbagha, R. E., Barton, F. B., and Barton, B. A.: Sonar biparietal diameter. I. Analysis of
percentile growth differences in two normal populations using same methodology, Am. J.
Obstet. Gynecol. **126:**479-484, 1976.)

bagha et al.: Sonar biparietal diameter. II. Predictive of three fetal growth patterns leading
to a closer assessment of gestational age and fetal weight, Am. J. Obstet. Gynecol. **126:**485-
490, 1976).

■ Bergsjo, P., Bakke, T. and Bjerkedal, T.: Growth of the fetal skull, with special reference
to weight-for-dates of the newborn child, Acta Obstet. Gynecol. Scand. **55:**53-57, 1976.

The authors looked at the biparietal diameter measurements in 165 women with normal
pregnancies, that is, without complications, and children born without malformations. They
looked at 131 pregnancies in women who had had regular menstrual periods who were not
taking oral contraceptive agents. Fifty-four pregnancies were examined in a retrospective way,
that is, constructing the curve from women who went into labor spontaneously and had
children compatible with their gestational dates. All the curves were relatively comparable
and all demonstrated the well known fact that there is considerable overlap in fetal biparietal
diameter with regard to using a single measurement for estimation of gestational age. Several
measurements were made serially in patients, and they did demonstrate progressive growth
of the biparietal diameter to the time of delivery. The correlation coefficient between birth
weight and biparietal diameter was relatively low. (See Table 11-2.)

TABLE 11-2

Coefficients of correlation (r) between the biparietal diameter measured during the last week before birth, and birth weight and length*

Condition	Number of observations	Biparietal diameter versus birth weight (r)	Biparietal diameter versus birth length (r)
Normal pregnancies	58	0.58	0.72
Preeclamptic pregnancies	15	0.63	0.37

*From Bergsjo, P., Bakke, T., and Bjerkedal, T.: Growth of the fetal skull, with special reference to weight-for-dates of the newborn child, Acta Obstet. Gynecol. Scand. 55:53-57, 1976.

COMMENT: This article, as have others, demonstrates the difficulty of using fetal biparietal diameter to estimate fetal weight. One must use other fetal diameters, that is, thorax or abdomen, to obtain acceptable limits of error.

■ Kurjak, A., and Breyer, B.: Estimation of fetal weight by ultrasonic abdominometry, Am. J. Obstet. Gynecol. **125**:962-965, 1976.

The authors examined 280 patients with singleton pregnancies within 2 days of delivery. They measured the diameter of the abdomen at its largest point. This was done by determining the entrance of the umbilical vein into the liver through B scan and measuring the anterior, posterior, and lateral diameter of this circumference. The results demonstrated that in 83% of cases the difference between actual and expected weight, taken from a curve constructed from their data, was within ±150 gm and in 94% was within ±250 gm. (See Fig. 11-5.)

COMMENT: These investigators obtained the best results of estimation of fetal weight from ultrasonic topography currently reported in the literature, the majority of the authors reporting ±400 to 500 gm (Willocks et al.: Foetal cephalometry by ultrasound, Obstet. Gynaecol. Br. Commonw. 71:11-20, 1964; Thompson et al.: Fetal development as determined by ultrasonic pulse echo techniques, Am. J. Obstet. Gynecol. 92:44-52, 1965, and Kohorn: An evaluation of ultrasonic fetal cephalometry, Am. J. Obstet. Gynecol. 97:553-559, 1967). This type of measurement would be of definite help to the clinician, particularly in the large-for-dates babies. Although this article does not include the diabetic pregnancies, if such calculations did hold true in the diabetic pregnancies, they would form a very valuable asset in the management of these patients, since one of the principal problems associated with vaginal delivery is the macrosomia found in some infants.

■ Lunt, R., and Chard, T.: A new method for estimation of fetal weight in late pregnancy by ultrasonic scanning, Br. J. Obstet. Gynaecol. **83**:1-5, 1976.

Sixty-eight patients were examined using ultrasound to determine the following: the biparietal diameter, the cross-sectional area of the fetal skull and of the fetal thorax, a multiple of the cross-sectional area of the fetal skull times that of the fetal thorax, and the log of the cross-sectional area of the fetal skull times that of the fetal thorax, the cross-sectional area of the fetal skull times the cross-sectional area of the fetal thorax raised to the third power and then taken to the fourth root. Correlation coefficients with actual weight were biparietal diameter, .62; skull area, .74; thorax area, .83; area of skull times area of thorax, .90; area of skull times area of thorax cubed and divided by the fourth power, .90, the log of the area of the skull times the area of thorax, .92.

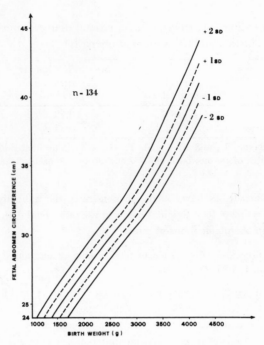

FIG. 11-5
Graphic representation of the dependence of abdominal circumference of the fetus on weight at delivery during the last 4 weeks of gestation. The graph was calculated from 134 cases measured within 2 days from delivery. (From Kurjak, A., and Breyer, B.: Estimation of fetal weight by ultrasonic abdominometry, Am. J. Obstet. Gynecol. **125:**962-965, 1976.)

■ Drumm, J. E., Clinch, J., and MacKenzie, G.: The ultrasonic measurement of fetal crown-rump length as a method of assessing gestational age, Br. J. Obstet. Gynaecol. **83:**417-421, 1976.

The authors made crown-rump length measurements on the fetuses of pregnant patients between 47 and 101 days from the onset of the last menstrual period. There are 253 patients who fulfilled criteria that would enhance the accuracy of the dates. There were a further forty patients in whom ovulation was judged by basal body temperature. In both groups, gestational dates could be estimated within ±3 days, using crown-rump length. There was a very small intrapatient variability of ±3 days. There was also an extremely small observation variability of the crown-rump length between two different observers, the mean difference being 1.1 mm, with a standard deviation of 0.99 mm. This difference in most instances would not affect the gestational age estimate more than 3 days.

COMMENT: This method of estimating gestational age is apparently extremely accurate; however, it relies on the relatively early assessment of the pregnancy using ultrasound (6 < 14 weeks). This technique would be particularly useful in the patient who is using oral contraceptives or has irregular cycles and becomes pregnant.

■ David, H., Weaver, J. B., and Pearson, J. F.: Doppler ultrasound and fetal activity, Br. Med. J. **2:**62-64, 1975.

These researchers studied 15 patients who had an ultrasonic device applied to the maternal abdomen. The mothers were asked to record fetal activity during the first 15 minutes of this study. The ultrasonic device was not turned on for the first 15 minutes, whereas it was during the last 15 minutes. Six patients were studied in which the ultrasonic device was not turned on at all. Fifteen patients were studied for three 15-minute periods. In the first period an ultrasonic device with a metal ring in contact with the mother's abdomen but with the transducer head shielded from the mother's abdomen by polyvinyl foam was placed on the abdomen and left this way for 15 minutes. During the second 15 minutes the device was turned on so that there was only electric contact with the head. Finally, during the third 15 minutes the insulating material was removed and then direct contact between the ultrasonic head that had been activated and the maternal abdomen was made. In each instance the mother was asked to count fetal movements. There was a statistically significant increase in the amount of fetal movement associated with the activated ultrasound.

COMMENT: If this should prove to be the case under more rigorous testing, that is, larger numbers, the absence of such activity would be indicative of some form of fetal distress, as has been demonstrated by others (Goodlin et al.: Human fetal arousal levels as indicated by heart rate recordings, Am. J. Obstet. Gynecol. 114:613-621, 1972). This may indeed be an excellent way for the obstetrician in the office to diagnose and evaluate fetal status. The trend seems to be toward evaluation of the reactive state of the fetus and the response of the fetal cardiovascular system to activity.

■ Hallman, M., Kulovich, M., Kirkpatrick, E., Sugarman, R. G., and Gluck, L.: Phosphatidylinositol and phosphatidylglycerol in amniotic fluid: indices of lung maturity, Am. J. Obstet. Gynecol. **125**:613-617, 1976.

The authors obtained amniotic fluid from twenty patients within 72 hours of birth. Of these, fifteen had lecithin/sphingomyelin (L/S) ratio of two or more and no respiratory distress syndrome (RDS) when born, five had an L/S ratio of less than 2, and four had RDS. In one category of cases the phosphatidylinositol (PI) concentration was less than 4% of the total. Phosphatidylglycerol (PG) was absent. In these instances the L/S ratio was exceedingly low. In the second category the phosphatidylinositol was more than 4% and phosphatidylglycerol less than 0.05%. Here the L/S ratios were between 1 and 3. In the third category the specimens had both phosphatidylglycerol and phosphatidylinositol, and the L/S ratios were in all cases mature.

COMMENT: The originators of the L/S ratio, Gluck et al., have looked at specific phospholipids. The problem with the L/S ratio is not in its incidence of false negatives defined as individuals with an L/S ratio of less than 2 in which there will not be difficulty with respiratory distress syndrome after the birth of the child. Perhaps the finding of phosphatidylglycerol could cut down somewhat on the incidence of false negatives, but the article does not clarify this. Another point brought out by Hallman et al. in their discussion is the fact that phosphatidylglycerol and phosphatidylinositol are found in very small quantities in blood. Thus one might get a better prediction from the L/S ratio after a bloody tap, using these two parameters rather than the L/S ratio, which is known to be influenced by blood.

■ Goldstein, P., Gershenson, D., and Hobbins, J. C.: Fetal biparietal diameter as a predictor of a mature lecithin/sphingomyelin ratio, Obstet. Gynecol. **48**:667-669, 1976.

The authors have looked at 148 patients who had undergone simultaneous determinations of fetal biparietal diameter and L/S. All these patients had both biparietal diameters and

L/S ratios done within a week of each other. They found that when a biparietal diameter of 8.7 was employed, the incidence of a false assumption of mature L/S ratio (greater than 2:1) was 34.5%, the incidence of a false assumption of an immature L/S ratio was 51.4%. Using a 9 cm biparietal diameter, the incidence of a false assumption of a mature L/S ratio was 29.5%, and the incidence of a false assumption of an immature L/S ratio was 56.4%.

COMMENT: The investigators point out in the discussion that in their experience they have never had the development of respiratory distress syndrome in newborns of nondiabetic mothers when the biparietal diameter was 9 cm or greater. Thus it would appear that babies who are from nondiabetic pregnancies but who do have biparietal diameters greater than 9 could be safely delivered. This is not surprising, since it is known that with L/S ratios less than 2, there are sizeable numbers of babies who will not develop respiratory distress, the incidence being 37% in one study (Donald et al.: Clinical experience with the amniotic fluid/sphingomyelin ratio. I. Antenatal prediction of pulmonary maturity, Am. J. Obstet. Gynecol. 115:547-552, 1973). Because of the possibility of morbidity such as fetal hemorrhage or amnionitis with amniocentesis, an accurate noninvasive technique is preferable for determining gestational age. Were such a technique to gain wide acceptance, it would prevent the loss of some babies that now occurs. Almost every series of elective repeat cesarean sections has a few unexpected prematures who die of respiratory distress. This could be almost totally avoided by use of biparietal diameters and/or amniocentesis prior to elective cesarean section. The same should be true for any elective induction of labor.

■ Staisch, K. J., Nuwayhid, B., Bauer, R. O., Welsh, L., and Brinkman, C.: Continuous fetal scalp and carotid artery oxygen tension monitoring in the sheep, Obstet. Gynecol. **47:** 587-592, 1976.

These researchers tested a newly developed oxygen electrode in both a fetal scalp electrode and an intra-arterial catheter. Studies were done on fetal sheep. An electrode was placed in the scalp and simultaneous samples were drawn, using the Saling scalp sampling technique. Another electrode was placed inside a catheter in the carotid artery of the fetal sheep. Samples were drawn simultaneously through the catheter and checked against the electrode in the carotid artery. Animals were given periods of hyperoxia (95% oxygen) lasting 20 minutes, normal oxygen for 20 minutes, hypoxia with 6% oxygen for 20 minutes, and then finally a 20-minute recovery period with hyperoxia. Correlation between the electrode and the actual blood sample was good in all situations, being plus or minus 1 or 2 mm of oxygen tension in the mean values. The values of the scalp electrode were consistently slightly lower by 1 to 5 mm below those of the carotid artery of the fetus.

COMMENT: The authors have tested an oxygen electrode that, if it continues to work well, might be beneficial, assuming reasonable flow through the vessels in the scalp. However, this electrode, as is true of scalp sampling, could get falsely low values if there is edema of the scalp. In situations of severe peripheral constriction and low fetal cardiac output one may also get extremely low oxygen tensions—lower than is true in carotid arterial blood. Neither of these situations was approached in the present article and should be tried before the electrode is considered suitable for clinical monitoring.

Assuming the electrode works perfectly, reflecting accurately the fetal P_{O_2}, one must ask what is abnormal and what does it mean? It is difficult to determine whether fetal tissue oxygen needs are being met by an arterial P_{O_2} value. For instance, a P_{O_2} of 15 mm may have one meaning with a normal pH and a much different meaning in the presence of acidosis.

■ Chang, A., Wood, C., Humphrey, M., Gilbert, M., and Wagstaff, C.: The effects of narcotics on fetal acid base status, Br. J. Obstet. Gynecol. **83:**56-61, 1976.

Two trials were conducted: in the first trial meperidine (pethidine) and nalorphine were used and in the second, morphine and heroin. In each of the two trials an intravenous infusion of 5% dextrose was started at 12 drops/min. Saline, morphine, demerol, nalorphine, or heroin was given intravenously. Amniotomy was done and fetal scalp samples were taken within 5 minutes of giving the drug and at 30 and 60 minutes. Blood samples were analyzed for P_{O_2}, P_{CO_2}, and pH. In the maternal blood the pH was lower and the P_{CO_2} higher in the nalorphine and heroin groups. The pH of the fetus in the nalorphine, morphine, and heroin groups was lower than those of the control groups, and the fetal base excess level of the morphine and heroin groups was lower than those of the control groups. There was no difference in maternal oxygen tension, base excess level, nor in fetal P_{O_2}, oxygen saturation, nor P_{CO_2} between the experimental and control groups.

COMMENT: Although it is true that the oxygen tension remained the same in those babies receiving narcotic, the pH did drop as compared to the saline controls.

Whether this is harmful is yet to be demonstrated; however, all too frequently this type of finding is clutched to the bosom of the zealot as absolute proof that any narcotic given to the mother must surely be bad for the fetus in all cases. Such a physician fails to realize that in some mothers the fear or pain of labor may cause them to excrete significant amounts of epinephrine, which could significantly reduce uterine blood flow and lead to fetal hypoxia. In such situations, maternal sedation may actually benefit the fetus. One message is, each situation must be examined on its own merits, taking into account all factors, and arriving at logical rather than emotional courses of action.

■ Keniston, R. C., Noland, G. L., and Pernoll, M. L.: The effect of blood, meconium, and temperature on the rapid surfactant test, Obstet. Gynecol. **48:**442-446, 1976.

The authors took pooled volumes of amniotic fluid from pregnancies with a mature fetus, a fetus intermediate maturity, and an immature fetus and added various quantities of maternal and fetal blood and serum as well as meconium, and altered the temperature. They have demonstrated that unless the hematocrit of the amniotic fluid is greater than 3, which can be determined from a nomogram that they have provided (Fig. 11-6), the value of the rapid surfactant test (shake test) is reliable. At values (Fig. 11-6) greater than 3, false positive values may be obtained.

The effect of meconium is similar. If there is a value greater than 50 mg/dl, a false positive result may be obtained. At concentrations less than 10 mg/dl, meconium contamination did not affect the rapid surfactant test result.

Temperature of the fluid likewise affected the validity of the results. The optimum temperature was between 20° and 30° C. If increasing temperatures were observed, the bubble stability test should be read more rapidly. It is suggested at 40° C to read after 5 minutes and at 50° C after 1 minute. At lower temperatures, that is, 10° C, the bubbles are more stable and the pattern should thus be read later, that is, after 30 minutes.

COMMENT: Blood or meconium may affect the L/S ratio. It likewise can affect the rapid surfactant test, as described by these investigators.

For small hospitals without 24-hour laboratories, the rapid surfactant test is a good one if properly done and should be more frequently utilized. The relatively low false positive rate with the test in general, if it is done correctly, is extremely encouraging, the major problem

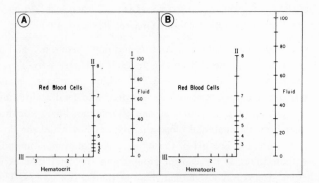

FIG. 11-6

Nomograms for estimating the hematocrit value of amniotic fluids contaminated with blood. **A,** Nomogram for 13 mm (11 mm inside diameter) culture tubes. **B,** Nomogram for 16 mm (14 mm inside diameter) culture tubes. *I,* Height of fluid in test tube; *II,* height of packed blood cells in millimeters; and *III,* hematocrit. (From Keinston, R. C., Noland, G. L., and Pernoll, M. L.: The effect of blood, meconium, and temperature on the rapid surfactant test, Obstet. Gynecol. 48:442-446, 1976.)

with this test being the relatively high false negative rate. The other problem with the test, of course, is that it must be done meticulously in terms of having absolutely clean test tubes and assurance that absolute alcohol is being used. Both these problems can be overcome with proper precautions.

■ Gabbe, S. G., Ettinger, B. B., Freeman, R. K., and Martin, C. B.: Umbilical cord compression associated with amniotomy: laboratory observations, Am. J. Obstet. Gynecol. 126:353-355, 1976.

The authors used the fetal monkey model: catheters and electrodes are attached to the fetus and then the fetus and mother are allowed to recover. Recordings have been made over several days. They demonstrated that removing roughly half the amniotic fluid is almost always associated with a variable deceleration type of change in the fetal heart rate. Infusion of normal saline, restoring the amniotic fluid volume, will decrease the frequency of these decelerations.

COMMENT: Severe variable decelerations may occur with oligohydramnios, and they are particularly prone to occur in severe postdatism. Removing fluid, as these investigators have demonstrated, may accentuate this cord compression. We frequently do try to tap away some small portion of the fluid, but perhaps fortunately for the fetus, it was almost impossible to get fluid in many of these oligohydramnic pregnancies; however, with amniocentesis directed by ultrasound, it may be possible to remove fluid. Serious consideration in these instances should be given to the authors' suggestion that perhaps normal saline be placed in the amniotic space to restore that amount of fluid which has been withdrawn in instances of oligohydramnios.

■ Raabe, N., and Belfrage, P.: Epidural analgesia in labour. IV. Influence on uterine activity and fetal heart rate, Acta Obstet. Gynecol. Scand. 55:305-310, 1976.

The authors recorded continuous uterine activity with an intrauterine catheter and continuous fetal heart rate on twenty-five healthy, nulliparous women, who were in established labor at term. Analgesia was started at between 4 and 5 cm. cervical dilatation, was given as a lumbar epidural block with bupivacaine, 0.25%, and epinephrine, 1:200,000. After an initial test dose of 2 ml, 8 ml were given as a final dose. The patients demonstrated a significant decrease in uterine activity during the first 30 minutes after the epidural blockade. The decrease in activity was fundamentally in the intensity of uterine contractions and appeared to be greater in those patients who had lower preblockade uterine activity. The decrease was 27% when the uterine activity was greater than 100 Montevideo units and 35% when activity was less than 100 Montevideo units. There were no significant changes in fetal heart rate.

COMMENT: These investigators have demonstrated what seemed to be clinically apparent, that is, some decrease in uterine activity following epidural analgesia. With this slight decrease in activity and some decrease in the patient's ability to push during the second stage, labor may be slightly prolonged. However, this is more than compensated for by relieving the discomfort, which may cut down on epinephrine secretion by the patient, increasing the speed of labor.

The fact that there was no change in heart rate recording simply reflects a very careful anesthesia team. If the anesthesia is too vigorous, there may be hypotension, which can lead to late decelerations. Since this is the case, it is particularly important not to use this type of anesthesia when one does not wish to alter the blood pressure, as in hypertensive vascular disease in pregnancy, that is, toxemia.

■ Tejani, N., Mann, L. I., and Bhakthavathsalan, A.: Correlation of fetal heart rate patterns and fetal pH with neonatal outcome, Obstet. Gynecol. 48:460-463, 1976.

The authors have examined the records of 200 consecutively monitored labors, looking at the second hour prior to delivery. They have codified heart rate pattern according to the criteria of Hon and looked at fetal scalp samples. These have been correlated with neonatal outcome in terms of 1-minute Apgar score and cord pH values. They found when the cord umbilical vein pH was greater than 7.25, 73% of the cases had an Apgar score between 7 and 10. When the Apgar score was between 4 and 6, the pH of the umbilical vein was less than 7.25 in 68% of cases. When the Apgar score was between 1 and 3, the pH of the umbilical vein and artery was less than 7.2 in 70% of the cases. If there were no periodic changes in the heart rate, the mean Apgar score at 1 minute was 8.2, and 92% of the infants had an Apgar score between 7 and 10. If there were accelerations or early decelerations, there was no change. In the presence of variable decelerations, the mean Apgar score was 7.9, and the Apgar score of 1 minute was ≤ 6 in 22% of cases. If there were late decelerations, the mean Apgar score at 1 minute was 6.8. Thirty-seven percent of cases had an Apgar score of less than 6 at 1 minute.

COMMENT: This is yet another article that indicates there is some correlation between fetal pH and fetal Apgar score. Since the immediate pH in the cord blood, and scalp pH and the Apgar score may or may not have correlation with subsequent neurologic development, the importance of long-term follow-up to determine the importance of such testing procedures is stressed. It would be a great tragedy to label an infant as potentially retarded due to low Apgar scores or low pH measurements, since simply the label can have significant consequences as to how that child is treated in the home and in the school. We may create a retarded child by the label, rather than by brain damage per se.

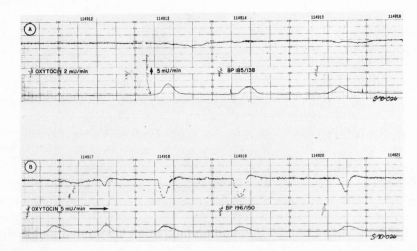

FIG. 11-7
OCT tracing for case 1 obtained with use of phonocardiographic signal and external tocograph (sequential strips). (From Freeman, R. K., and James, J.: Clinical experience with the oxytocin challenge test. II. An ominous atypical pattern, Obstet. Gynecol. **46:**255-259, 1975.)

■ Freeman, R. K., and James, J.: Clinical experience with the oxytocin challenge test. II. An ominous atypical pattern, Obstet. Gynecol. **46:**255-259, 1975.

Three cases are reported. The patients were pregnant with chronic hypertension, severe intrauterine growth retardation, and chronically low 24-hour urinary estriol excretion. The oxytocin challenge test pattern demonstrated repeated variable deceleration with the contractions and concomitant loss of baseline irregularity. The pattern was seen only three times in over 1500 oxytocin challenge tests and was associated with three stillbirths. (See Fig. 11-7.)

COMMENT: This pattern pointed out by Freeman and James is seldom seen; however, when it is seen in conjunction with oligohydramnios, it does indeed indicate a severe problem that should not be overlooked. Simply the fact that it is a variable deceleration type of pattern—and we usually associate variable decelerations with mild-to-moderate fetal asphyxia at most—should not lead the observer to the assumption that the pattern is less than ominous. It should be regarded as most ominous, certainly more so than the majority of the late decelerations seen with the contraction stress test, and should make the physician seriously consider delivery by cesarean section.

■ Saldana, L. R., Schulman, H., and Lin, C.-C.: Routine amnioscopy at term, Obstet. Gynecol. **47:**521-524, 1976.

These researchers studied 508 patients registered in a prenatal clinic, doing amnioscopy at 37 weeks of gestation and then weekly until the onset of labor. The patients were divided into four groups: group I, no meconium-stained amniotic fluid before or during labor; group II, no antepartum meconium staining by amnioscopy but meconium detected during labor; group III, antepartum meconium but clear fluid during labor; and group IV, meconium-stained amniotic fluid before and during labor. The results indicated that the majority of the patients (82.3%) fell into group I. There were two patients in this group who had a perinatal mortality. One patient had felt no movement for a week prior to amnioscopy and the second baby developed a fulminating meningitis at 5 days of age. In group II there were two antepartum deaths not forecast by amniscopy. One of these patients had clear amniotic fluid a few hours prior to fetal death. In group IV there were no perinatal losses.

COMMENT: This article, as did the article of Miller et al. (Transfer of lidocaine across the sheep placenta to the fetus, Am. J. Obstet. Gynecol. 122:573-580, 1975), questions the value of meconium staining of the amniotic fluid as an indicator of fetal distress. When we had few other clinical measures to guide us, meconium staining could be used, but it is apparent that meconium staining is a relatively poor indicator and certainly should not take the place of more sophisticated monitoring techniques such as fetal heart rate monitoring.

Although meconium staining may be a poor indicator of fetal distress, it may be extremely important at delivery to the subsequent newborn course (Chapter 12).

■ Haverkamp, A. D., Thompson, H. E., McFee, J. G., and Cetrulo, C.: The evaluation of continuous fetal heart rate monitoring in high-risk pregnancy, Am. J. Obstet. Gynecol. **125**:310-320, 1976.

The authors studied 483 patients who were classified as high-risk pregnancies. Randomly 242 patients were assigned to a monitored group and 241 patients to an auscultated group. Monitored patients were monitored directly with scalp electrode and intrauterine catheter. Auscultated patients also had a scalp electrode and an intrauterine catheter. The bedside unit was cut off and they were monitored on a remote monitor in the hall. The auscultated patients also had a nurse at the bedside who listened for the fetal heart rate 20 seconds after contractions every 30 minutes during the first stage of labor and every 5 minutes during the second stage of labor. There were thirty-nine monitored and thirty auscultated patients who had late decelerations or severe variable decelerations at some time during labor. Cesarean section rate for fetal distress in the monitored group was significantly higher than that of the auscultated group. Postpartum infection rate was significantly higher in the monitored group than for the auscultated group, even correcting for the higher cesarean section rate. There were no differences in arterial and venous cord blood pH, P_{CO_2} and P_{O_2} in the two groups. Five-minute Apgar scores were similar in the two groups.

■ Renou, P., Chang, A., Anderson, I., and Wood, C.: Controlled trial of fetal intensive care, Am. J. Obstet. Gynecol. **126**:470-476, 1976.

The authors studied 350 high-risk patients admitted to a high-risk unit. The patients were randomly allocated to an intensive care or control group. In the intensive care group there were continuous fetal heart rate monitoring and fetal scalp sampling for blood pH when necessary. The control patients were managed by the nursing and medical staff without the aid of fetal heart rate monitoring or scalp sampling. The babies were examined at the time of discharge from the hospital. Those found to be normal did not have further examinations. Any with abnormalities were seen for at least 3 months. The incidence of primary cesarean section was the same in both groups. The Apgar scores were the same in the two groups. There was a higher incidence of neurologic abnormalities in the control group, thirteen compared to two in the intensive care group. Four babies in the control group were diagnosed as having brain damage. The cord blood pH, P_{O_2}, and P_{CO_2} were significantly better in the intensive care group than in the control group.

COMMENT: These two articles present somewhat divergent results in that Haverkamp et al. point out the higher incidence of cesarean section in the monitored group compared to

the control and the similarity of the Apgar scores. Also the two groups of Renou et al. did have similar Apgar scores, but their primary cesarean section rate was identical. Perhaps this can be explained best by the use of fetal scalp pH recording where necessary. The decisions of Haverkamp et al. for cesarean section were based on fetal heart rate patterns alone, whereas those of Renou et al. were based on fetal scalp pH. The controls in the former were also more closely clinically monitored than is usually done. It is apparent from both studies that one must use all modalities of fetal monitoring, including the patient's, history, fetal heart rate patterns, and fetal scalp pH, if a correct diagnosis is to be achieved and proper therapy pursued. The long-term follow-up in the study by Renou et al. is crucial and brings out a potentially important difference in his two groups, that is, brain damaged children. However, the numbers in this study are small (four children) and may or may not be significant. The study to demonstrate a significant difference would be difficult to undertake in this country, requiring large numbers of babies and long-term follow-up. Many instances of apparent brain damage diagnosed at 1 year of age disappear by age 7 in the proper environment.

■ Duenhoelter, J. H., and Pritchard, J. A.: Fetal respiration: quantitative measurements of amnionic fluid inspired near term by human and rhesus fetuses, Am. J. Obstet. Gynecol. **125:**306-309, 1976.

The authors injected ^{51}Cr-labeled maternal red cells into the amniotic sac of three fetuses with severe congenital anomalies incompatible with life. The cells were injected for 24 to $24\frac{1}{2}$ hours prior to delivery. When the live born fetuses had died and autopsy was done, the lungs were examined for chromium-labeled red cells. Using this technique, it was calculated that the fetus inhaled 370 to 510 ml of amniotic fluid. Similar studies were done in pregnant rhesus monkeys utilizing the injection of chromium-labeled red cells approximately 24 hours prior to delivery and red blood cells labeled with radioactive iron immediately prior to delivery. The fetal monkey also demonstrated inhalation of the chromium-labeled red cells in significantly larger amounts than that of the iron labeled cells, indicating that normal respiration went on prior to delivery and that the trapping of the chromium-labeled cells in the lungs was not just a phenomenon of the stress of delivery. In one monkey, microspheres labeled with radiostrontium were also injected, and these too appeared in the lungs in equal proportion, although not in as great numbers, to the chromium-labeled red cells. The studies did demonstrate that the minimum amount of amniotic fluid inspired is approximately 189 ml/kg/24 hr in the human and 224 ml/kg/24 hr in the rhesus monkey.

■ Patrick, J. E., Dalton, K. J., and Dawes, G. S.: Breathing patterns before death in fetal lambs, Am. J. Obstet. Gynecol. **125:** 73-78, 1976.

These observations were made on sixteen fetal lambs who died before the onset of labor. Continuous records were kept of carotid arterial pressure, tracheal pressure, amniotic pressure, and heart rate. In contrast to the normal lamb, in which, during the last third of gestation, episodes of rapid irregular breathing movements are present about 40% of the time, in six of these lambs fetal breathing was continuous, in eight apnea was present with gasping respirations, and in two lambs brief episodes of breathing were associated with gasping. In all situations there was a prolonged period of apnea before the onset of continuous respiration or the onset of gasping.

■ Piercy, W. N., Day, M. A., Neims, A. H., and Williams, R. L.: Alteration of ovine fetal respiratory-like activity by diazepam, caffeine, and doxapram, Am. J. Obstet. Gynecol. **127:**43-49, 1977.

These investigators used a chronic sheep preparation and ewes that were 90 to 130 days' pregnant. The fetus had been previously instrumented with carotid arterial and tracheal catheters as well as a catheter in the amniotic cavity. Maternal infusions of diazepam, 0.18 to 0.22 mg/kg, were followed by quiescent periods in all fetuses. The average time lag between the drug injection and the cessation of respiratory activity was 4.4 minutes. The average duration of cessation of respiratory activity was 57 minutes. With fetal intravenous injections of diazepam, 1 to 5 mg/kg, there was an abrupt cessation of fetal respiratory activity. Intravenous caffeine stimulated fetal activity in 37% of cases; when given by intercarotid infusion, 90% of cases responded with increase in fetal respiratory activity. Doxapram was an effective stimulant of respiratory activity in the sheep fetus.

■ Manning, F. A., and Feyerabend, C.: Cigarette smoking and fetal breathing movements, Br. J. Obstet. Gynaecol. **83:**262-270, 1976.

These authors used an A scan ultrasound method to record continuous fetal wall chest movements in sixty-four women in the third trimester of pregnancy. All these women were chronic smokers. A portion of these women, sixteen in number, had normal pregnancies. Eight had preeclampsia, ten had diabetes, and five delivered small-for-date infants. Fetal breathing movements were present 69.7% of the time prior to smoking. There was a significant reduction in the proportion of time during which fetal breathing movements were present within 5 minutes after the start of smoking. The maximum reduction was reached at 30 minutes, the fetus breathing approximately 50% of the time. Recovery was not complete until 90 minutes after smoking. In the preeclamptic patients fetal breathing prior to smoking was present 77.2% of the time. There was no significant reduction in the fetal breathing after smoking. In the diabetic prior to smoking the fetal breathing was present 74.8% of the time; following smoking there was a significant reduction in fetal breathing. In the small-for-dates infant initial fetal breathing movements were present 56% of the time. There was progressive fall after smoking, reaching a maximum at 15 minutes when fetal breathing was only presented 24% of the time.

The investigators then attempted to determine whether the reduction in fetal breathing movements was due to the carboxyhemoglobin present when a patient smoked or to the nicotine. They used herbal cigarettes and found that the carboxyhemoglobin was roughly the same as with regular cigarette smoking. In these patients there was no reduction in fetal breathing. However, in the patients who chewed gum containing 8 mg of nicotine, which would elevate the blood level to approximately that of the smoking mother, there was a significant reduction in fetal breathing movements.

COMMENT: Since the studies of Dawes (Respiratory movements and paradoxical sleep in foetal lamb, J. Physiol. 210:47P, 1970) intrauterine fetal thoracic motion has been a reasonably well-established phenomenon. As was pointed out by Dawes in 1970 and is further reinforced in this article by Patrick et al., severe acidosis does alter the fetal thoracic movement pattern. Unfortunately there are a series of other situations that alter the patterns demonstrated by Manning and Feyerabend and by Piercy et al. The type of thoracic movement, percentage of time it is present, and its presence or absence may all prove to be valuable in the assessment of the antepartum fetus. However, significantly more basic information is necessary, such as what is the pattern in the normal human fetus, what are its variants, and what other drugs or activity will alter its pattern. Only then can we have a better idea of indications of hypoxia. In all probability, the procedure for obtaining more basic information will resemble the fetal activity test and the contraction stress test in that the incidence of false negatives will be relatively low and the incidence of false positives will be relatively high.

■ Aubry, R. H., Rourke, J. E., Almanza, R., Cantor, R. M., and Van Doren, J. E.: The lecithin/sphingomyelin ratio in a high-risk obstetric population, Obstet. Gynecol. **47**:21-27, 1976.

The authors analyzed 501 amniotic fluid samples from 308 high-risk obstetrics patients for the L/S ratio. The gestational ages of the patients were documented by menstrual dates, appearance of fetal heart rate sonography, and neonatal maturity assessment. L/S ratios were obtained by using the Borer-Gluck method. They found that the L/S ratio near term was lower than expected in the presence of class A diabetes; however, when chronic hypertension was present, the values were greater than 2 by 37 weeks' gestation. They also found a delay in rise of the L/S ratio in the insulin requiring–diabetic, class B through F, unless there was a superimposition of hypertension; then the values were normal by 37 weeks. In the chronic hypertensives, there was a trend towards an early rise in the L/S ratio. None of their infants with an L/S ratio over 2 developed severe respiratory distress syndrome, and 5.6% developed a mild form of it. It was also noted that one third of the neonates, who had a L/S ratio of less than 1 within 10 days of delivery, did not develop any respiratory problems.

COMMENT: These investigators bring to our attention again the fact that the L/S ratio may be somewhat retarded in the diabetic patient unless hypertension is superimposed, in which case the values will apparently be normal. In the chronic hypertensive, they report that there is a trend toward an early rise in the L/S ratio. The results in this situation are not uniform. The Los Angeles County/University of Southern California Medical Center statistics show there is apparently no significant retardation of the L/S ratio in the diabetes, nor was there a significant acceleration demonstrated in our hypertensives, although it is clinically apparent that in the hypertenssive population the incidence of respiratory distress syndrome is significantly lower than we would expect for given gestational ages. It is difficult to explain the discrepancy in the various series in this regard; however, it does point out the fact that investigators should look at their own population statistics carefully and determine normal values for their population and their laboratory.

Another area of change in pulmonary maturity recently discussed has been the association of increased pulmonary maturity and rupture of the membranes. Gluck and Kulovich (Lecithin/sphingomyelin ratios in amniotic fluid in normal and abnormal pregnancy, Am. J. Obstet. Gynecol. **115**:539-546, 1973) believes that when the membranes have been ruptured longer than 24 hours, the pulmonary maturity is accelerated. Jones et al. (Failure of association of premature rupture of membranes with respiratory-distress syndrome, N. Engl. J. Med. **292**:1253-1257, 1975) could not confirm the finding in his study. Obviously, there are profound clinical reasons for wanting to know the correct answer, that is, the risk of fetal infection from remaining in the uterus versus the risk of respiratory distress syndrome in the newborn from a too hasty delivery.

CHAPTER 12

Neonatal physiology

Oxygen toxicity

■ Crapo, J. D., and McCord, J. M.: Oxygen-induced changes in pulmonary superoxide dismutase assayed by antibody titrations, Am. J. Physiol. **231**:1196-1203, 1976.

Rats exposed to 100% oxygen generally die between 60 and 72 hours of exposure. However, when the rats are first exposed to sublethal doses of oxygen for 5 to 7 days, they acquire tolerance to 100% oxygen. In this study, pulmonary superoxide dismutase (SOD) in control rats and rats adapted to high oxygen was measured by means of an antibody titration technique. The antibodies were prepared using rat liver cuprozinc SOD. In rats exposed to 85% oxygen for 5 days, cuprozinc SOD was 41% higher than in the controls. The results also suggest the presence of a manganese SOD in the lungs, but its role in oxygen tolerance has not been established.

■ Northway, W. H., Rezeau, L., Petriceks, R., and Bensch, K. G.: Oxygen toxicity in the newborn lung: reversal of inhibition of DNA synthesis in the mouse, Pediatrics **57**:41-46, 1976.

Continuous exposure to 100% oxygen at atmospheric pressure at sea level for 2 weeks causes significant alterations in the growth of the lung and the body of newborn mice. These changes can be divided into three phases. In the first 96 hours of exposure to 100% oxygen there is inhibition of lung DNA synthesis, diminished total lung DNA, and a decrease in the lung DNA/body weight ratio (phase 1). The intermediate phase from 96 to 144 hours is characterized by a sharp increase in mortality and, in the surviving mice, a plateau in body weight and a minimal lung DNA/body weight ratio. In this period the inhibition of DNA synthesis in the lungs begins to subside. The third phase occurs after 144 hours and is characterized by a continued increase in DNA synthesis and total lung DNA, a gain in body weight, and a sharp decline in mortality. Of the newborn mice (total number, 496), 54% survived exposure to 100% oxygen for 2 weeks. This survival contrasts with a mortality rate of almost 100% in adult animals similarly exposed. Perhaps some newborn animals are inherently resistant to oxygen toxicity or are capable of developing an adaptive process.

■ Autor, A. P., Frank, L., and Roberts, R. J.: Developmental characteristics of pulmonary superoxide dismutase: relationship to idiopathic respiratory distress syndrome, Pediatr. Res. **10**:154-158, 1976.

Pulmonary SOD activity was determined in human fetuses, infants, and adults. Enzyme activity was found to increase with age from 17 U/mg of DNA in fetal lungs to 49 U/mg of DNA in adult lungs ($p < .05$). No difference in lung SOD activity was demonstrated between normal infants and those with idiopathic respiratory distress syndrome. SOD activity in lung tissue from both rats and rabbits was found to increase with age from a low value in the fetus to a maximum activity in adults ($p < .05$). Exposure of rabbits prematurely delivered by cesarean section to 80% oxygen for 24 hours resulted in a 42% increase in lung SOD activity. Similar results were obtained in 7-day-old rats, but no increase was observed when adult rats were exposed to 85% oxygen for 24 hours. Rat lung incubated in vitro and exposed to 100% oxygen showed a 30% increase in SOD activity after 2 hours. The capacity to increase SOD in response to hyperoxia was age dependent. The effect was maximal in lungs from 10- to 12-day-old rats and disappeared by 19 or 20 days of age.

COMMENT: It is generally recognized that the lungs can be damaged by prolonged exposure to high oxygen tensions. A current theory of oxygen toxicity postulates that the damage is due to production within lung tissues of the free radical O_2^-, which is known as superoxide. The production rate of superoxide radicals increases as the oxygen pressure increases. The presumption is that normal oxygen tensions are not toxic because tissues have an enzyme, SOD, that converts the superoxide free radical to hydrogen peroxide and water. In some bacteria, exposure to high oxygen tensions leads to increased tolerance and increased production of SOD.

A similar ability to increase SOD activity in response to high oxygen tensions is present in mammalian lungs (Crapo and Tierney: Superoxide dismutase and pulmonary oxygen toxicity, Am. J. Physiol. 226:1401-1407, 1974). The article by Crapo and Tierney shows that this increase of SOD activity is due, in fact, to an increase in the quantity of enzyme present in the tissues.

In the lungs of the newborn, oxygen toxicity can be manifested by a decrease in pulmonary growth, as shown in the report of Northway et al. Their report describes an unexpected result: that a fairly large proportion of newborn mice can survive prolonged exposure to 100% oxygen. The result is more surprising in view of the finding by Autor et al. that pulmonary SOD activity is relatively low in fetal and neonatal humans, rats, and rabbits. On the other hand, increased SOD activity appears to be more easily induced in the young animal.

Clearly, much more remains to be learned about the effects of high oxygen on the developing lungs, how tolerance could be induced without damage, whether there are substantial differences among individuals of the same species in the ability to develop tolerance, and whether the clear relationship between oxygen tolerance and SOD activity, which has been demonstrated in bacteria, can be demonstrated for the lungs of newborn mammals.

Calcium metabolism in the neonatal period

■ Garel, J., and Barlet, J.: Calcium metabolism in newborn animals: the interrelationship of calcium, magnesium, and inorganic phosphorus in newborn rats, foals, lambs, and calves, Pediatr. Res. 10:749-754, 1976.

This study presents data on the changes in calcium, inorganic phosphorus, magnesium concentration, and calcitonin and parathyroid hormone in the plasma of newborn animals from four different species; rats, horses, sheep, and cattle. The study demonstrates that magnesium concentration does not change significantly in the neonatal period. The changes in calcium concentration varied, depending on the species. Calcium concentration during the newborn period fell in rats and foals. There were no significant changes in calcium concentration in lambs and calves. In all species, inorganic phosphorus concentration increased after birth. The changes in both calcitonin and parathyroid hormone were more variable among the four species.

■ Stimmler, L., Snodgrass, G. J. A. I., Gupta, Y., Stothers, J. K., and Brown, D.: Relation between changes in plasma calcium in first week of life and renal function, Arch. Dis. Child. 50:786-790, 1975.

This study presents data on plasma calcium and creatinine concentrations and plasma osmolality in infants fed cow's milk or human breast milk. The excretion of calcium/creatinine in urinary solutes was measured over a 24-hour period. Those infants fed a cow's milk formula who experienced a fall in plasma calcium concentration during the first week of postnatal life were also infants who had significantly higher plasma creatinine concentrations and serum osmolalities and significantly lower creatinine excretion and urinary solute excretion.

■ Kooh, S. W., Fraser, D., Toon, R., and DeLuca, H. F.: Response of protracted neonatal hypocalcaemia to 1-α,25-dihydroxyvitamin D₃, Lancet 2:1105-1107, 1976.

This study reports the use of either intravenous or oral 1-α,25-dihydroxyvitamin D, the probable hormonal form of vitamin D, in six newborn infants with protracted hypocalcemia. It should be emphasized that these were newborn infants with a particularly protracted hypocalcemia. The dose varied from 0.2 to 0.05 μg/kg/24 hr. The response seemed equally well-defined and of equally rapid onset with oral as with intravenous administration. The data establish that in these six newborn infants, protracted hypocalcemia could be corrected rapidly and with no apparent complications by the administration of the hormonal form of vitamin D.

COMMENT: The report by Garel and Barlet is largely descriptive and presents information regarding some aspects of interspecies differences in calcium metabolism. Studies on the comparative physiology and biochemistry of neonatal development are relatively rare. Such studies ultimately should help us understand the factors responsible for the postnatal changes in calcium concentration that occur in man.

The report of Stimmler et al. demonstrates that one additional factor which contributes to the fall in plasma concentration in infants fed cow's milk formulas is the difference in neonatal renal function and, specifically, in glomerular filtration rate. Glomerular filtration rate increases rapidly in early postnatal life. Those infants in whom the changes in glomerular filtration rate is less rapid might be more prone to neonatal hypocalcemia, secondary to a dietary intake of a cow's milk formula presenting a high phosphate load for renal excretion.

The report by Kooh et al. extends studies on the hormone 1-α,25-dihydroxyvitamin D and begins to consider its therapeutic usage in newborn infants with hypocalcemia. The use of this hormone in newborn infants with hypocalcemia would avoid the necessity for large supplements of calcium and the restriction of dietary phosphate. It should also provide additional information regarding the role of vitamin D together with parathyroid function in regulating the postnatal fall in calcium concentration during the neonatal period.

Follow-up studies of low birth weight infants

■ Davies, P. A., and Tizard. J. P. M.: Very low birthweight and subsequent neurological defect, Dev. Med. Child Neurol. 17:3-17, 1975.

This report presents a review of the literature regarding incidence, severity, and type of defects in children of very low birth weight. It also presents new data on low birth weight infants in relation to the incidence of spastic diplegia. The outcome of 165 infants born between 1961 and 1970 weighing less than 1500 gm at birth was reviewed. All infants were cared for at the Hammersmith Hospital in London. Fifty-eight were born between 1961 and 1964, and 107 between 1965 and 1970. There was a highly significant decrease in the incidence of cerebral palsy in the 1965-1970 group. Other differences between these two groups of infants are presented in Table 12-1 taken from their report.

TABLE 12-1

Significant differences between surviving babies of < 1500 gm in 1960–1964 compared with 1965–1970*

	1961-1964	*1965-1970*	χ^2	T	p
Total	58	107			
Born outside Hammersmith Hospital	15	54	8.37		0.004
Birth asphyxia (intubated)	11	36	4.23		0.04
Fits	9	3	7.23		0.007
Symptomatic hypoglycaemia	4	0	4.93		0.03
Mild recurrent apnoea	25	20	10.10		0.001
Mean maximum bilirubin (mg)	15.0 (±4.4)	11.7 (±4.3)		3.98	<0.001
Mean lowest rectal temperature (° C)	33.2 (±1.3)	34.7 (±1.2)		7.30	<0.001

*From Davies, P. A., and Tizard, J. P. M.: Very low birthweight and subsequent neurological defect, Dev. Med. Child Neurol. **17**:3-17, 1975.

TABLE 12-2

Findings at follow-up in neonatal hypoglycemia*

Category of neonatal hypoglycemia	*Number of cases*	*Normal findings*	*Severe mental retardation*	*Minor developmental defects*	*Cerebral palsy*	*Abnormal EEG findings*	*Squint*	*Later convulsions*	*Hypoglycemic episodes*
Asymptomatic	7	5	—	1	—	2	—	—	—
Symptomatic, transient									
Convulsion group	6	1	1	1	2	4	2	3	2
Non-convulsion group	3	—	—	1	2	1	1	1	—
Secondary									
Convulsion group	4	1	—	—	1	1	—	—	—
Non-convulsion group	17	9	—	4	—	2	3	—	—

*From Fluge, G.: Neurological findings at follow-up in neonatal hypoglycaemia, Acta Paediatr. Scand. **64**:629-634, 1975.

■ Fluge, G.: Neurological findings at follow-up in neonatal hypoglycaemia, Acta Paediatr. Scand. **64**:629-634, 1975.

This article reports follow-up data in children between the ages of 2 years 6 months and 4 years 9 months. Of sixty-seven newborn infants identified with hypoglycemia during the 3-year period from 1967 to 1969, thirty-seven patients were maintained in a follow-up study. Table 12-2 presents the follow-up data on the thirty-seven infants subdivided into those who had hypoglycemia recognized by glucose determinations without symptoms, those who had symptomatic hypoglycemia, and those in whom hypoglycemia occurred along with other neonatal complications such as asphyxia and respiratory distress. A worse clinical course was found in the groups with symptomatic hypoglycemia. Four of the

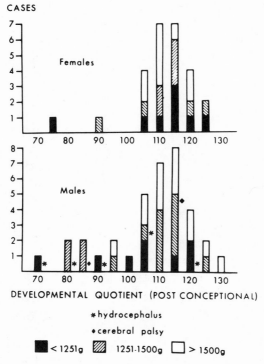

CASES

DEVELOPMENTAL QUOTIENT (POST CONCEPTIONAL)

＊hydrocephalus

◆cerebral palsy

■ < 1251g ▨ 1251-1500g □ > 1500g

FIG. 12-1
The DQ using the postconceptional age is depicted for the girls and boys of the three weight groups. Asterisks, scores of children with major neurologic defects. (From Fitzhardinge, P. M.: Early growth and development in low-birthweight infants following treatment in an intensive care nursery, Pediatrics **56**:162-172, 1975.)

nine patients with symptomatic transient hypoglycemia continued to have seizures after the neonatal period. Other neurologic problems were recognized in eight out of the nine patients.

■ Fitzhardinge, P. M.: Early growth and development in low-birthweight infants following treatment in an intensive care nursery, Pediatrics **56**:162-172, 1975.

This study presents follow-up data over a 12-month period for infants who were preterm AGA infants of less than 32 weeks' gestation. All the infants were born between October 1, 1970, and September 1, 1972. All the infants were delivered at other obstetric services and referred for care after birth to the neonatal intensive care unit at the Montreal Children's Hospital. During the follow-up a variety of anthropomorphic measurements and neurologic evaluations, as well as a measurement of developmental quotient, were made on the children. The measurements of linear growth, height indices, and head circumference were similar for the preterm AGA infants at 12 months of age and for a control group of twenty-four full-term infants. The only differences in body proportions were found among female infants who had a slower weight gain during the 12-month follow-up period. However, a high incidence (22.5%) of gross central nervous system defects was found among the male infants. Over 50% of these abnormalities were due to hydrocephalus. The distribution of the developmental quotients for male and female infants is shown in Fig. 12-1 taken from the report.

■ Goldstein, G. W., Chaplin, E. R., and Maitland, J.: Transient hydrocephalus in premature infants: treatment by lumbar punctures, Lancet 1:512-514, 1976.

This report consists of the description of the clinical course in three premature babies treated for posthemorrhagic hydrocephalus by removing large volumes of cerebrospinal fluid with repeated lumbar punctures. The diagnosis of hydrocephalus was made with computer-assisted tomography (CAT-scan). The hydrocephalus was considered a posthemorrhagic complication of intracranial hemorrhage in premature infants on the basis of both the clinical history and the character of the spinal fluid removed. Two of the infants were treated with two lumbar punctures and a third required eleven lumbar punctures over 17 days. In each lumbar puncture, from 5 to 15 ml of cerebrospinal fluid was removed. At the end of the procedures in all three infants, head growth was normal and normal ventricular size was confirmed by CAT-scan. The authors suggest the posthemorrhagic hydrocephalus may be a frequent complication following intracranial hemorrhage in preterm babies. The diagnosis may be made with assurance far more frequently, since CAT-scans are used more widely in intensive care nurseries. This report suggests that infants may be helped through a relatively short time period in the management of hydrocephalus by lumbar puncture rather than resorting directly to ventricular shunts.

COMMENT: These reports describe a few of the extensive efforts being made in many countries to document whether the increasing survival rate of low birth weight infants is associated with a higher percentage of infants showing significant neurologic damage in later childhood. The issue itself is extremely important because this information is necessary for physicians working in intensive care nurseries to make proper and informed decisions conjointly with the parents regarding appropriate limits to the support offered very low birth weight infants. It is also important in providing us with some insight into which aspects of the total package of supportive care have been most effective in eliminating certain specific neurologic handicaps.

The report by Davies and Tizard documents an important observation: that the incidence of one specific neurologic problem, spastic diplegia, has fallen dramatically in the decade of the 1960s. They review some of the factors that may be responsible. Many factors have been suggested as contributing to the elimination of this severe neurologic handicap from nurseries. It seems to us that Davies and Tizard might have commented on the possible relationship of early hydration to the prevention of hypoglycemia and spastic diplegia.

In the earlier studies of the 1950s, which examined changes in serum osmolality or sodium concentration when preterm babies were fasted and thirsted for varying periods of time up to 3 days, it was shown that invariably the infants developed severe hypertonicity and hypernatremia. The first reports of hypoglycemia as a problem of newborn infants appeared in the late 1950s and early 1960s. Those reports gave a strong impetus to a liberal use of intravenous or intra-arterial infusions of 5% or 10% glucose to newborn infants for the prevention of hypoglycemia. The prevention of hypoglycemia also prevented hypertonicity and hypernatremia. The suggestion that hypertonicity may have contributed to the incidence of spastic diplegia is supported by observations of a fall in hematocrit coincident with a decrease in the incidence of spastic diplegia.

The report by Fluge shows that the infants who had symptomatic hypoglycemia continued to have neurologic problems after the neonatal period. It is not surprising that symptomatic infants would have more difficulty subsequently, since the central nervous system signs in the nursery must be a reflection of glucose supply to the brain. In that regard, glucose supply to the brain would reflect the product of cerebral plasma flow × the glucose concentration. In clinical practice we measure the glucose concentration but have no information regarding cerebral blood flow. It is for this reason that most centers have attempted to maintain glucose concentrations considerably above the earlier limits of 20 mg/dl in preterm babies and 30 mg/dl in term infants, recognizing that an arterial glucose concentration of 30 mg/dl may mean an extremely different arterial glucose flow to the brain in two newborn infants varying markedly in cerebral blood flow. For further discussion regarding the importance of glucose to cerebral metabolism, see the Comments in Chapter 1.

Fitzhardinge's careful study regarding the growth and development of low birth weight infants is not at all reassuring. He reported a moderately high incidence of serious neurologic problems in the infants, particularly in the male. An important part of that report was the observation that half the central nervous system abnormalities were accounted for by hydrocephalus.

The report of Goldstein et al. is encouraging in that it provides an attempt to correct transient hydrocephalus by repeated lumbar punctures instead of moving directly to a neurosurgical procedure for the placement of a shunt. This approach may have applicability, especially as computer-assisted tomography becomes increasingly available for the diagnosis of intracranial hemorrhage in preterm infants. Certainly, the early reports reviewing the use of CAT-scans in nursery services have documented the fact that significant intracranial hemorrhage is often overlooked in the nursery. This is particularly important, since it can lead to progressive hydrocephalus, which is easily diagnosed by CAT-scan long before an increase in head circumference or changes in the character of the fontanel. One can only hope that an early approach to therapy in these infants may avoid some of the neurologic handicaps observed in Fitzhardinge's study.

Neonatal glucose homeostasis

■ Lind, T., Gilmore, E. A., and McClarence, M.: Cord plasma glucose and insulin concentrations and maternal-fetal relations, Br. J. Obstet. Gynaecol. 82:562-567, 1975.

The concentrations of glucose and insulin in umbilical cord plasma from 854 pregnancies were compared with those in 503 maternal blood samples. The fetal cord blood insulin concentrations were skewed; that is, there was a mean value of approximately 8 μU/ml plasma in umbilical samples, but twelve infants had insulin concentrations exceeding 30 μU/ml. The mode of delivery had little appreciable effect on plasma insulin level in the fetus. Since fetal glucose concentrations were lower than maternal concentrations, it is clear that neither fetal plasma glucose concentrations nor stress of delivery is an adequate explanation for the high levels of circulating insulin in some fetuses. A significant positive correlation was found between cord plasma insulin levels and the infant's birth weight. This is shown in Table 12-3.

■ Wu, P. K., Modanlou, H., and Karelitz, M.: Effect of glucagon on blood glucose homeostasis in infants of diabetic mothers, Acta Paediatr. Scand. 64:441-445, 1975.

Thirty infants who were born at term of insulin-dependent diabetic mothers were divided into three groups. The first group served as control, the second received 300 μgm of glucagon per kilogram intramuscularly at the time of birth, and the third received the same

TABLE 12-3

Correlations between selected variables for the 490 paired maternal and fetal samples for which all data were available*

Variables		"No fluid"	"Fluid"	Significance of differences between the two groups
Log cord				
insulin	× birthweight	0.268§	0.285§	NS
	× cord glucose	0.119	0.197‡	NS
	× maternal glucose	0.126†	0.022	NS
	× log maternal insulin	0.228§	0.267§	NS
Cord glucose				
	× birthweight	−0.092	−0.021	NS
	× maternal glucose	0.714§	0.421§	1%
	× log maternal insulin	0.322§	0.510§	5%
Log maternal				
insulin	× nonpregnant weight	0.231§	0.123	NS
	× maternal glucose	0.504§	0.318§	5%
Maternal glucose				
	× nonpregnant weight	0.054	−0.042	NS

*From Lind, T., Gilmore, E. A., and McClarence, M.: Cord plasma glucose and insulin concentrations and maternal-fetal relations, Br. J. Obstet. Gynaecol. 82:562-567, 1975.
The significant level of individual correlation is indicated as follows: †, 5%; ‡, 1%; and §, 0.1%.

dose of glucagon intravenously at birth. Fig. 12-2 taken from their report summarizes the results. The third group did not develop significant hypoglycemia and stabilized their blood glucose concentration rapidly. The report did not present data beyond 4 hours after birth, nor did it present their subsequent course relative to total caloric intake; however, one assumes that normal glucose concentrations persisted. This suggests that infants treated with intravenous glucagon at birth may be managed by oral milk intake alone and still avoid the initial hypoglycemia that occurs in most infants of insulin-dependent mothers.

COMMENT: The study of Lind et al. is important in demonstrating that the fetus has a relative hyperinsulinism compared to the mother and that this pertains to women both without and with diabetes. These data support similar data in animals: that at the same plasma glucose concentration, fetal plasma tends to have higher insulin concentrations than maternal plasma. The fetal hyperinsulinism could not be explained by either the plasma glucose concentration or the mode of delivery. Their observation of a positive correlation between plasma insulin levels in the fetus and the infant's birth weight supports the hypothesis that insulin may be acting to regulate fetal growth rate. The report of Wu et al. confirms earlier observations made by Cornblath et al. (Studies of carbohydrate metabolism in the newborn infant. IV. The effect of glucagon on the capillary blood sugar in infants of diabetic mothers, Pediatrics 28:592-601, 1961) many years ago that infants of diabetic mothers will respond by elevating their plasma glucose concentrations when given intravenous glucagon. The study of Wu et al. does not resolve the question that has persisted in perinatology: whether it is safer and more appropriate in babies of insulin-dependent

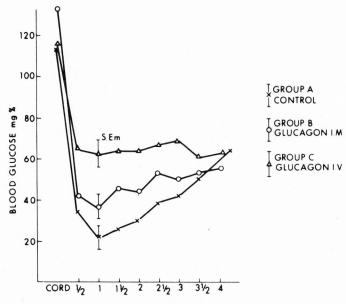

FIG. 12-2
Mean blood glucose levels during the first 4 hours in the three groups of infants. (From Wu, P. K., Modanlou, H., and Karelitz, M.: Effect of glucagon on blood glucose homeostasis in infants of diabetic mothers, Acta Paediatr. Scand. **64:**441-445, 1975.)

mothers and other infants at risk of neonatal hypoglycemia to provide additional glucose by intravenous or intra-arterial infusions or to stimulate an increase in plasma glucose concentration by the administration of either glucocorticoids or glucagon. This question still needs resolution, and the effect of hormones on other organ metabolism, including the lung and the heart, may determine the answer.

Neonatal myotonic dystrophy

- Sarnat, H. B., and Silbert, S. W.: Maturational arrest of fetal muscle in neonatal myotonic dystrophy, Arch. Neurol. **33:**466-474, 1976.

This report presents the findings from muscle biopsies or postmortem examination of muscles in four newborn infants with severe clinical manifestations of myotonic muscular dystrophy. Three of the four infants died and were studied at autopsy. In addition to the muscle groups involved with arthrogrypotic joints, other muscles severely affected included pharyngeal muscle and diaphragm. This explains many of the most critical management problems of the infants presenting in the newborn period, including difficulties with swallowing, handling secretions, and respiration. The findings on muscle biopsy helped explain the prominent differences between the clinical features of myotonic dystrophy in the neonatal period versus the adult form. The findings of the biopsies were consistent with those of muscle tissue that was arrested in development at an early fetal stage. The findings included the presence of fetal myotubes, poorly formed Z bands, simple mitochondria, and the presence of many satellite cells, suggesting an arrest of muscle development rather than presenting any evidence of the kind of muscle fiber degeneration seen in adult muscle from patients with this disease. The authors speculate that this may be due to the fact that the sarcolemma in myotonic dystrophy is abnormal and unresponsive to normal trophic influences of innervation. Thus, during embryonic and fetal development, there was a delay in muscle development unaccompanied by delays in neural development.

■ Sarnat, H. B., O'Connor, T., and Byrne, P. A.: Clinical effects of myotonic dystrophy on pregnancy and the neonate, Arch. Neurol. **33:**459-465, 1976.

This companion article to the previous report describes the clinical signs associated with myotonic dystrophy present in the mother during pregnancy and in the newborn infant at the time of delivery. The report presents a description of the course of the pregnancy and labor in five women with myotonic dystrophy and in four severely affected newborn infants.

COMMENT: The companion articles of Sarnat et al. describe a comparatively rare disease in the newborn infant, neonatal myotonic dystrophy. It is one of the causes of marked hypotonia of the newborn that is present at the time of delivery and thus becomes part of the differential diagnosis of "floppy baby" syndrome. The reports are of particular interest in that approaching the disease from the point of view of fetal development makes the apparent discrepancy in clinical course understandable. Older children and adults with myotonic dystrophy show clinical signs of hypertonia, not hypotonia. These reports make evident the fact that the pathology characteristic of myotonic dystrophy in the adult is not present in the newborn, but rather there is an arrest in a normal maturational sequence of muscle. The arrest in muscle development leads to muscle tone consistent with the earlier stage of development, rather than with the chronologic age of the newborn infant at the time of delivery. Not surprisingly, the hypotonia regresses during postnatal life as muscle maturation continues.

In their clinical review, the authors stress the interesting fact that despite an autosomal pattern of inheritance, the mother rather than the father has been the affected parent in over 90% of instances when the target case was a newborn infant with myotonic dystrophy. Additionally, they point out that myotonic dystrophy is another disease of women that may have as an associated complication polyhydramnios, perhaps due to abnormal swallowing of amniotic fluid during fetal life. As newer techniques are introduced in obstetrics to evaluate fetal swallowing, abnormalities in fetal swallowing may permit a high suspicion of this disease prior to delivery.

Respiratory disease other than hyaline membrane disease in newborn infants

■ Krauss, A. N., Klain, D. B., and Auld, P. A. M.: Carbon monoxide diffusing capacity in newborn infants, Pediatr. Res. **10:**771-776, 1976.

The diffusing capacity of the lung for carbon monoxide was measured in twenty-one infants without respiratory distress. The infants ranged in birth weight from 765 to 4720 gm. Eight infants with hyaline membrane disease (HMD) were also studied. Fig. 12-3 demonstrates a highly significant correlation between diffusing capacity of the lung for carbon monoxide and functional residual capacity in healthy newborn infants. No such relationship was seen in the infants with HMD. In these infants, diffusing capacity varied over a wide range at the same functional residual capacity. When the diffusing capacity for carbon monoxide was compared to arterial P_{O_2} in healthy newborn infants, there was a slight corre-

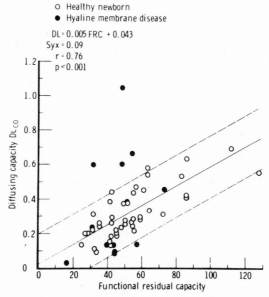

FIG. 12-3

Diffusing capacity for carbon monoxide (DL$_{CO}$) versus functional residual capacity (FRC) in cubic centimeters. DL$_{CO}$ units are cubic centimeters per minute per mm Hg of carbon monoxide. (From Krauss, A. N., Klain, D. B., and Auld, P. A. M.: Carbon monoxide diffusing capacity in newborn infants, Pediatr. Res. **10:**771-776, 1976.)

lation (r = .391, p < .01). Most of the infants with hyaline membrane disease showed normal or increased diffusing capacities for carbon monoxide. In both groups of infants no significant correlation could be found between diffusing capacity of the lung per milliliter functional residual capacity versus arterial oxygen tension. This study supports the two concepts that lung volume is the major determinant of diffusing capacity of the lung and that a diffusion limitation is a minor component in etiology of arterial hypoxemia in the newborn.

■ Krauss, A. N., Klain, D. B., and Auld, P. A. M.: Chronic pulmonary insufficiency of prematurity (CPIP), Pediatrics **55:**55-58, 1975.

This study presents some relatively late respiratory complications occurring in very immature babies. The complications reported developed primarily during the second and third week of postnatal life in premature appropriately grown infants with birth weights less than 1200 gm. The gestational ages were not given, but the infants were described as AGA. They began postnatal life without evidence of respiratory distress and tolerated room air oxygen concentrations well. However, starting between the fourth and seventeenth days, the infants gradually showed a decrease in lung volume. These data are presented in Fig. 12-4 from the original report, which compares the infants having chronic pulmonary insufficiency of prematurity with very low birth weight infants and with larger preterm babies. The striking decrease in functional residual capacity during the second and third weeks of postnatal life in the infants with chronic pulmonary insufficiency of prematurity (CPIP) is clearly demonstrated. There was a fall in arterial oxygen tension and an increase in Pa$_{CO_2}$

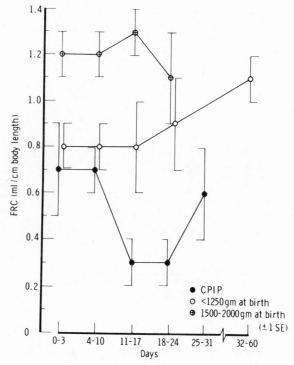

FIG. 12-4

FRC determined by helium dilution versus age in days in infants with CPIP, nondistressed premature infants weighing less than 1250 gm at birth, and nondistressed infants weighing 1500 to 2000 gm at birth. (From Krauss, A. N., Klain, D. B., and Auld, P. A. M.: Chronic pulmonary insufficiency of prematurity [CPIP], Pediatrics **55**:55-58, 1975.)

associated with a decrease in lung volume. The mean Pa_{O_2} fell to approximately 24 mm Hg during the second week of life, and the Pa_{CO_2} rose to 70 mm Hg concurrently. After the third and fourth weeks of life, the infants showed a gradually increasing functional residual capacity and a return of respiratory gas tensions to normal.

■ Ablow, R. C., Driscoll, S. G., Effmann, E. L., Gross, I., Jolles, C. J., Uauy, R., and Warshaw, J. B.: A comparison of early-onset group B streptococcal neonatal infection and the respiratory-distress syndrome of the newborn, N. Engl. J. Med. **294**:65-70, 1976.

This report reviews the signs and symptoms in thirteen newborn infants who were admitted with antemortem blood cultures positive for group B streptococci. Eight of the thirteen infants with positive group B streptococci blood cultures died. The eight fatal cases were compared with nine babies having severe HMD. The authors believed that group B streptococcal pneumonia could be distinguished from HMD as follows: (1) an association with premature rupture of membranes, (2) the early onset of apnea and shock, and (3) better pulmonary compliance. Four of the eight fatal cases of group B streptococcal infection had chest x-ray films that were read as indistinguishable from hyaline membrane disease; however, the radiograph reproduced in the report did not demonstrate a pattern consistent with classic HMD. Additionally, the infants with respiratory distress syndrome were reported

TABLE 12-4

Comparison of the incidence and severity of MAS among three groups
of infants in which meconium staining was managed differently*

	Group I	Group II	Group III
Term births	7585	2320	1681
Meconium staining (percent incidence)	947 (12.5%)	381 (16.4%)	273 (16.2%)
MAS, total cases	18	7	1
Mild	9	4	1
Moderate	3	2	0
Severe	6	1	0
MAS deaths	5†	0	0

*From Carson, B. S., Losey, R. W., Bowes, W. A., and Simmons, M. A.: Combined obstetric
and pediatric approach to prevent meconium aspiration syndrome, Am. J. Obstet. Gynecol.
126:712-715, 1976.
†Twenty-eight percent of MAS cases (0.52% of all with meconium staining).

to require much higher ventilating pressures than have been necessary at the University of
Colorado Medical Center. On pathologic examination of the lungs, group B streptococci
were identified in areas with hyaline membranes, in addition to their presence in abundance
in inflammatory exudate.

■ Carson, B. S., Losey, R. W., Bowes, W. A., and Simmons, M. A.: Combined obstetric and
pediatric approach to prevent meconium aspiration syndrome, Am. J. Obstet. Gynecol.
126:712-715, 1976.

This prospective study presents data on the incidence of severe meconium aspiration
pneumonitis after the introduction of a new obstetric approach to the management of the
delivery of newborn infants whenever meconium-stained amniotic fluid is observed. Essentially the procedure consists of suctioning the nasopharynx thoroughly with a DeLee catheter
before delivery of the thorax with the head still on the perineum. This procedure takes
advantage of the fact that during vaginal delivery the thorax of the infant is markedly
compressed and secretions are pushed into the pharynx. Once delivery of the thorax has
occurred with thoracic recoil, these secretions are sucked into the tracheobronchial tree and
further suctioning of the tracheobronchial tree after delivery is made more difficult. Table
12-4 illustrates the fact that when this obstetric procedure was introduced (group III of
their study), only one case of meconium aspiration syndrome (MAS) of mild degree occurred among 273 pregnancies complicated by meconium-staining of the amniotic fluid.
This represents a striking reduction in the frequency of this complication. The authors
recommend that one continue the pediatric practice of routine suctioning of the trachea
under direct visualization of the vocal cords if meconium is visualized at the level of the
cords. However, they do point out that this procedure is rarely required with the introduction of the previously described obstetric procedure. Pulmonary lavage, which had been
recommended by some centers in the past, was no longer necessary, and severe meconium
aspiration syndrome was effectively prevented on the service. Table 12-5 from their report
presents the protocol from their combined obstetric and pediatric management.

**COMMENT: There are many reasons why newborn infants may show the clinical signs of
tachypnea and oxygen dependency during the newborn period. In many instances the cause**

TABLE 12-5

Protocol for combined obstetric and pediatric management*

1. As soon as the baby's head appears on the perineum, the obstetrician passes a DeLee suction catheter through the nares to the level of the nasopharynx and aspirates any mucus or meconium, then suctions the mouth and hypopharynx.
2. Immediately after delivery the pediatrician suctions the oropharynx with a bulb and, if meconium is present, inspects the cords by direct laryngoscopy while an assistant monitors the heart rate.
3. If meconium is present at the cords, direct suctioning of the trachea with either a DeLee catheter or mouth–endotracheal tube is performed.
4. Usual measures of ventilation and resuscitation are carried out.

*From Carson, B. S., Losey, R. W., Bowes, W. A., and Simmons, M. A.: Combined obstetric and pediatric approach to prevent meconium aspiration syndrome, Am. J. Obstet. Gynecol. 126:712-715, 1976.

may lie outside the lungs and even outside the cardiovascular system and represent problems of metabolism, central nervous system disease, and so forth. Even within the lungs, proper gas exchange requires adequate perfusion of the lungs as well as adequate ventilation. Thus, over the last 5 or 6 years in neonatology, we have seen the description of disease problems such as hyperviscosity syndrome, transient persistence of the fetal circulation, wet lung syndrome, and so forth—problems in which effective gas exchange has been blocked by problems within the circulation. This has become an important clinical distinction, since therapy in the latter conditions must be directed at improving perfusion rather than focused on improvement in ventilation.

The study by Krauss et al. on the carbon monoxide diffusing capacity in newborn infants continues the careful work by this group in documenting conditions in which ventilation is a primary cause of inadequate gas exchange. Their data certainly support the concept that a diffusion limitation to oxygen transport remains a minor component in most conditions producing arterial hypoxemia in the neonatal period. Their second report describes a newly recognized condition in preterm infants. The striking findings are a reduction in functional residual capacity associated with hypercapnia and hypoxemia. This condition occurred late in the neonatal course of preterm babies (second and third weeks of postnatal life) and in this respect differed from hyaline membrane disease. It also differed in that the typical radiographic changes of diffuse atelectasis consistent with the diagnosis of HMD was not found in these infants. It is of considerable interest because it is one of the very few conditions in newborn infants other than HMD associated with striking decrease in functional residual capacity. It would be of considerable interest to know whether these preterm babies gave evidence of marked changes in behavioral states associated with the hypercapnia and hypoxemia.

The report by Ablow et al. points out that group B streptococcal infection in the neonatal period can mimic HMD. It confirms the extremely high mortality rate in infants with group B streptococcal sepsis. It makes evident the fact that it may be extremely hazardous to withhold antibiotic therapy because of a presumptive diagnosis of HMD at a time when a nursery service may be experiencing a marked increase in the frequency of group B streptococcal infections.

The article by Carson et al. describes a new management approach to the prevention of meconium aspiration syndrome and is important for two reasons. First, it describes a relatively simple step that can be taken by obstetricians prior to the delivery of the infant which effectively prevents a disease, meconium aspiration syndrome, that has a high mortality in newborn infants. Second, it lengthens the list of procedures and techniques that obstetricians can use in the course of delivering an infant which will significantly reduce neonatal morbidity and mortality. In that regard, it encourages us to think of re-suscitation as an event beginning with the onset of parturition and involving a total approach by obstetricians and pediatricians to "perinatal resuscitation," rather than continuing to center our thinking around the care and support of the newborn infant after the completion of delivery.

Breast-feeding

■ Teicher, M. H., and Blass, E. M.: Suckling in newborn rats: eliminated by nipple lavage, reinstated by pup saliva, Science **193**:422-425, 1976.

This study demonstrated that attachment of pups to the mother's teats could be eliminated virtually completely by chemical lavage of the nipples. The studies were carried out on 4- or 5-day-old pups of maternal rats. A normal suckling pattern could be reinstated by painting the teats with a vacuum distillate of either the wash from the breasts or a vacuum distillate of pup saliva. Thus one or more substances necessary to release and direct suckling appeared to coat the nipple surface. These substances may have as their origin pup saliva, maternal saliva, or a product produced on the teat itself (Fig. 12-5). This work confirmed the earlier work of Kovach and Kling (Mechanisms of neonate sucking behaviour in the kitten, Anim. Behav. **15**:91-101, 1967) and Tobach et al. (Development of olfactory function in the rat pup [abstr.], Am. Zool. **7**:792-793, 1967) who have demonstrated that they could eliminate suckling in young kittens and rats by making them anosmic. Thus, taken together, the three studies support olfactory clues as essential for attachment and normal suckling.

■ Downham, M. A. P. S., Scott, R., Sims, D. G., Webb, J. K. G., and Gardner, P. S.: Breast-feeding protects against respiratory syncytial virus infections, Br. Med. J. **2**:274-276, 1976.

This study reports the incidence of breast-feeding in two different populations: one consisting of 115 infants admitted to the hospital during the winter of 1973-1974 with respiratory syncytial (RS) virus infection and the other consisting of 157 infants whose mothers were interviewed without selection after appearing at Newcastle City Child Health Clinics (Newcastle upon Tyne, England) during the same time period. There was a significant difference in the percentage of infants who had been breast-fed for at least 1 month among those admitted with respiratory syncytial virus infection and those infants coming to the clinic for other reasons. Only eight out of 115 infants admitted with respiratory syncytial viral infection had been breast-fed, compared with forty-six out of 167 controls. Table 12-6 taken from this report presents the data for the children with RS virus infection versus the controls against the age at which breast-feeding was discontinued. Twenty-one samples of human colostrum were examined and all contained RS virus–neutralizing activity. In eighteen of the twenty-one samples, specific IgA and IgG were detected. The authors postulate that the infants may have inhaled their early milk feedings. In regurgitating them through the nose, they coated the respiratory tract of the nasopharynx with specific IgA, which might then protect against a severe RS virus infection. An alternate hypothesis proposed is that breast-feeding may have protected the infant from an early mild, but sensitizing, infection.

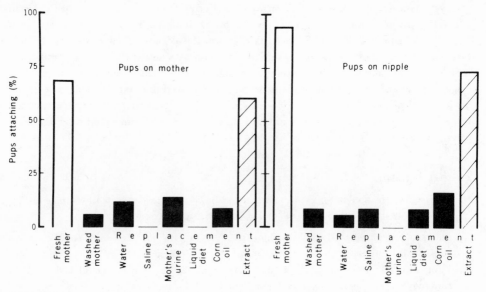

FIG. 12-5

Percentage of pups attaching to the unwashed mother, to washed mother, and to washed mother following replacement with water, isotonic saline, maternal urine, a milk-based liquid diet, corn oil, or nipple wash extract. (From Teicher, M. H., and Blass, E. M.: Suckling in newborn rats: eliminated by nipple lavage, reinstated by pup saliva, Science **193:**422-425, July 30, 1976; copyright 1976 by the American Association for the Advancement of Science.)

TABLE 12-6

Age at which breast-feeding was discontinued*

	Age (mo)				
	< 1	1-2	3	4	> 4
Children admitted with RS virus	5	1		1	1
Controls	24	9	7	4	2

*From Downham, M. A. P. S., Scott, R., Sims, D. G., Webb, J. K. G., and Gardner, P. S.: Breast-feeding protects against respiratory syncytial virus infections, Br. Med. J. **2:**274-276, 1976.

COMMENT: These two reports illustrate some of the diverse research activity centered around breast milk feeding. The one by Teicher and Blass is of particular interest, considering the large number of studies currently under way that attempt to evaluate the quality of mothering and infant bonding. The study clearly demonstrates the importance of olfactory clues in establishing normal suckling in newborn rats. Olfactory clues may be important in higher mammals as well. Recently, a number of studies have established the importance of olfactory clues in directing mounting behavior in subhuman primates. The substances acting as sexual pheromones in primates have been relatively short-chain fatty acids produced by the action of bacteria on vaginal secretion.

Downham et al. report still another potential role of breast milk feedings in protecting newborn infants from infection. In this case their data suggest a protective role against one of the viruses causing respiratory disease in early infancy, respiratory syncytial virus infection. Breast milk feedings were shown to have a protective effect for the gastrointestinal tract in that breast milk feeding tends to encourage the colonization of the bowel with lactobacilli rather than other gram-negative organisms. Since many of the gram-negative organisms are now being identified by various bioassay techniques as specific pathogens for the gastrointestinal tract, the importance of this role for breast milk feedings has received increasing attention. The report of Downham et al. is of special interest today with attention focused on the role of respiratory viral infections, particularly RS virus infections, in triggering respiratory arrests at home. The question of whether infants with immaturity of the autonomic nervous system or with specific sleep disturbances evident even in the immediate neonatal period might be particularly prone to sudden infant death syndrome brought about by upper respiratory viral infections makes this report intriguing.

Thyroid function in the newborn

- Sack, J., Beaudry, M., DeLamater, P. V., Oh, W., and Fisher, D. A.: Umbilical cord cutting triggers hypertriiodothyroninemia and non-shivering thermogenesis in the newborn lamb, Pediatr. Res. **10**:169-175, 1976.

This study was undertaken to clarify the mechanisms responsible for the early increases in serum thyroid hormone concentrations in the newborn. Six groups of newborn lambs were studied to determine the influence of neonatal cooling, cord cutting, and the effects of thyrotropin-releasing hormone (TRH) and triiodothyronine (T_3) injections. The results indicate that the newborn lamb's response to parturition is similar to that of the human newborn. There are marked increases in mean serum T_3 and FFA levels during the first hour, with only a transient fall in body temperature, indicating effective nonshivering thermogenesis. Serum thyroxin (T_4) concentrations do not increase significantly during this time. Warming the lamb in a water bath at 39° C prevented the FFA and T_3 responses. Delayed cord cutting while the fetus was delivered into room air produced marked hypothermia and no increase in serum FFA and T_3. Concentrations of thyroid-stimulating hormone (TSH) increased after parturition, irrespective of cord cutting. Injection of TRH did not increase T_3 levels during the first hour, but a significant 4-hour response was observed. Injection of T_3 did not stimulate FFA or thermogenic response directly, but significantly augmented both responses to cord cutting.

The results indicate that umbilical cord cutting, rather than cooling, stimulates FFA release, T_3 production, and thermogenesis.

- Walfish, P. G.: Evaluation of three thyroid-function screening tests for detecting neonatal hypothyroidism, Lancet **1**:1208-1211, 1976.

This study compared three thyroid function screening tests for possible application on a routine basis in the early diagnosis of neonatal hypothyroidism. The three methods were (1) the measurements of T_4 on dried capillary blood by the method of Dussault and Laberge (Dosage de la thyroxine [T_4] par méthode radio-immunologique dans l'éluat de sang séché: nouvelle méthode de dépistage de l'hypothyroïdie néonatale, Union Med. Can. **102**:2062-2064, 1973), (2) the measurements of T_4 determined by standard double-antibody radioimmunoassay on blood collected from the umbilical cord at the time of delivery, and (3) the measurement of TSH concentrations using equilibrium double-

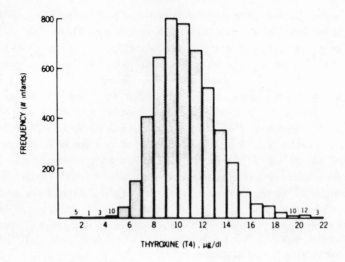

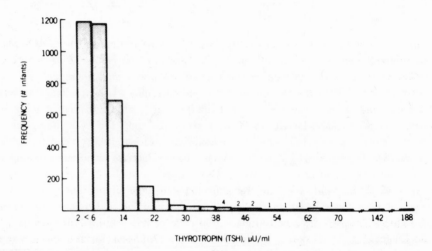

FIG. 12-6

Observed distribution of values for cord blood serum using T_4 assay (upper) compared to TSH measurements (lower). Upper panel: n = 4911, + = 10.7 µg/dl, SD = +2.5. Lower panel: n = 3773, median = 8.4 µU/ml. (From Walfish, P. G.: Evaluation of three thyroid-function screening tests for detecting neonatal hypothyroidism, Lancet **1**:1208-1211, 1976.)

antibody radioimmunoassay also on umbilical cord blood. The false positive recall incidence was approximately 90% with both measurements of thyroxin concentration, either on drug capillary blood or umbilical cord blood. Fig. 12-6 presents the results for the cord blood T_4 and TSH concentrations. Umbilical cord blood TSH concentrations had a higher specificity and sensitivity for the diagnosis of primary hypothyroidism. Less than 1% (0.24%) of the population had values greater than 50 µU of TSH per milliliter and the two affected cases had values greater than 70 µU/ml. The author recommends that initial screening be done with dried capillary blood T_4 measurements and that to avoid a very high recall rate, those with a low T_4 level be screened with TSH measurements.

■ Cuestas, R. A., Lindall, A., and Engel, R. R.: Low thyroid hormones and respiratory-distress syndrome of the newborn: studies on cord blood, N. Engl. J. Med. **295:**297-302, 1976.

This study demonstrated a relationship between T_3, T_4, and TSH concentrations on cord blood versus the frequency of the respiratory distress syndrome (RDS). The data demonstrate that infants who developed RDS had significantly lower umbilical cord T_3 and T_4 concentrations and higher TSH concentrations than those of newborns who did not develop the syndrome. Conversely, a higher frequency and severity of RDS was observed in infants with low umbilical cord T_3 and T_4 concentrations and high TSH levels when compared with infants whose umbilical cord thyroid hormone concentrations were normal. This study, together with several other reports in the literature, makes a strong case for a relationship between thyroid function and pulmonary maturation. Redding and Pereira (Thyroid function in respiratory distress syndrome [RDS] of the newborn, Pediatrics **54:** 423-428, 1974) had shown that infants with RDS failed to develop the normal postnatal increase in T_4 concentration during the first 2 days of life. More recently, Fisch et al. (Physical and mental status at 4 years of age of survivors of the respiratory distress syndrome: follow-up report from the collaborative study, J. Pediatr. **86:**497-503, 1975) presented data showing a significantly higher incidence of clinical hypothyroidism in children surviving the RDS compared with the general population (2.3% vs 0.006%). The authors suggest that until mass screening for neonatal hypothyroidism is introduced, it may be appropriate to make certain that children with RDS have normal TSH or T_4 concentrations during the newborn period.

COMMENT: In recent years there has been a moderate amount of research carried out on large animals that has had as its goal defining to what extent fetal thyroid metabolism is independent of maternal control. Sack et al. report part of an interesting series of studies from Fisher's laboratory on the physiology of thyroid hormones in fetal and neonatal life. According to these investigators, there is a rapid increase in the serum levels of TSH, T_3, and T_4 after birth. Because of these events, there is effective nonshivering thermogenesis and only a moderate fall in body temperature in the transition from intrauterine to extrauterine life. Thus it may seem that cooling of the body surface should be the most important stimulus for the postnatal elevation of thyroid hormones. Contrary to this expectation, the experiments by Sack et al. show that cutting the cord is essential in triggering the nonshivering thermogenesis of the newborn and the elevation of T_3. If the fetus is delivered in room air but the cord is left intact, the temperature of the fetus continues to decrease and the concentration of T_3 remains at the fetal level. It is not clear why separation of the fetus from the placenta rather than a thermal stimulus is important in initiating thermal adaptation to the extrauterine environment.

The report by Walfish continues a series of clinical studies published from a number of centers that attempt to evaluate the best approach to mass screening of newborn infants for congenital hypothyroidism. This study clearly points out that measurements of TSH concentration in umbilical cord blood provided the greatest specificity and sensitivity for the diagnosis of primary congenital hypothyroidism. Ample justification has been provided in the pediatric literature to support the establishment of mass screening programs in the neonatal period for congenital hypothyroidism. At Colorado General Hospital, we have

used the measurement of TSH concentration on umbilical cord blood for screening. However, it is likely that measurements of T_4 concentrations on dried capillary blood samples obtained from the newborn infants will be more widely used principally because the samples can be collected at the same time as are the screening blood samples for phenylketonuria. As mass screening for hypothyroidism with T_4 measurements becomes widely used, we should have additional information concerning the precise incidence of congenital hypothyroidism and perhaps additional clues concerning the effect of certain drugs taken or dietary fads followed by the mother on neonatal thyroid metabolism.

The report by Cuestas et al. strengthens the evidence in favor of the association of low thyroid hormone concentrations in infants with RDS. Their suggestion that all infants with RDS should be screened for neonatal hypothyroidism should be supported. In fact, until mass screening for hypothyroidism is developed, any neonatal problem associated with hypothyroidism should prompt T_4 and TSH concentration measurements on the newborn infants. This would include unexplained jaundice as well as RDS.

Estimation of gestational age

■ Nicolopoulos, D., Perakis, A., Papadakis, M., Alexiou, D., and Aravantinos, D.: Estimation of gestational age in the neonate: a comparison of clinical methods, Am. J. Dis. Child. **130:**477-480, 1976.

This report continues a series of studies that have appeared in the literature attempting to evaluate various neurologic and morphologic criteria that can be used in the examination of newborn infants for an estimate of their gestational ages. A total of 710 infants of varying gestational ages, from 28 to 44 weeks, were examined. The criteria examined included those evaluated in studies by Farr et al. (The value of some external characteristics in the assessment of gestational age at birth, Dev. Med. Child. Neurol. **8:**657-661, 1966), Dubowitz et al. (Clinical assessment of gestational age in the newborn, J. Pediatr. **77:**1-10, 1970), Petrussa (A scoring system for the assessment of gestational age of newborn infants. In Proceedings of the Second European Congress in Perinatal Medicine, Basel, 1971, S. Karger AG), and Robinson (Assessment of gestational age by neurologic examination, Arch. Dis. Child. **47:**437-447, 1966). Table 12-7 taken from the report of Nicolopoulos et al. gives the correlation coefficients for each of the ten neurologic criteria and eleven morphologic criteria. The table demonstrates that two neurologic criteria, arm and leg recoil, and two morphologic criteria, genital examination and degree of edema, showed a poor correlation with gestational age. The authors stressed the difficulty of using neurologic criteria in examining infants who are receiving respirator care and other forms of intensive care. For this reason, they evaluated the use of nine morphologic criteria alone and found that these gave a correlation coefficient of .878 with the estimation of gestational age.

■ Malan, A. F., and Higgs, S. C.: Gestational age assessment in infants of very low birthweight, Arch. Dis. Child. **50:**322-324, 1975.

This report makes an important contribution in extending the evaluation of the neurologic and morphologic criteria applied by Dubowitz to infants with birth weights less than 1500 gm. The correlation coefficient found between the scored gestational age after the neurologic and morphologic examination and the calculated gestational age was .915 with 95% confidence limits of approximately 2 weeks. The study suggests that the neurologic and morphologic criteria used in the assessment of more mature, larger infants can be applied to very low birth weight babies.

TABLE 12-7
Correlation of scores with gestational age*

Criteria	Correlation coefficient (r)	Criteria	Correlation coefficient (r)
Neurologic		Morphologic	
Popliteal angle	0.757	Skin texture	0.767
Heel-to-ear	0.755	Plantar creases	0.766
Dorsiflexion	0.742	Breast size	0.764
Square window	0.725	Ear firmness	0.756
Posture	0.724	Ear form	0.755
Ventral suspension	0.718	Skin color	0.755
Scarf sign	0.716	Lanugo	0.731
Head lag	0.710	Nipple formation	0.723
Arm recoil	0.651	Skin opacity	0.719
Leg recoil	0.545	Genitals	0.651
		Edema	0.642

*From Nicolopoulos, D., Perakis, A., Papadakis, M., Alexiou, D., and Aravantinos, D.: Estimation of gestational age in the neonate: a comparison of clinical methods, Am. J. Dis. Child. **130:**477-480, May, 1976; copyright 1976, American Medical Association.

COMMENT: The study of Nicolopoulos et al. should prove useful for the estimation of gestational age in critically ill preterm infants. It should be stressed that any attempt to equate changes in body composition or function, as represented by the neurologic or morphologic criteria, with gestational age implies that all these characteristics should change at the same chronologic time in newborn infants in the absence of disease. This is a simplification of the true variability in biology. After a child is born and during the child's subsequent growth (childhood and adolescence), we have no trouble recognizing great variability in maturation indices even among healthy, normal children. For instance, we do not presume to correct a child's birth date by the time of appearance of various stages of puberty during early adolescence. Rather we accept the variability in the sequential appearance of puberty staging in early adolescence as representing the normal spectrum in biology and not representing errors in the child's birth date. It is likely that similar variability occurs during intrauterine development. Thus, all attempts to "age" newborn infants by the examination of the infant, although very useful clinically, should not obscure thinking about what these differences may imply concerning intrauterine development and organ maturation.

The study of Malan and Higgs extends the evaluation of gestational age to the very low birth weight baby. Part of the study deals with a gestational age range also included in the study of Nicolopoulos. However, attention in the Malan and Higgs study is devoted to the 26- to 32-week gestational age group. It should also be emphasized that Malan and Higgs eliminated attempts to evaluate infants who had respiratory distress, congenital anomalies, or obvious infection. Furthermore, in both studies the evaluations were carried out on the second or third day of life.

Both studies are significant in that they point out that a reasonable assessment of gestational age can be made even in very small infants. However, it has been our clinical experience that evaluations of the very low birth weight, very immature infant are extremely difficult at the time of delivery or in the first few hours after delivery. The Apgar scoring system, so useful in older preterm babies, can be misleading in the very immature infant in whom immaturity of the neuromuscular system rather than any disease may produce some degree of hypotonia and inadequate initial respiratory efforts. For this reason it is hazardous to attempt to make predictions of viability within the first few hours after delivery of the very low birth weight infant. Such assessments are better made after the initial support is provided, the infant is stabilized, and a more thorough and complete medical examination, including the neurologic examination, is made.

Respiratory distress syndrome

■ Smith, B. T., Giroud, C. J. P., Robert, M., and Avery, M. E.: Insulin antagonism of cortisol action on lecithin synthesis by cultured fetal lung cells, J. Pediatr. **87**:953-955, 1975.

This study demonstrates that cortisol administered to monolayer cell cultures prepared from late-gestation rabbit fetal lung stimulates lecithin synthesis and reduces cell growth. When insulin is added in a concentration from 25 to 100 μU/ml, it blocks the stimulatory effect of cortisol on lecithin synthesis (see Table 12-8 from their report). In contrast, insulin has no effect on altering the cortisol-induced inhibition of cellular growth. The authors speculate that this apparent antagonism of insulin versus cortisol on surfactant synthesis may have clinical significance in explaining the increased incidence of RDS associated with infants of diabetic mothers.

■ Robert, M. F., Neff, R. K., Hubbell, J. P., Taeusch, H. W., and Avery, M. E.: Association between maternal diabetes and the respiratory-distress syndrome in the newborn, N. Engl. J. Med. **294**:357-360, 1976.

This study presents a retrospective review of the incidence of RDS in newborn infants born to mothers with diabetes (805 infants) and to nondiabetic mothers (10,152 infants). The study was conducted on patients delivered between 1958 and 1968. There was a significantly higher incidence of RDS in infants born to mothers with diabetes than in those born to nondiabetic mothers. When gestational age, a major determinant of the incidence

TABLE 12-8
Effect of insulin and cortisol on lecithin synthesis*

Insulin† (µU/ml)	^{3}H-choline incorporated into lecithin (pmol/flask)‡	
	Control	Cortisol§
0	10.2 ± 0.9	26.1 ± 3.5
1	10.9 ± 1.1	19.0 ± 2.0
10	12.2 ± 1.3	17.9 ± 1.9
25	13.9 ± 0.4	15.3 ± 1.7
100	13.8 ± 1.0	15.3 ± 1.4

*From Smith, B. T., Giroud, G. J. P., Robert, M., and Avery, M. E.: Insulin antagonism of cortisol action on lecithin synthesis by cultured fetal lung cells, J. Pediatr. **87**:953-955, 1975.
†Mean umbilical cord blood levels of immunoreactive insulin are 14 μU/ml in the normal infant and 83 μU/ml in the infant of the diabetic mother (Jorgensen et al., 1956).
‡Each value represents the mean (± SD) recovery of ^{3}H-lecithin from triplicate cultures prepared from each of two litters at 28 days' gestation (n = 6), following incubation with ^{3}H-choline.
§5.5 × 10^{-6}M. The normal umbilical cord blood level of cortisol is 1.9 × 10^{-7}M (Murphy, 1974).

of RDS, was controlled, infants born to mothers with diabetes still had 5.6 times the incidence of RDS as infants born to mothers without diabetes.

■ Moss, G., and Stein, A. A.: The centrineurogenic etiology of the respiratory distress syndrome: induction by isolated cerebral hypoxemia and prevention by unilateral pulmonary denervation, Am. J. Surg. **132:**352-357, 1976.

This study describes experiments in adult animals aimed at clarifying the role of the central nervous system in producing "shock lung." The report demonstrates that when cerebral perfusion is carried out with hypoxemic blood, a syndrome develops that is similar to the adult form of RDS, including congestion, edema, hemorrhage, and atelectasis. This syndrome in the lung triggered by cerebral hypoxia can be prevented by reimplantation of the lung, a procedure that severs all neurogenic connections to the lung. When this is done unilaterally in one lung and then cerebral hypoxic perfusion is performed, the pulmonary changes consistent with RDS develop only in that lung that has maintained its neurogenic connections. These lesions do not develop in dogs in which cerebral perfusion is carried out with normoxemic blood. This study raises questions concerning the level of hypoxemia and shock at which cerebral hypoxia would be introduced in man and thus trigger the neurogenic mechanisms leading to the adult form of the RDS.

■ Gottuso, M. A., Williams, M. L., and Oski, F. A.: The role of exchange transfusions in the management of low-birth-weight infants with and without severe respiratory distress syndrome. II. Further observations and studies of mechanisms of action, J. Pediatr. **89:**279-285, 1976.

The effect of exchange transfusion on two groups of infants was studied. The first group consisted of infants with birth weights between 700 and 1000 gm with and without respiratory distress; the second consisted of infants with birth weights between 1000 and 2000 gm, all of whom had severe RDS. The study demonstrated that there was no significant improvement in infant mortality in the infants under 1000 gm; however, in the infants with severe RDS the mortality rate was 41% in those receiving exchange transfusions and 80% in those not so treated. There did not seem to be any relationship between clinical improvement in the course of RDS and changes in coagulation factors or in red cell concentrations of 2,3-diphosphoglycerate. There was a significant decrease in the required F_{IO_2}/Pa_{O_2} with exchange transfusion. The study could not distinguish whether this reflected an improvement in pulmonary perfusion or in ventilation. No data were provided to distinguish the causes of death in both groups.

■ Kroushkop, R. W., Brown, E. G., and Sweet, A. Y.: The early use of continuous positive airway pressure in the treatment of idiopathic respiratory distress syndrome, J. Pediatr. **87:**263-267, 1975.

Twenty-one preterm babies with RDS were divided into two groups. One group of ten infants was treated with continuous positive airway pressure (CPAP) early (the criterion for entry being successive Pa_{O_2} values < 60 mm Hg while the infant was provided with an F_{IO_2} of < 0.4, or a right-to-left shunt $> 40\%$). A second group of 11 infants were managed by adjustments of F_{IO_2} until the F_{IO_2} exceeded 0.7 to maintain an arterial Pa_{O_2} between 60 and 100 mm Hg. Fig. 12-7 taken from their study shows that the infants receiving early CPAP were exposed to significantly lower F_{IO_2}'s throughout the course of the illness. However, there were no differences in survival within the two groups. Even for the infants < 1500 gm, CPAP did not significantly affect survival. Those infants had a high mortality rate regardless of when CPAP was applied.

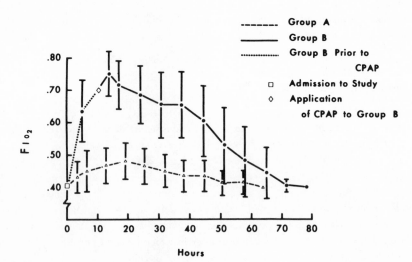

FIG. 12-7

The mean $F_{I_{O_2}}$ ($\pm$ 1 SD) of infants in each treatment group from the time of admission to the study until CPAP therapy was discontinued. (From Krouskop, R. W., Brown, E. G., and Sweet, A. Y.: The early use of continuous positive airway pressure in the treatment of idiopathic respiratory distress syndrome, J. Pediatr. 87:263-267, 1975.)

COMMENT: The two reports by Smith et al. and Robert et al. from the same center attempt to evaluate the relationship between maternal diabetes and the RDS in newborn infants. The report of Smith et al. demonstrates an apparent antagonism between insulin and cortisol on lecithin synthesis. However, their in vitro studies may not bear much relevance to in vivo conditions. The changes in cortisol concentration and insulin concentration follow very different time courses in fetal development. An infant of an insulin-dependent mother is exposed to a chronic hyperinsulinemia, whereas cortisol concentration increases sharply in late gestation. Furthermore, the work reviewed in Chapter 4 points out the fact that the increase in surfactant occurs prior to the surge in cortisol concentration. The report by Roberts et al. supports the view that hyperinsulinemia in the infant of a diabetic mother may contribute to a higher incidence of RDS by its antagonistic effect on cortisol induction of surfactant synthesis. However, it is somewhat disturbing that this applies only to infants delivered vaginally. When one restricts the review to infants delivered by cesarean section, no differences between infants born to mothers with or without diabetes were apparent. Fig. 12-8 taken from their report demonstrates that the striking difference in incidence of RDS is due to the fact that infants born *vaginally* to nondiabetic mothers had an extremely low incidence of RDS compared with all other infants.

The report by Moss and Stein is of interest because of its emphasis on the role of neuroreflexes in the initiation of the adult form of the RDS. Given the changes that must occur in every organ system, including the central nervous system, at the time of birth, it may be that neuromechanisms are involved in some of the pulmonary pathology in the neonatal period, particularly when one considers the high incidence of intracranial hemorrhage in preterm babies and the frequency with which intracranial hemorrhage occurs in infants manifesting one or another form of respiratory distress.

The study by Gottuso et al. raises more questions than it answers. It would be interesting

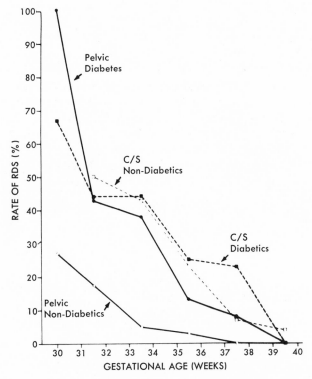

FIG. 12-8

Rate of RDS versus gestational age according to route of delivery—pelvic (vaginal) or C/S (cesarean section). Each point represents the rate of RDS for all the infants born in the week before and the week after the gestational age designated. (From Robert, M. F., Neff, R. K., Hubbell, J. P., Taeusch, H. W., and Avery, M. E.: Association between maternal diabetes and the respiratory-distress syndrome in the newborn, reprinted by permission of The New England Journal of Medicine **294:**357-360, 1976.)

to pursue the causes of death in the groups of infants studied. It is possible that exchange transfusions were reducing the risks of intracranial hemorrhage, a frequent terminal complication in infants with severe RDS. The difficulty in the study rests with the fact that nursery care can never be completely standardized from one nursery to another. The data from this study and the previous studies of Delivoria-Papadapoulos et al. (The role of exchange transfusion in the management of low-birthweight infants with and without severe respiratory distress syndrome. I. Initial observations, J. Pediatr. 89:273-278, 1976) demonstrate that in those nurseries exchange transfusions significantly reduced mortality in preterm babies with RDS. Whether this would apply to other nurseries is conjectural. The initial hypothesis that motivated the exchange transfusion studies is probably not the basis for any physiologic improvement. Initially the study was launched on the premise that transfusion with adult blood of low oxygen affinity would improve the release of oxygen to tissues reflected in an increased venous P_{O_2}. The importance of this phenomenon is doubtful considering the fact that no evidence of a release problem of oxygen to tissues can be demonstrated in fetal life, despite very low arterial and venous P_{O_2}s. Recent physiologic studies have tended to discount the advantage of a low oxygen affinity in blood in improving tissue oxygenation. Definitive evidence that there is, in fact, a release problem for oxygen delivery to tissues in the face of a high oxygen affinity has not been provided in animal experimentation. It seems possible that the introduction of exchange transfusions in these nurseries may have altered other forms of therapy, including the administration of salt solutions or colloid, and thus have contributed to the improved survival rate.

The study by Kroushkop et al. illustrates an application of CPAP in the early treatment of idiopathic RDS. As with many other therapeutic procedures introduced shortly after birth, it increases the pressure on the physician for a more precise diagnosis of pulmonary disease in the first few hours after birth. The article by Ablow et al. reviewed in this chapter, illustrating the fact that group B streptococcal pneumonia may present early and with a clinical course that is indistinguishable from hyaline membrane disease, further accentuates the difficulties posed by early intervention and the risks of an improper diagnosis.

CHAPTER 13

Water and electrolyte balance

■ Baum, J. D., and Robertson, N. R. C.: Immediate effects of alkaline infusion in infants with respiratory distress syndrome, J. Pediatr. **87**:255-261, 1975.

In this study nineteen infants were treated with either 7% tromethamine (THAM) or 8.4% sodium bicarbonate for correction of acidosis associated with respiratory distress syndrome. The THAM solution had an osmolality of 708 mOsm/kg of water and the sodium bicarbonate solution, 1680 mOsm/kg of water. Infants were divided into subgroups according to which buffer was used and how rapidly it was given. Length and rapidity of injections varied from 30 seconds to 5-minute infusions. In all infants the pH rose quickly and remained elevated for the 10 minutes following the termination of the THAM or bicarbonate administration. The changes in hematocrit and colloid osmotic pressure of the plasma were similar; both fell to ~20% from preinfusion values, changes consistent with an expansion of blood and plasma volume. Plasma osmolality increased markedly in all groups, the changes being most striking when hypertonic bicarbonate solutions were given for 2 minutes or less. The authors comment that six of the nineteen infants had intraventricular hemorrhage, an incidence which they did not regard as excessive in infants with respiratory distress syndrome and acidemia.

COMMENT: The article by Baum et al. makes one wonder how often it is necessary to reinvent the wheel. It is a classic experiment in physiology, well described in Gamble's original text (Gamble: Chemical anatomy, physiology and pathology of extracellular fluid: a lecture syllabus, ed. 6, 1954, Harvard University Press) demonstrating that if a hypertonic sodium solution is given to a patient, the hypertonicity of the extracellular fluid will pull water from the intracellular space, diluting the red cells and plasma proteins with a fall in hematocrit and colloidal osmotic pressure. The sodium concentration initially will be elevated and then gradually will return toward normal as water is pulled from the intracellular compartment. It is not clear why this experiment needs to be repeated. The approximately 30% incidence of intraventricular hemorrhage in the nineteen infants studied seems high by any standard.

Water and electrolyte balance in preterm infants

■ Aperia, A., Broberger, O., Thodenius, K., and Zetterström, R.: Renal control of sodium and fluid balance in newborn infants during intravenous maintenance therapy, Acta Paediatr. Scand. **64**:725-731, 1975.

Water and sodium balance studies were carried out over a short term in thirty-eight newborn infants varying in gestational ages from 28 to 42 weeks. The infants had a variety of clinical disorders. All had received intravenous fluid therapy for at least 24 hours, with the exception of two infants studied on the first day of life. The infants received a water intake of 60, 80, 90, and 100 ml/kg/24 hr on the first, second, third, and fourth days,

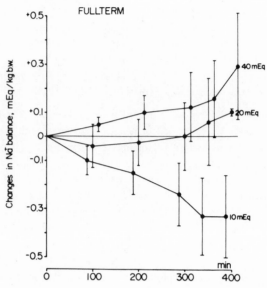

FIG. 13-1

The accumulated changes in sodium balance in infants born after 36 weeks of gestation when receiving the three different saline solutions. ●, mean values of sodium balance. Range bar represents SEM. (From Aperia, A., Broberger, O., Thodenius, K., and Zetterström, R.: Renal control of sodium and fluid balance in newborn infants during intravenous maintenance therapy, Acta Paediatr. Scand. **64:**725-731, 1975.)

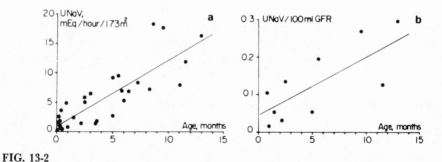

FIG. 13-2

a, Average hourly urinary sodium excretion, *UNaV,* during first year of life. The correlation coefficient (r = 0.764) is highly significant (p < 0.001). **b,** The development of *UNaV* in relationship to glomerular filtration rate. The correlation coefficient (r = 0.755) is significant (0.01 > p > 0.001). (From Aperia, A., Broberger, O., Thodenius, K., and Zetterström, R.: Development of renal control of salt and fluid homeostasis during the first year of life, Acta Paediatr. Scand. **64:**393-398, 1975.)

respectively. The solutions contained sodium at a concentration of 10, 20, or 40 mEq/L. Fig. 13-1 illustrates the data obtained in infants over 36 weeks' gestation. It should be emphasized that the data were collected over a relatively short time period of ~6 to 7 hours. A sodium concentration of 20 mEq/L at these infusion rates provided ~2 mEq/kg/24 hr and achieved sodium balance. In the preterm babies less than 36 weeks' gestational age, a larger quantity of sodium was lost in the urine during the course of the study, and sodium balance showed a much greater variance at each sodium concentration used. However, even with the maximum sodium load provided by the 40 mEq/L sodium concentration, there was a negative sodium balance in the early part of the study.

- Aperia, A., Broberger, O., Thodenius, K., and Zetterström, R.: Development of renal control of salt and fluid homeostasis during the first year of life, Acta Paediatr. Scand. **64:** 393-398, 1975.

This study presents data on the glomerular filtration rate, excretion of an oral sodium or water load, and diluting capacity in twenty-three infants studied between 3 weeks and 13 months of age. The study demonstrated that the glomerular filtration rate increased exponentially during the first year of life. In contrast, sodium excretion increased linearly. These are shown in Fig. 13-2. Water excretion, on the other hand, remained unchanged per unit of surface area during the first year of life. The authors hypothesize that the decreased ability of infants to concentrate the urine, coupled with their enhanced ability for renal reabsorption of sodium, will predispose infants to hypertonic dehydration. This situation can be complicated by excessive water losses in the stool or a disproportionate intake of sodium to water in the diet.

- Mestyán, I., Horváth, M., and Mestyán, J.: Plasma osmolality in the early and late neonatal period with particular reference to low birthweight infants, Biol. Neonate **28:**303-316, 1976.

In this study sodium concentrations in the plasma and plasma osmolality were determined in two groups of infants: one consisted of 114 normal full-term infants and another consisted of a variety of infants, including preterm and term babies with mild neonatal problems. The infants showed a steady fall in plasma osmolality demonstrated in Fig. 13-3. Although the osmolality fell steadily over the first month of life, the wide variance in plasma osmolality at each age is also apparent. The investigators demonstrated that the fall in osmolality was significantly correlated with the fall in plasma/sodium concentration.

COMMENT: During the last 2 years there has been a large number of studies from many centers evaluating water and sodium balance in newborn infants of varying gestational age and birth weights. The studies from different centers have been in remarkably good agreement and are well represented by the data presented in the first report by Aperia et al. Essentially, all reports have shown that there is a higher obligatory sodium loss in the urine expressed in mEq/kg/24 hr for preterm babies than for term infants. In the very immature infant, sodium intakes as high as 3 mEq/kg/24 hr are required to maintain sodium balance. This is demonstrated nicely in the data of the first report of Aperia et al. for the preterm infants given solutions containing sodium at a concentration of 40 mEq/kg. Obviously, such studies provide a basis only for the initial fluid and electrolyte orders that are written for preterm infants. The more immature the infant, the more frequently one must reassess the actual needs of a particular infant and adjust appropriately water and electrolyte intake. For the infants under 1000 gm, these readjustments normally must be made approximately every 8 hours.

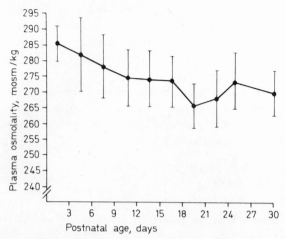

FIG. 13-3

Mean plasma osmolality (± SD) corresponding to the different age groups of infants (full-term and preterm) followed after admission to the referral unit. (From Mestyán, I., Horváth, M., and Mestyán, J.: Plasma osmolality in the early and late neonatal period with particular reference to low birthweight infants, Biol. Neonate **28**:303-316, 1976; S. Karger AG, Basel.)

The study of Mestyán et al. clearly demonstrates the hypertonicity and hyponatremia that frequently develops in preterm babies given sodium and water intakes appropriate for larger, more mature infants. There was no suggestion in this study that marked changes in plasma osmolality occur in low birth weight infants independent of changes in plasma sodium concentration. In this regard, it would be useful to have more information on the large group of infants described by Thomas (see review of his article later in this chapter), who had marked hypertonicity without hypernatremia and who, in association with hypertonicity, developed intracranial hemorrhage.

Hypernatremia and intracranial hemorrhage

■ Robertson, N. R. C., and Howat, P.: Hypernatraemia as a cause of intracranial haemorrhage, Arch. Dis. Child. **50**:938-942, 1975.

The authors carried out a retrospective study on all infants born at their hospital who had (1) developed hypernatremia (sodium concentration ≥ 150 mEq/L), (2) received more than 8 mEq/kg/24 hr of sodium, or (3) developed any form of intracranial hemorrhage detected clinically or at postmortem examination during the neonatal period. The study period encompassed 25 months ending July 31, 1974. There were 188 high-risk infants (that is, infants between 1 and 2 kg birth weights). In these 188 infants, six developed documented hypernatremia, and one of the six developed intraventricular hemorrhage, an incidence of 17%. In the remaining 182 infants without hypernatremia, there were fourteen cases of intraventricular hemorrhage, an incidence of 8%.

■ Anderson, J. M., Bain, A. D., Brown, J. K., Cockburn, F., Forfar, J. O., Machin, G. A., and Turner, T. L.: Hyaline-membrane disease, alkaline buffer treatment, and cerebral intraventricular haemorrhage, Lancet **1**:117-119, 1976.

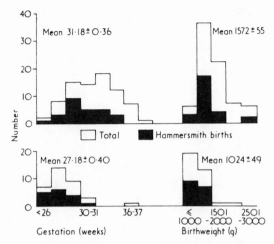

FIG. 13-4

Frequency distribution by gestation and birthweight of babies with intraventricular hemorrhage, *IVH*, with and without hyaline membrane disease, *HMD*. Differences in birth weight and gestation distributions are highly significant (p $<$ 10^{-6} for each comparison). (From Wigglesworth, J. S., Keith, I. H., Girling, D. J., and Slade, S. A.: Hyaline membrane disease, alkali, and intraventricular haemorrhage, Arch. Dis. Child. **51**:755-762, 1976.)

This article reviews the findings in fifty-five preterm babies dying from hyaline membrane disease, with or without cerebral intraventricular hemorrhage. The infants dying with both hyaline membrane disease and intraventricular hemorrhage had received more sodium bicarbonate during their nursery course than those with hyaline membrane disease alone. However, the infants dying with hyaline membrane disease alone had received as much bicarbonate therapy at birth as those dying with combined hyaline membrane disease and intraventricular hemorrhage. The incidence of intraventricular hemorrhage among live-born infants under 2500 gm remained the same in the two time periods, 1956 through 1959 versus 1971 through 1974. The former represented a time period when buffer therapy for metabolic acidosis was not used on their service. The authors conclude there is no association between hypernatremia and the incidence of intraventricular hemorrhage.

■ Thomas, D. B.: Hyperosmolality and intraventricular hemorrhage in premature babies, Acta Paediatr. Scand. **65**:429-432, 1976.

This report presents data on plasma sodium concentrations and plasma osmolality measurements in infants cared for in an intensive care nursery whose gestational ages were less than 33 weeks. Twenty-eight infants were studied. In six of the twenty-eight infants, intraventricular hemorrhage occurred that was fatal. In nine other infants, deaths occurred unassociated with intraventricular hemorrhage, and all the remaining infants survived. There was no association between intraventricular hemorrhage and hypernatremia documented in this study.

■ Wigglesworth, J. S., Keith, I. H., Girling, D. J., and Slade, S. A.: Hyaline membrane disease, alkali, and intraventricular haemorrhage, Arch. Dis. Child. **51**:755-762, 1976.

This report presents a retrospective survey of necropsy findings for the years 1966 through 1973 on patients cared for at the neonatal unit at Hammersmith Hospital. It in-

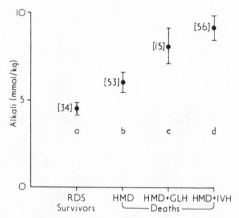

Fig. 13-5
Maximum 12-hour alkali dosage expressed as mean ± SEM of survivors of severe respiratory
distress syndrome, *RDS* (ventilated), compared to deaths with *HMD, HMD + GLH*
(germinal layer hemorrhage), and *HMD +IVH*. Numbers in each group in parentheses.
Statistical comparisons (Wilcoxon's Rank Sum test) a : b and c : d, not significantly different;
a : c, p = 0.0012; a : d, p < 0.0001; b : c, p = 0.02; b : d, p < 0.0001. (From Wigglesworth,
J. S., Keith, I. H., Girling, D. J., and Slade, S. A.: Hyaline membrane disease, alkali, and
intraventricular haemorrhage, Arch. Dis. Child. **51**:755-762, 1976.)

cluded 176 cases with intraventricular hemorrhage and 285 with hyaline membrane disease.
The study compared infants who had intraventricular hemorrhage and hyaline membrane
disease with those who had intraventricular hemorrhage alone in terms of their birth weight
and gestational age distribution. Fig. 13-4 taken from their report illustrates the striking
differences in both birth weight and gestational age for the infants with intraventricular
hemorrhage plus hyaline membrane disease. Those infants were both more mature and of
larger birth weight than the infants with intraventricular hemorrhage alone, strongly suggesting some factor or factors associated with hyaline membrane disease that contributed
to the higher incidence of intraventricular hemorrhage in large babies near term.

The authors compared the infants with intraventricular hemorrhage and hyaline disease
with those who had hyaline membrane disease alone in terms of respiratory gas measurements. There were no significant differences in the lowest Pa_{O_2}, highest Pa_{CO_2}, lowest pH,
or standard bicarbonate concentrations in the two groups, suggesting no difference in the
severity of hyaline membrane disease within the two groups. Figs. 13-5 and 13-6 taken
from their report clearly demonstrate that the infants with germinal layer hemorrhage and
hyaline membrane disease or with intraventricular hemorrhage and hyaline membrane disease
had received larger total doses of alkali in mmol/kg than infants with respiratory distress
syndrome who survived or those who died. In addition, at each gestational age group above
30 weeks, the infants with any intracranial hemorrhage plus hyaline membrane disease had
received significantly greater amounts of alkali therapy than those having hyaline membrane
disease alone, with mean values of approximately 8 to 80 mmol/kg.

■ Turbeville, D. F., Bowen, F. W., and Killam, A. P.: Intracranial hemorrhages in kittens:
hypernatremia versus hypoxia, J. Pediatr. **89**:294-297, 1976.

This study compares the effects of acute hypoxia or acute hypernatremia either alone
or in combination on the incidence of intracranial hemorrhage in kittens. Hypernatremia

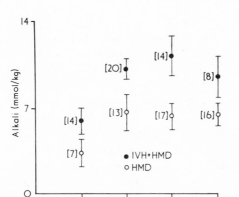

FIG. 13-6

Maximum 12-hour alkali dosage, expressed as mean ± SEM in IVH + HMD and HMD groups, by gestation. Numbers in each group in parentheses. (From Wigglesworth, J. S., Keith, I. H., Girling, D. J., and Slade, S. A.: Hyaline membrane disease, alkali, and intraventricular haemorrhage, Arch. Dis. Child. **51:**755-762, 1976.)

TABLE 13-1

Statistical analysis by Student's t test of the group means*

Group	Weight	Blood pressure	Hematocrit	Pa_{CO_2}	Pa_{O_2}	pH	Base deficit	Sodium	Central nervous system hemorrhage
I vs II	NS	NS	NS	NS	< 0.001	< 0.001	< 0.001	NS	NS
I vs III	NS	NS	NS	NS	NS	NS	NS	< 0.001	< 0.001
I vs IV	NS	NS	NS	NS	< 0.001	< 0.001	< 0.001	< 0.001	< 0.001
II vs III	NS	NS	NS	NS	< 0.001	< 0.001	< 0.001	< 0.001	< 0.001
II vs IV	NS	NS	NS	NS	NS	NS	NS	< 0.001	< 0.001
III vs IV	NS	NS	NS	NS	< 0.001	< 0.001	< 0.001	NS	NS
Hemorrhage vs no hemorrhage	NS	NS	NS	NS	NS	NS	NS	< 0.001	< 0.001

*From Turbeville, D. F., Bowen, F. W., and Killam, A. P.: Intracranial hemorrhage in kittens: hypernatremia versus hypoxia, J. Pediatr. **89:**294-297, 1976.

was produced by the intra-arterial injection of 5 ml/kg of a solution containing sodium bicarbonate in a concentration of 0.89 mEq/ml. The intra-arterial injections were given on three occasions at 90-minute intervals. Hypoxia was produced by adjusting FI_{O_2} to 0.1. At the end of the experiments the animals were sacrificed and the brains were fixed, examined, and graded for evidence of central nervous system hemorrhage. Table 13-1 taken from their report summarizes their results and demonstrates that central nervous system hemorrhage developed only in those kittens in which iatrogenic hypernatremia was produced either alone or in combination with acute hypoxia. Acute hypoxia, per se, in the absence of iatrogenic hypernatremia, did not produce central nervous system hemorrhage.

COMMENT: These articles represent a trend of reports that followed the publication of Simmons et al. (Hypernatremia and intracranial hemorrhage in neonates, N. Engl. J. Med. 291:6-10, 1974), in which the authors reported an association between hypernatremia and intracranial hemorrhage in newborn infants. Perhaps an appropriate beginning to a comment would be to emphasize that hypertonicity is one of a group of environmental changes that produces cell death in all living things, whether studied in vivo or in vitro. The addition of salt to foodstuffs has been used as a method of food preservation by preventing bacterial growth. Cell death occurs when tissues are presented with a sufficiently hypertonic medium in vitro. Stated crudely, then, one could say that brine is good for pickles, not people. Therefore the reluctance to accept the fact that hypertonicity may be associated with an increased mortality rate in newborn infants and specifically may increase the risk of intracranial hemorrhage is probably based on the assumption that the hypertonicity created by clinical intervention is quantitatively negligible.

The reports by Robertson and Howat and Anderson et al., which purport to show no association between hypernatremia and intracranial hemorrhage, included in their studies a large group of infants who were at no risk of intracranial hemorrhage. For example, Robertson and Howat studied all infants born at their hospital, which would include a large group of infants who were born at term. If we restrict the review to the 188 high-risk infants in the study of Robertson et al., then twenty infants received an excess of 8 mEq/kg/24 hr over a 24-hour period with ten cases of intraventricular hemorrhage, an incidence of 50%. In the remaining 168 infants who received less than 8 mEq/kg/24 hr, there were five cases of intraventricular hemorrhage, an incidence of 3%. For reasons that are not clear, the authors concluded that there was no evidence of a causal relation between intraventricular hemorrhage and either hypernatremia or large sodium intakes.

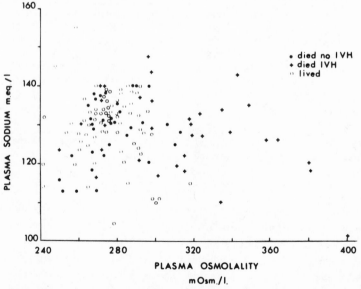

FIG. 13-7

Absence of relationship between sodium concentrations and osmolality in all specimens tested from the twenty-eight babies. (From Thomas, D. B.,: Hyperosmolality and intraventricular hemorrhage in premature babies, Acta Paediatr. Scand. 65:429-432, 1976.)

In the study by Thomas, hypernatremia was avoided by the water and sodium intake provided these preterm babies. Fig. 13-7 taken from this report illustrates the fact that only one infant had a serum sodium greater than 150 mEq/L. Thus a lack of association between hypernatremia and intraventricular hemorrhage could not be established in this study, since hypernatremia was effectively avoided. Fig. 13-7 also points out the interesting observation that all but one of the infants who died with intraventricular hemorrhage had marked elevations in plasma osmolality. Thus hypertonicity was clearly evident in the group with intraventricular hemorrhage, in contrast with the other preterm babies. No data are provided describing the solutes contributing to the marked rise in plasma osmolality. Some of these infants may have had significant hyperglycemia, but this would hardly explain osmolalities as high as 380 mOsm/L. Regardless of the solutes contributing, osmolalities above 320 represent severe hypertonicity, and it is not surprising that intraventricular hemorrhage occurred in those infants.

One can draw erroneous conclusions from a study design in which there is a dilution of a group of patients at risk for a particular problem by a much larger number of patients at no risk for that problem. This is a frequent hazard in clinical studies. Fifteen or 20 years ago there was considerable confusion about the repercussions of adolescent pregnancy on infant outcome. All the early studies tended to demonstrate no increase in preterm delivery or in perinatal mortality in adolescent pregnancies. However, the early studies included teenagers up to the age of 19; and thus, in the study population there was a large percentage of adolescents between the ages of 17 and 19, at which age, in fact, reproductive outcome was very good. This group masked the pregnancy outcome in the smaller number of pregnancies occurring in 13-, 14-, and 15-year-old girls, at which age pregnancy was associated with a marked increase in prematurity and perinatal mortality. A similar problem arises in these first three reports. The report of Thomas exemplifies the problem most clearly; certainly if a study includes no patients with hypernatremia, it is unlikely that there will be an incidence of a disease problem associated with hypernatremia.

The report by Wigglesworth et al. presents data similar to those reported by Simmons et al., confirming an association between hypernatremia and intracranial hemorrhage. The study by Turbeville et al., describing the association of intracranial hemorrhage in kittens with the administration of sodium bicarbonate rather than with hypoxia, further strengthens this supposition. Certainly intracranial hemorrhage occurs associated with hypernatremia in many markedly preterm babies. However, hypernatremia should be regarded as only one of several potential etiologic agents.

CHAPTER 14

Chemical and physical hazards

■ Ráliš, Z. A.: Birth trauma to muscles in babies born by breech delivery and its possible fatal consequences, Arch. Dis. Child. **50:**4-13, 1975.

This study documents extensive damage to the skin and muscles of the lower extremities and the back. It is known that there is a much higher perinatal mortality in babies born by breech presentation, particularly in preterm deliveries. This study consists of a pathologic examination of the soft tissues with special attention to the skin and muscles of the lower extremities in all infants dying after breech delivery. The study clearly demonstrates that massive hemorrhage and necrosis of muscle tissue of the lower extremities occur frequently in infants dying after breech delivery. Fig. 14-1 presents a microscopic appearance of damaged muscle of the lower extremity in a preterm baby. The massive hemorrhage is obvious. Table 14-1 points out that this complication occurred in its severe form most frequently in the preterm infant.

■ Douek, E., Bannister, L. H., Dodson, H. C., Ashcroft, P., and Humphries, K. N.: Effects of incubator noise on the cochlea of the newborn, Lancet **2:**1110-1113, 1976.

This study measured the variable noise level within incubators in regular use within nurseries. The noise level was applied to guinea pigs during their second week after birth and also to adult guinea pigs. After continuous treatment for 7 days, the animals were allowed 3 weeks without exposure to the noise level for scar formation from any damage to the cochlea. The animals were then sacrificed and the cochleas examined histologically. Table 14-2 presents their data and demonstrates that outer hair cell loss was confined to the exposed newborn guinea pigs. Hair cell loss did not occur in either the control newborn animals or the adult animals exposed to the noise. Micrographs of the surface preparations from the cochleas of the exposed newborn animals frequently demonstrated scar formation. The authors point out that previous work to evaluate the potential danger of noise levels in incubators may have been falsely reassuring, since studies were often carried out on adult or mature animals.

Twelve children varying in age from 4 to 20 years were selected for audiograms. All the children had been low birth weight infants and had been cared for in incubators for at least one week. Fig. 14-2 presents audiograms from six of the patients. Audiograms of all twelve children showed the same characteristics, mainly severe high-tone hearing deficit characteristic of traumatic deafness. This was consistent with the location of the principal pathology in the newborn guinea pigs exposed to the same level of noise. These observations, coupled with the fact that patients who were of low birth weight show a much higher percentage of unexplained deafness compared with the general population, strongly suggest that the noise level within incubators, together with other trauma, such as that induced by drugs, to the cochlea, would be sufficient to cause deafness.

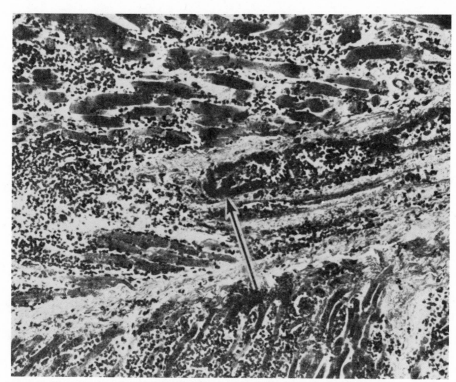

FIG. 14-1

Microscopic appearance of the damaged gracilis muscle in a premature baby who died 5 days after breech delivery. Damage to muscle fibers and hemorrhage of third degree. The vessel in the center of the figure (arrow) contains an adherent fibrin-positive thrombus. (Goldner's trichrome, ×85.) (From Ráliš, Z. A.: Birth trauma to muscles in babies born by breech delivery and its possible fatal consequences, Arch. Dis. Child. 50:4-13, 1975.)

TABLE 14-1

Severity of trauma in 86 breech-born babies: significance of prematurity*

	No injury (% cases)	Slight injury (% cases)	Severe injury (% cases)
Preterm babies	5	8	87
Term babies	4	54	42

*From Ráliš, Z. A.: Birth trauma to muscles in babies born by breech delivery and its possible fatal consequences, Arch. Dis. Child. 50:4-13, 1975.

COMMENT: The article by Ráliš is important in directing attention to the fact that what would appear to be superficial bruising of the lower part of the body may, in fact, represent massive hemorrhage in infants. Ráliš points out that one could expect this complication in its most severe form in the very low birth weight infant because soft tissues of the preterm baby would be particularly prone to direct trauma by apparently "minor" pressure

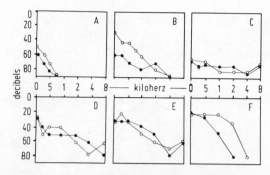

FIG. 14-2
Audiograms of six patients who had been of low birth weight. (From Douek, E., Bannister, L. H., Dodson, H. C., Ashcroft, P., and Humphries, K. N.: Effects of incubator noise on the cochlea of the newborn, Lancet 2:1110-1113, 1976.)

TABLE 14-2
Comparison of outer hair cell loss in 8 control and 8 experimental neonatal guinea pigs (Wilcoxon's rank sum test)*

Cochlear turn	% outer hair cell loss in control neonatal animals		% outer hair cell loss in sound-exposed neonatal animals		Probability
	Mean	SD	Mean	SD	
3½	1.1	±0.9	10.4	±6.0	< 0.01
3	0.8	±0.7	3.6	±3.3	< 0.01
2½	0.4	±0.4	2.3	±3.1	NS
2	0.3	±0.4	2.6	±2.6	< 0.05
1½	0.6	±0.7	1.4	±1.5	< 0.05
1	0.5	±0.8	1.9	±4.5	NS
½	0.03	±0.1	1.1	±2.8	NS

*From Douek, E., Bannister, L. H., Dodson, H. C., Ashcroft, P., and Humphries, K. N.: Effects of incubator noise on the cochlea of the newborn, Lancet 2:1110-1113, 1976.
NS: not significant.
SD: standard deviation.

and handling during delivery. The study presents a convincing case that massive hemorrhage and muscle destruction could trigger a clinical picture compatible with a crush syndrome and disseminated intravascular coagulation. Certainly it should stimulate further studies that attempt to document the degree of hemorrhage and muscle necrosis in all infants after breech delivery.

Douek et al. present convincing evidence of another kind of trauma imposed on newborn infants. This time the trauma is imposed by the environmental noise level within incubators and leads to traumatic deafness. Such studies are extremely important, not only in the impact they should have on incubator design but also in warning us of cumulative damage to specific organs such as the ear. If we superimpose on the trauma induced by noise that produced on neural tissue by various drugs frequently used in the nursery, the cumulative effect on hearing may be marked. Since a significant loss in hearing or vision acuity would certainly affect subsequent neurologic development in the child, one can see how we might ascribe subsequent neurologic handicaps to the wastebasket diagnosis of "complications of prematurity" without recognizing that these were entirely avoidable complications.

■ Hanson, J. W., and Smith, D. W.: The fetal hydantoin syndrome, J. Pediatr. **87:**285-290, 1975.

Five children born to women treated with hydantoin anticonvulsants for epilepsy are reported. The cases illustrate the broad involvement of many organ systems in the pattern of abnormalities seen in children exposed during fetal life to hydantoin anticonvulsants. The features of this syndrome, which occurred almost without exception in these five cases, included the following:

Motor or mental deficiency

Microcephaly

Postnatal growth retardation

Short nose with low nasal bridge

Hypertelorism

Low-set and/or abnormal ears

Hypoplasia of the nails and distal phalanges

Fingerlike thumb

Short or webbed neck ± low hairline

Additionally, the authors comment that they are aware of one set of dizygotic twins born to a woman taking hydantoin in whom many features of the syndrome appeared in both twins.

■ Hanson, J. W., Myrianthopoulos, N. C., Harvey, M. A. S., and Smith, D. W.: Risks to the offspring of women treated with hydantoin anticonvulsants, with emphasis on the fetal hydantoin syndromes, J. Pediatr. **89:**662-668, 1976.

This report presents data on the frequency of abnormalities that have been associated with fetal hydantoin syndrome. The clinical data were obtained from thirty-five children studied prospectively who were born to twenty-three women receiving hydantoin anticonvulsants during pregnancy. A second part of the study included a comparison of the findings in 104 children whose mothers were treated with hydantoins throughout pregnancy compared with a control group whose mothers neither had seizures nor received anticonvulsants during pregnancy. The control subjects were matched for socioeconomic status, age, race, and hospital of birth. These latter data were obtained from the Collaborative Perinatal Project of the National Institute of Neurological and Communicative Disorders and Stroke. The abnormalities found most frequently in the children exposed to hydantoins prenatally included:

Microcephaly

Ridging of the metopic suture

Inner epicanthic folds

Broad and/or depressed nasal bridge

Nail and/or distal phalangeal hypoplasia

As in the fetal alcohol syndrome (Jones and Smith: Recognition of the fetal alcohol syndrome in early infancy, Lancet **2:**999-1001, 1973; Greene: Infants of alcoholic mothers, Am. J. Obstet. Gynecol. **118:**713-716, 1974), there was evidence of prenatal growth retardation that involved body weight, length, and head circumference. The authors present data suggesting that the microcephaly is associated with some degree of mental retardation.

COMMENT: The fetal hydantoin syndrome and the fetal alcohol syndrome are similar in presenting a fairly broad spectrum of distortions in normal growth introduced by prenatal exposure to these drugs. As in the case in the fetal alcohol syndrome, both head circumference and body length have been proportionately reduced and in both syndromes the authors have made the suggestion that the microcephaly is associated with mental retardation. This suggestion is worth a cautionary note, however, principally in light of the experience now well-documented in the literature regarding long-term follow-up studies with infants showing the congenital rubella syndrome. In that disease as well, microcephaly had been associated with a reduction in intrauterine growth and intrauterine body length. However, the microcephaly was not associated with mental retardation, although that had been ascribed to the congenital rubella syndrome in the initial report. It is at least possible that the same will hold true for the disturbances of growth seen with the fetal alcohol and fetal hydantoin syndrome: that when head circumference and body length and weight are reduced, the implication to later mental development may not be as serious as microcephaly unassociated with a generalized retardation of growth.

Aspirin ingestion in pregnancy

■ Slone, D., Siskind, V., Heinonen, O. P., Monson, R. R., Kaufman, D. W., and Shapiro, S.: Aspirin and congenital malformations, Lancet 1:1373-1375, 1976.

This brief report presents the data on a retrospective review of 50,282 women and their children who were seen in twelve hospitals throughout the United States. The data were collected as part of the collaborative perinatal project. Aspirin was taken by 32,164 women; 14,864 women ingested aspirin during the first 4 lunar months of pregnancy, and 5128 of these women were classified as having "heavy exposure"; that is, they had taken aspirin for at least 8 days during this time period. For all pregnancies, there were 1393 major malformations, an incidence of 2.8%. No significant differences were found between the malformation rates in children heavily exposed during the first 4 lunar months of pregnancy when compared to children who were moderately exposed or children who were not exposed to aspirin at all. This study did not support one earlier report (Nelson and Forfar: Associations between drugs administered during pregnancy and congenital abnormalities of the fetus, Br. Med. J. 1:523-527, 1971) that found an increased incidence of congenital anomalies associated with maternal aspirin ingestion.

■ Shapiro, S., Siskind, V., Monson, R. R., Heinonen, O. P., Kaufman, D. W., and Slone, D.: Perinatal mortality and birthweight in relation to aspirin taken during pregnancy, Lancet 1: 1375-1376, 1976.

The same authors were unable to find any association of aspirin ingestion in pregnancy with an increased incidence of stillbirth, neonatal death, or reduced birth weight. In this regard, their findings conflict with the Australian study that documented an increased fetal wastage when pregnant women were ingesting much larger amounts of aspirin. That study was unable to evaluate the length of gestation or labor. Those potential complications of maternal aspirin ingestion related to its role as a prostaglandin synthesis–inhibitor could not be tested in this report of Shapiro et al.

TABLE 14-3

Fetal wastage: present + past pregnancies*

	Group 1	Group 2	Controls
Stillbirth rate†	58‖	24	12
Neonatal mortality rate‡	31	39	16
Perinatal mortality rate§	87‖	62	27

*From Turner, G., and Collins, E.: Fetal effects of regular salicylate ingestion in pregnancy, Lancet 2:338-339, 1975.
†Fetal deaths at 20 weeks' gestation or later (or birth weight greater than 400 gm) per 1000 total births.
‡Deaths within first 28 days of life per 1000 live births.
§Stillbirths—neonatal deaths per 1000 total births.
‖Significantly increased over controls (P < .01 and < .005, respectively).

■ Turner, G., and Collins, E.: Fetal effects of regular salicylate ingestion in pregnancy, Lancet 2:338-339, 1975.

This report consists of 146 infants born to 144 mothers who had reported taking salicylates during pregnancy. In the sixty-four infants who were born to mothers taking salicylates daily a significant decrease was found in birth weight of approximately 300 gm (mean birth weight of 3283 gm at term). There was no significant decrease in birth weight in the eighty-two infants whose mothers were taking salicylate at least once a week. Despite an increase cord blood salicylate concentration in many of the infants, no clinical evidence was found of bleeding or hypoglycemia nor any increased incidence of congenital anomalies. Table 14-3 presents the data on fetal and neonatal mortality rates among the controls and two groups of patients. Only the stillbirth rate was significantly increased over the control group. This increase occurred in the patients whose mothers were taking salicylate daily. There was no significant change in neonatal mortality rate. The preparations consumed in Australia included aspirin, salicylamide, caffeine, and phenacetin.

■ Collins, E., and Turner, G.: Maternal effects of regular salicylate ingestion in pregnancy, Lancet 2:335-337, 1975.

This study compared women who were taking salicylate preparations every day during pregnancy with a group of pregnant women who were intermittent users of salicylate (at least once a week) and with a control group of nonusers. These women were followed in the same antenatal clinics and were matched for age, parity, and gravity. All the women included in the study in both the experimental and control groups were from lower socioeconomic groups. Other factors (including smoking, which would have a higher frequency among the salicylate users, psychic stress, or family disruption) were not controlled between the experimental and control groups. The women who were chronically self-administering aspirin preparation were identified by urine testing of all prenatal patients with 10% ferric chloride solution. The maternal complications that were identified among regular salicylate takers included an increased incidence of anemia, antepartum and postpartum hemorrhage, prolonged gestation, complicated deliveries, and an increased perinatal mortality. The preparations consumed in Australia included aspirin, salicylamide, caffeine, and phenacetin.

COMMENT: The role of aspirin ingestion during pregnancy in altering mortality rate or morbidity in the infants is not well-established by these additional clinical reports. If there

is any effect of maternal ingestion of aspirin early in pregnancy on fetal congenital anomaly rates, it is certainly not impressive. Similarly, the role of aspirin ingestion in late pregnancy on the progress of labor deserves further careful study. Collins and Turner confirm earlier reports that aspirin ingestion is associated with prolonged gestation. This effect and that on the duration of labor may represent effects of aspirin as an inhibitor of prostaglandin synthesis. The higher perinatal mortality noted by Turner and Collins may reflect the continuous use of aspirin preparations in large amounts in contrast to intermittent use in the studies by Slone et al. and Shapiro et al.

Anesthesia and newborn behavior

■ Tronick, E., Wise, S., Als, H., Adamson, L., Scanlon, J., and Brazelton, T. B.: Regional obstetric anesthesia and newborn behavior: effect over the first ten days of life, Pediatrics 58:94-100, 1976.

This study describes the behavioral characteristics of a group of newborn infants evaluated by the Neurobehavioral Examination of Scanlon and the Neonatal Behavioral Assessment Scale of Brazelton. The infants were studied within the first 12 hours after birth and on days 1 through 10 of postnatal life. The behavioral state of the infant was compared with the obstetric anesthesia that the mothers received. The data were carefully controlled

TABLE 14-4

The eight drug groups in the study and the circulating anesthetic drug levels in the neonates*

Group	Medication	Number of subjects	Mean umbilical cord level	24-hour heel-stick level
Minimal drug groups				
1	No medication at all	6	—	—
2	Lidocaine spinal only (within 1 hour of delivery; no premedication)	4	0.10 µg/ml	0.04 µg/ml
3	Lidocaine local (just prior to delivery for episiotomy; no premedication)	10	0.00 µg/ml	0.04 µg/ml
Analgesic groups				
4	Alphaprodine and/or promazine ≤ 60 mg total	4	—	—
5	Alphaprodine and/or promazine ≤ 60 mg total and lidocaine spinal as in group 2	7	0.04 µg/ml	0.00 µg/ml
6	Alphaprodine and/or promazine ≤ 60 mg total and lidocaine local as in group 3	9	0.63 µg/ml	0.01 µg/ml
Epidural groups				
7	Mepivicaine or lidocaine epidural within 4 hr of delivery	10	1.58 µg/ml of mepivicaine; 0.55 µg/ml of lidocaine	0.46 µg/ml of mepivicaine; 0.05 µg/ml of lidocaine
8	Mepivicaine or lidocaine epidural within 4 hr of delivery and alphaprodine and/or promazine as in group 4	4	—	—

*From Tronick, E., Wise, S., Als, H., Adamson, L., Scanlon, J., and Brazelton, T. B.: Regional obstetric anesthesia and newborn behavior: effect over the first ten days of life, Pediatrics 58: 94-100, 1976.

for other factors that may occur during delivery, altering behavioral state, such as any abnormalities of parturition. With the moderate obstetric anesthesia used in this study (Table 14-4), effect on newborn behavior was minimal. There were few significant behavioral changes in the infants following local anesthesia or analgesic premedication.

COMMENT: This study provides strong support for a clinical observation apparent to all who work in high-risk obstetric services: that obstetric anesthesia, when well-done and carefully controlled, presents no risk to the infant, nor need it interfere in any significant way with initial parenting and contact with the infant soon after birth. In the current wave of enthusiasm among health professionals to encourage "natural" childbirth, one should be careful not to impart guilt feelings to parents who elect other support during labor and delivery. Careful obstetric anesthesia implies no additional hazard to the fetus.

Exposure to organic chemicals

■ Hillman, L. S., Goodwin, S. L., and Sherman, W. R.: Identification and measurement of plasticizer in neonatal tissues after umbilical catheters and blood products, N. Engl. J. Med. **292:**381-386, 1975.

This study presents data on the concentrations in neonatal tissues of a plasticizer frequently utilized in polyvinyl tubing in current medical use. The plasticizer, di-(2-ethylhexyl) phthalate (DEHP), was identified by gas chromatography mass spectrometry. The study was carried out principally on left ventricular tissue from the heart, although a few observations on tissue from the gastrointestinal tract were also made. Seventeen infants who had umbilical catheterization with or without the administration of protein-containing solutions were compared with thirteen stillborn infants or older control infants. The concentrations of DEHP in the left ventricular tissue were significantly higher than in tissue from the control groups of infants. Similarly the concentrations of DEHP in gastrointestinal tissue from three infants with enterocolitis were significantly higher than tissue obtained from three infants without neonatal entercolitis.

■ Dowty, B. J., and Laseter, J. L.: The transplacental migration and accumulation in blood of volatile organic constituents, Pediatr. Res. **10:**696-701, 1976.

This study used the very sensitive analytical technique of gas chromatography combined with mass spectrometry to obtain a chemical profile on maternal and umbilical cord blood samples. Eleven pairs of maternal and umbilical cord blood samples were obtained from term pregnancies at the time of vaginal delivery. All infants were normal by physical examination except for one with a lumbosacral meningomyelocele. This descriptive study of some trace organic compounds in the blood of the mother and newborn infant revealed the presence of a number of halogenated hydrocarbons and components of plastics, including xylene and styrene. Some of the compounds were present in higher concentration in the umbilical cord blood compared to the maternal blood samples. Acetone was present in most of the maternal cord blood pairs and was in extremely high concentration in the one infant with a lumbosacral meningomyelocele. The presence of such compounds as dichloromethane, chloroform, benzene and carbon tetrachloride, methyl ethyl ketone, and methyl cyclopentane raised questions concerning tissue toxicity, particularly liver toxicity, and potential carcinogenic or teratogenic effects.

COMMENT: The study by Hillman et al. continues the documentation that DEHP will leach out of polyvinyl tubing, particularly when exposed to protein-containing solutions.

This was a major contribution by Jaeger and Rubin (Plasticizers from plastic devices: extraction, metabolism, and accumulation by biological systems, Science 170:460-462, 1970) when they first reported its potential accumulation in tissues. Following their initial report, Jaeger and Rubin presented a series of articles over the next four or five years that thoroughly documented the accumulation of this plasticizer in liver and other tissues when patients had received extensive transfusion of blood- or protein-containing solutions by way of polyvinyl tubing. The current study simply confirms this in infants who have been exposed to umbilical catheterization. It is still conjectural whether such exposure triggers any acute or chronic organ dysfunction or carries any significant morbidity to the patients.

The study of Dowty and Laseter presents the same dilemma in interpretation as do other more recent studies. The application of gas chromatography–mass spectroscopy to umbilical cord blood samples, for example, has shown that a large number of organic compounds can be identified in the umbilical cord blood. However, the technique of gas chromatography–mass spectroscopy provides a sensitivity that is several orders of magnitude greater than that of previous techniques. Further thorough investigation is necessary to determine the effects of exposure to trace amounts of such organic compounds on developing tissues of the fetus and newborn infant.

■ Beck, S. L., and Gavin, D. L.: Susceptibility of mice to audiogenic seizures is increased by handling their dams during gestation, Science **193**:427-428, 1976.

This study reports the effect of 50 mg of beta-2-thienylalanine given to the mother on the incidence of audiogenic seizures in mice 23 days after birth. During the course of the study it was found that all the mice born to mothers who had been handled during the pregnancy, and thus given a maternal stress induced by handling, had a higher incidence of audiogenic seizures than did a control group who were not handled. This applied equally to the group treated with β-2-thienylalanine or solvent or sham injection.

COMMENT: The authors note that a psychic stress such as that induced by handling of the pregnant animals produces a variety of effects in the newborns after birth. They point out that other studies reported effects of handling pregnant animals on the newborn's behavior, body weight, or adrenal function. Handling pregnant animals may increase fetal or embryonic mortality. The importance of the observation is that it demonstrates the caution that must be used in interpreting effects of prenatal manipulations on postnatal behavior and emphasizes the profound effect on perinatal biology of apparently minor stress of the pregnant animal.

■ Guerrero, R., and Rojas, O. I.: Spontaneous abortion and aging of human ova and spermatozoa, N. Engl. J. Med. **293**:573-575, 1975.

Data from 1980 basal body temperature conception charts were analyzed in relation to the time of insemination and the outcome of 965 pregnancies. Of these, 890 ended in term deliveries and seventy-five in spontaneous abortions. Fig. 14-3 demonstrates that there was an increased probability of abortion at both extremes away from the date of the temperature shift. There was a marked increase in the incidence of abortions when fertilization occurred with aging spermatozoa (indicated by insemination taking place 4 days or more prior to the day of the thermal shift) or with aging ova (that is, inseminations taking place 3 days after the thermal shift). The authors point out that aneuploidy is frequently described as a chromosomal abnormality associated with postovulatory overripeness in animals. Similarly, Mikamo (Anatomic and chromosomal anomalies in spontaneous abortion. Effect of the

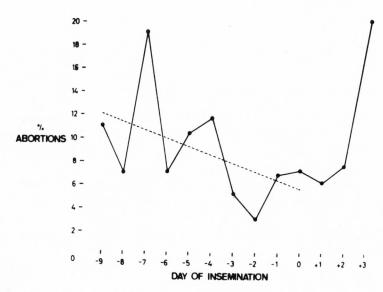

FIG. 14-3
Probability of abortion according to the day of insemination in relation to the day of the thermal shift in basal body temperature. The broken line represents a regression line fitted with the data from days −9 to 0. Observe the high probability for day +3. (From Guerrero, R., and Rojas, O. I.: Spontaneous abortion and aging of human ova and spermatozoa, reprinted by permission of The New England Journal of Medicine **293**:573-575, 1975.)

day of ovulation and the time of insemination, Am. J. Obstet. Gynecol. **106**:243-254, 1970) had shown an increased incidence of aneuploidy in human abortions.

COMMENT: This study demonstrates not only that postovulatory aging in human ova leads to aneuploidy, but also that it leads to postimplantation losses. Taken together with the previous studies such as that of Guerrero (Association of the type and time of insemination within the maternal cycle with the human sex ratio at birth, N. Engl. J. Med. 291: 1056-1059, 1974), which was reviewed in the first volume of *Perinatal Medicine* (pp. 21-22), this study would help explain a preponderance of males in human abortions, which has been frequently described. In addition, it raises questions about the basis for the effectiveness of the rhythm method in birth control. This study would suggest that some of the effectiveness of the rhythm method stems from the high spontaneous abortion rate of conceptions occurring at either end of the time spectrum from the time of ovulation.

Theophylline and phenobarbital in infants

■ Shannon, D. C., Gotay, F., Stein, I. M., Rogers, M. C., Todres, I. D., and Moylan, F. M. B.: Prevention of apnea and bradycardia in low-birthweight infants, Pediatrics **55**:589-594, 1975.

Theophylline was administered by nasogastric tube as a 10% alcohol elixir to seventeen low birth weight infants with apnea. The drug was given at 6-hour intervals in a dose of 4 mg/kg. Theophylline concentration was measured by a macrochemistry technique requiring 4 ml of blood, and thus only a 2-hour blood sample was obtained for theophylline concentration. Given in this dosage schedule in these seventeen infants, theophylline prevented all apneic spells greater than 20 seconds' duration and reduced the frequency of 10- to 20-second apneic episodes. No obvious complications were observed in the infants from the theophylline administration.

■ Uauy, R., Shapiro, D. L., Smith, B., and Warshaw, J. B.: Treatment of severe apnea in prematures with orally administered theophylline, Pediatrics **55:**595-598, 1975.

Twelve infants with apnea severe enough to be a major clinical management problem were studied; that is, infants who had two or more episodes of apnea of such severity to require assisted ventilation within 24 hours. Theophylline was given as a 20% alcohol solution in a dose of 4 ml/kg every 6 hours. In all infants there appeared to be a reduction in both the number of daily apneic episodes and in the number of episodes requiring assisted ventilation. No obvious complications were observed, although there was a significant increase in heart rate. No changes in serum glucose concentration or arterial pressure were found.

■ Aranda, J. V., Sitar, D. S., Parsons, W. D., Loughnan, P. M., and Neims, A. H.: Pharmacokinetic aspects of theophylline in premature newborns, N. Engl. J. Med. **395:**413-416, 1976.

Theophylline concentrations were measured in whole blood of six premature infants varying in gestational age between 25 and 32 weeks and in birth weights from 624 to 1200 gm. The infants were treated first with intravenous theophylline and then arterialized capillary blood samples were obtained beginning at time 0. Thereafter, blood samples were obtained frequently during the first hour, sporadically through the first 8 hours, and every 12 hours thereafter for 1 to 3 days. The half-life of theophylline in premature infants was markedly increased, the values being approximately nine times longer than those of children 1 to 4 years of age. The percentage of theophylline bound to plasma proteins was significantly lower in cord plasma than that in adult plasma; the mean values were 36.4% ± 3.8% for cord plasma and 56.4% ± 3.8% for adult plasma. Table 14-5 presents the information on plasma clearance and half-life of theophylline in three groups of patients.

■ Jalling, B.: Plasma concentrations of phenobarbital in the treatment of seizures in newborns, Acta Paediatr. Scand. **64:**514-524, 1975.

TABLE 14-5
Theophylline disposition as a function of age*†

Group	Age (range)	Number of subjects	Clearance (ml/kg/hr)	Half-life‡ (hr)
Premature infants	3-15 days	6	17.6 (12.1-25.9) §	30.2 (14.4-57.7)
Children	1-4 yr	10	100 (67-163)	3.4 (1.9-5.5)
Adults	23-79 yr	19	66 (29-124)	6.7 (3.6-12.0)

*From Aranda, J. V., Sitar, D. S., Parsons, W. D., Loughnan, P. M., and Neims, A. H.: Pharmacokinetic aspects of theophylline in premature newborns, reprinted by permission of The New England Journal of Medicine **395:**413-416, 1976.
†Calculations relating to premature infants based on blood concentrations; others on plasma concentrations.
‡Values refer to beta-phase half-lives.
§Range.

The plasma phenobarbital concentration was determined in eighteen infants during the neonatal period. All were being treated for overt or suspected seizures. Two of the eighteen infants were treated with repeated daily doses approximating 17.5 mg/kg/24 hr, which was the current routine on that nursery service. These two infants demonstrated that drug concentrations increased throughout the first 5 days of administration when daily administration was used. In the remaining sixteen infants a single intramuscular injection was given. The half-life of phenobarbital concentration was found to vary between 59 and 182 hours. Of even greater clinical significance was the fact that the phenobarbital half-life varied within the same infant from day to day. Thus, for seriously ill infants with seizures it was difficult, if not impossible, to construct a rational maintenance dosage; the physician could not be assured that phenobarbital concentrations were being maintained in a therapeutic range without determination of plasma phenobarbital concentrations. The frequency with which phenobarbital concentrations would need to be determined could not be defined in this study.

COMMENT: The articles of Shannon et al. and Uauy et al. present data demonstrating an effect of theophylline on the frequency and severity of apneic episodes. However, in neither study was a proper control group included. Since the incidence of apnea tends to decrease as infants get older, one is not certain to what extent the results represent increasing maturity or therapy over the 6 days the infants were treated. In neither study were careful measurements of blood levels of theophylline done, and no plasma clearance data were provided for the infants.

The much lower clearance rate and prolonged half-life of theophylline in preterm babies is evident in the report of Aranda et al. In addition, the data establish a variability among the six preterm babies of almost 400% to 500% in the theophylline half-life. A similar study from this same group of investigators (Parsons et al.: Elimination of transplacentally-acquired caffeine in full-term neonates, Pediatr. Res. 10:333 [Abst. No. 195], 1976) established similar findings for another related methylxanthine—caffeine. In that study, half-lives varying from 36 to 144 hours were found for caffeine in premature and newborn infants. From the studies on the prolonged half-life of both theophylline and caffeine, it would appear that deficiencies in the cytochrome P-450 mono-oxygenase complex in liver may be responsible for the slow metabolism of these related drugs.

Jalling's report emphasizes that plasma clearance varied tremendously not only for theophylline but also for phenobarbital and that this variability occurs even within the same infants from day to day. The wide range of plasma clearances obtained in infants of the same age makes it clear that a rational approach to the use of these drugs in prematures or older children requires frequent determination of blood concentrations.

Mercury levels

■ Wannag, A., and Skjaeråsen, J.: Mercury accumulation in placenta and foetal membranes. A study of dental workers and their babies, Environ. Physiol. Biochem. 5:348-352, 1975.

This study presents interesting data on the mercury levels in the placenta and in maternal and fetal membranes of two groups of pregnant women. One group consisted of nineteen women who worked in dental offices and were exposed in the course of that work to elemental mercury. A control group of twenty-six pregnant women unexposed to that environmental hazard were compared to this experimental group. At the time of delivery, blood samples were taken for analysis from the mother and baby, as well as tissue from the membranous portion of the placenta, including the chorion, amnion, and amniotic fluid, as well as from the main portion of the placenta. Mercury levels were measured by atomic absorption spectrophotometry. There were no differences in the mercury concentration in the blood of the mother and babies of exposed mothers compared to the control group. However, all the placenta tissues studied had an increased concentration of mercury compared with blood and plasma samples.

COMMENT: The observation that placental tissues, including the membranous portion of the placenta, accumulated mercury above the plasma concentrations was true for both the exposed and unexposed women. There was a significant elevation of mercury concentrations in the tissues of the placenta in the exposed group. Thus the study documented that blood samples from the mothers or the babies did not indicate increased exposure to mercury as an environmetal hazard. Furthermore, it demonstrated that, regardless of the degree of environmental exposure to mercury, the placental tissues accumulated mercury. This suggests that analysis of placental tissue may offer a more accurate reflection of total exposure during pregnancy to some toxins than does analysis of blood concentrations. Unfortunately, data on tissue concentrations of mercury for other fetal organs was not presented so that we cannot say at this point whether the placenta was acting as a barrier to the transfer of mercury to the fetus or whether it reflected an accumulation in mercury that occurred in other fetal tissues as well.

Congenital anomalies and drug ingestion

■ Safra, M. J., and Oakley, Jr., G. P.: Association between cleft lip with or without cleft palate and prenatal exposure to diazepam, Lancet 2:478-480, 1975.

The clinical data analyzed in this report were obtained from 278 histories of women who had delivered infants with selected major congenital anomalies. Table 14-6 taken from their report presents the list of congenital anomalies used for identification of the indexed cases. It also presents the data relating diazepam (Valium) ingestion in the first trimester to these various anomalies. Interviews were conducted 4 months after delivery of the affected infant. Table 14-7 demonstrates the fact that prenatal exposure to diazepam carried a fourfold increase in relative risk for cleft lip deformities, with or without cleft palate, compared to infants with all other defects who did not experience fetal exposure to the drug.

■ McLachlan, J. A., Newbold, R. R., and Bullock, B.: Reproductive tract lesions in male mice exposed prenatally to diethylstilbestrol, Science 190:991-992, 1975.

This study reports the outcome in twenty pregnant mice treated with approximately 100 μg/kg of maternal weight of diethylstilbestrol (DES) on days 9 through 16 of gestation. All the male mice that were delivered of the DES-treated mothers were sacrificed at 9 to 10 months of age and examined for lesions of the reproductive tract. Sixty percent of the males were sterile. Fifteen of the twenty-four animals were found to have testicular changes. A frequent lesion was a retained intra-abdominal testis firmly attached to the posterior pole of the kidney. Epididymal cysts and other testicular lesions were also present. The fibromuscular growths and nodular masses found in some of the male offspring of DES-treated mice are consistent with the anatomic locations of vestigial tissue of Müllerian duct origin. Thus these lesions found in the male offspring support the hypothesis offered for the lesions in females: that DES is affecting Müllerian duct tissue in the fetus.

TABLE 14-6

First-trimester diazepam use by mothers of children with various malformations (ascertained by interviews using drug sample card)*

Type of malformation	No.	Diazepam in first trimester		Relative risk†	χ^2‡
		No.	%		
All cases	278	16	6.1		
Neural-tube defects	57	1	1.8	0.25	1.28
CL ± CP	49	7	14.3	4.07	6.18
CP alone	20	1	5.0	0.85	0.12
Down syndrome	52	2	3.9	0.61	0.10
Esophageal atresia	9	1	11.1	2.12	0.00
Small-bowel atresia	8	0	0.0	0.00	0.00
Rectal and anal atresia	15	0	0.0	0.00	0.17
Omphalocele	17	0	0.0	0.00	0.26
Diaphragmatic hernia	10	0	0.0	0.00	0.01
Limb reductions	42	3	7.1	1.32	0.00

*From Safra, M. J., and Oakley, Jr., G. P.: Association between cleft lip with or without cleft palate and prenatal exposure to diazepam, Lancet 2:478-480, 1975.
†By comparison to all other interviews.
‡Chi-square with Yates' correction and 1 degree of freedom.

TABLE 14-7

First-trimester diazepam exposure: mothers of infants with CL ± CP vs mothers of infants with other serious malformations (controls)*

Com- parisons†	Cases CL ± CP		Controls		Relative risk	95% confidence interval of relative risk
	Exposed	Unexposed	Exposed	Unexposed		
1	7	42	9	220	4.1	1.5-11.5
2	6	38	9	220	3.9	1.3-11.6
3	6	30	9	220	4.9	1.6-14.7
4	6	29	9	162	3.7	1.2-11.2
5	6	25	9	162	4.3	1.4-13.2

*From Safra, M. J., and Oakley, Jr., G. P.: Association between cleft lip with or without cleft palate and prenatal exposure to diazepam, Lancet 2:478-480, 1975.
†(1) Includes data from all interviews with drug sample card; (2) excludes 5 interviews of mothers of infants with CL ± CP associated with trisomy D; (3) further excludes 8 interviews because infants with CL ± CP had other major malformations; (4) includes only white members of comparison 2; and (5) includes only white members of comparison 3.

■ Herbst, A. L., Poskanzer, D. C., Robboy, S. J., Friedlander, L., and Scully, R. E.: Prenatal exposure to stilbestrol: a prospective comparison of exposed female offspring with unexposed controls, N. Engl. J. Med. **292:**334-339, 1975.

This study presents the results of gynecologic examinations that were carried out in a group of women who had been exposed prenatally to DES. All the women were 18 years of age or older. The group of infants was compared with a control group of unexposed female infants who were born on the clinic service of the hospital closest in time to each exposed female infant. Table 14-8 taken from their report demonstrates that the women

TABLE 14-8

Results of pelvic examinations*

Group	Number examined	Failure of part of vagina to stain with iodine (%)	Vaginal adenosis identified in biopsy specimen (%)†	Failure of part of cervix to stain with iodine (%)	Cervical erosion identified in biopsy specimen (%)†	Vaginal or cervical fibrous ridges (%)
Exposed	110	56	35	95	85	22
Control	82	1	1	49	38	0
Chi-square		64.8	33.4	52.5	47	20.4
p value		< 0.0001	< 0.0001	< 0.0001	< 0.0001	< 0.0001

*From Herbst, A. L., Poskanzer, D. C., Robboy, S. J., Friedlander, L., and Scully, R. E.: Prenatal exposure to stilbestrol: a prospective comparison of exposed female offspring with unexposed controls, reprinted by permission from The New England Journal of Medicine 292: 334-339, 1975.

†Biopsies taken from areas that appeared red or failed to stain with iodine solution.

who were exposed prenatally to DES had a markedly increased incidence of a variety of changes in the cervix and vagina. It illustrates the impact of prenatal exposure to DES on the reproductive tissues of the fetal birth canal and points out that this occurred in a high frequency (that is, abnormal vaginal mucosa was seen in 56% of the exposed women). These changes in the reproductive tissues of the birth canal did not produce significant clinical problems, since no significant difference in health histories of the mothers in each group were found.

COMMENT: The report of Safra and Oakley confirms the association of the ingestion of benzodiazepine in the first trimester with an increased risk of cleft lip, with or without cleft palate. The first report was presented by Saxén and Saxén (Association between maternal intake of diazepam and oral clefts, Lancet 2:489, 1975). A previous study covered in volume 1 of *Perinatal Medicine* (p. 65) reviewed the first trimester ingestion of meprobamate and chlordiazepoxide (Librium) and the incidence of major congenital anomalies. The earlier report found no association between the ingestion of chlordiazepoxide and an increased incidence of cleft lip or palate. Thus, if diazepam has a teratogenic effect leading to an increased incidence of cleft lip and/or palate, it does not seem to be associated with the broad group of drugs, the benzodiazepines. The authors are careful to point out that this study does not establish a causal relationship between diazepam and cleft lip or palate. Furthermore, even if the increased risk is established, the risk would be in the order of 0.4% against a 2% background risk for major congenital defects.

The report by Herbst et al. continues the studies relating prenatal exposure to stilbestrol to later development. It illustrates the very general impact this drug had on reproductive tissues. McLachlan et al. demonstrates that this broad impact on reproductive tissues is not confined to females, but produced dystrophic changes in male reproductive tissues as well.

CHAPTER 15

Complications of intensive care

■ Gassner, C. B., and Ledger, W. J.: The relationship of hospital-acquired maternal infection to invasive intrapartum monitoring techniques, Am. J. Obstet. Gynecol. **126**:33-37, 1976.

The authors studied 5240 patients who delivered at Women's Hospital, Los Angeles County–University of Southern California Medical Center, from March 1 through August 31, 1973. The cesarean section rate for the monitored patients was 15.3% and for the unmonitored patients 7.4%. The hospital-acquired infection rate in those patients undergoing a cesarean section who were monitored was 40.4% and in those not monitored who had a cesarean section 20.4%. In those patients who had a vaginal delivery who were monitored, the infection rate was 2.7%, and in the nonmonitored 1.4%. Both differences were statistically significant. The investigators also examined the concept that the duration of monitoring would have an effect on the incidence of infection; as Fig. 15-1 shows, this was not the case.

■ Campbell, H., and Turnbull, A. C.: Use of oxytocin and incidence of neonatal jaundice, Br. Med. J. **2**:116-118, 1975.

The records of 11,192 infants and mothers were examined. The records were divided into three categories: (1) those mothers whose labors were either accelerated or induced with oxytocin; (2) those whose labors were of spontaneous onset in which no oxytocin was given, and (3) those whose labors were induced by amniotomy. Jaundice was defined as a plasma bilirubin in the infant of 10 mg/dl or greater. In the infants whose mothers had received oxytocin, the incidence of neonatal jaundice was 12.4% and in the spontaneous labor group it was 8.1%. This difference was significant. The authors then looked at various factors that might affect neonatal jaundice, such as birth weight, Apgar score, length of labor, and method of feeding. The significantly higher incidence of jaundice persisted in infants weighing over 3500 gm, those who had an Apgar score of 7 or greater, and those whose gestational age was greater than 36 weeks. There was no significant difference in the length of labor in the first two groups. There was an increased incidence of jaundice in those mothers who breast-fed and received oxytocin compared to those who breast-fed and did not receive oxytocin.

COMMENT (Campbell and Turnbull): **The investigators examined the majority of the factors that might be responsible for the increased jaundice in the infants of patients receiving oxytocin, such as hypoxia examined by Apgar score at birth and gestational age, and have found that oxytocin itself does seem to play a major role in the onset of this neonatal jaundice. The etiology of this neonatal jaundice at present must remain obscure; however, it would be most interesting to see if the same type of findings occur when labor is induced with prostaglandin, perhaps implicating the induction of the labor rather than the drug itself.**

■ Gassner, C. B., and Paul, R. H.: Laceration of umbilical cord vessels secondary to amniocentesis, Obstet. Gynecol. **48**:627-630, 1976.

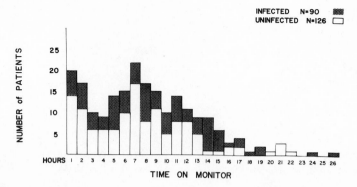

FIG. 15-1

Length of time of internal monitoring and the number of women with or without infection who delivered by cesarean section. Each bar represents the total number of women monitored for that time interval. For example, the bar above hour *1* represents the total number of women monitored for 1 hour or less, the bar above hour *2* represents the total number of women who were monitored for an interval of 1 to 2 hours. (From Gassner, C. B., and Ledger, W. J.: The relationship of hospital-acquired maternal infection to invasive intrapartum monitoring techniques, Am. J. Obstet. Gynecol. **126:**33-37, 1976.)

The authors report three cases of umbilical cord laceration as a complication of amniocentesis. Of these three and six additional cases previously reported in the literature, there were six live births delivered following this complication and three fetal deaths. Two deaths were associated with bloody taps and a third had blood fluid on amniotomy 7 hours after amniocentesis. There was no evidence of abnormal fetal heart tones. In one of the three, indirect fetal heart rate was judged to be normal for 5 hours after amniocentesis.

COMMENT: In the presence of bloody amniotic fluid, the source of blood should be determined by an Apt or Kleihauer-Betke test. If it is fetal blood, continuous fetal heart rate monitoring should be done. If the fetal heart rate shows a persistent bradycardia, immediate delivery should be performed. If the fetal heart rate is normal and the baby is mature, that is, greater than 35 weeks, it should be delivered; if it is less than 35 weeks, observation is indicated.

- Fernandez-Rocha, L., and Oullette, R.: Fetal bleeding: an unusual complication of fetal monitoring, Am. J. Obstet. Gynecol. **125:**1153-1155, 1976.

This is a report of a case of a patient who was admitted with a diagnosis of postterm gestation intrauterine growth retardation and premature rupture of the membranes. Labor was induced; an intrauterine pressure catheter was inserted with the use of a semirigid guide, and a scalp electrode was placed. The baby's heart rate slowed to 90, the baby was immediately delivered by cesarean section, and a significant tear of a fetal vessel was noted on the fetal surface of the placenta. Fetal hemoglobin and hematocrit were 13.9 gm/dl and 43, respectively.

COMMENT: The obstetrician placing an intrauterine catheter must remember that the catheter guide is relatively rigid and can cause penetration of the uterus or a tear of vessels in a placenta that is in the lower uterine segment. The catheter going through the guide into the uterine cavity is relatively flexible and should not be associated with either pene-

tration or tear. Although it is not specified in this article exactly what was responsible for the tear, the physician placing the catheter did state that he inserted the catheter guide well beyond he tip of his examining fingers. This should never be done. Another unusual complication has been reported: leakage of cerebrospinal fluid, this occurring after placement of the spiral electrode in the anterior fontanelle (Burnett et al.: Intra-amniotic urea as a midtrimester abortifacient: clinical results and serum and urinary changes, Am. J. Obstet. Gynecol. **121**:7-16, 1975).

■ Gottdiener, J. S., Ellison, R. C., and Lorenzo, R. L.: Arteriovenous fistula after fetal penetration at amniocentesis, N. Engl. J. Med. **293**:1302-1303, 1975.

The authors report a case in which the mother had undergone amniocentesis. At delivery the infant's right anterior chest wall had a penetrating wound in the sixth intercostal space. There was a systolic ejection murmur at the left sternal border. Angiocardiography demonstrated a branch from the thoracic aorta at the level of the tenth thoracic segment that joined the right lower lobe pulmonary vein.

COMMENT: This is an extremely unusual case; however, penetration of the fetus with a needle used for amniocentesis is not at all uncommon, and virtually every site in the fetus' body has been penetrated. Fortunately, in most instances there is little if any damage; however, it is important that the obstetrician take every precaution to prevent fetal penetration. The performance of amniocentesis under ultrasonic direction may help to reduce this type of injury.

■ Plavidal, F. J., and Werch, A.: Fetal scalp abscess secondary to intrauterine monitoring, Am. J. Obstet. Gynecol. **125**:65-70, 1976.

During the period under observation, 7200 patients were delivered. There were thirty-one cases of fetal scalp abscess found secondary to monitoring, or an incidence of one in 230 patients monitored—roughly four per 1000 cases. Of the twenty-nine abscesses cultured, ten had no growth; however, anaerobic cultures were not performed. The organisms cultured from these cases are seen in Table 15-1.

TABLE 15-1
Culture data*

Organism cultured	Number times cultured	Positive cultures (%)
Staphylococcus epidermidis	11	58
Staphylococcus aureus	1	5
Alpha-*Streptococcus*	2	10
Beta-*Streptococcus*	2	10
Enterococcus	1	5
Anaerobic *Streptococcus*	2	10
Aerobic gram-negative bacilli	3	15
Klebsiella	2	10
Proteus	1	5
Citrobacter	1	5
Diphtheroids	1	5
Candida (not *Albicans*)	1	5

*From Plavidal, F. J., and Werch, A.: Fetal scalp abscess secondary to intrauterine monitoring, Am. J. Obstet. Gynecol. **125**:65-70, 1976.

COMMENT: Scalp abscess is one of the more frequent complications of fetal monitoring, and yet even its incidence is extremely low. As noted in this article and as stated in a previous comment, the incidence from our own hospital is roughly four per 1000 cases. Some institutions have found a signficantly higher rate in the past (Winkel et al.: Scalp abscess: a complication of the spiral fetal electrode, Am. J. Obstet. Gynecol. 126:720-722, 1976). This seemed to be related to an electrode that is no longer on the market. Another unusual complication has been reported: leakage of cerebrospinal fluid, this occurring after placement of the spiral electrode in the anterior fontanelle (Burnett et al.: Am. J. Obstet. Gynecol. 121:7-16, 1975).

■ Gibbs, R. S., Listwa, H. M., and Read, J. A.: The effect of internal fetal monitoring on maternal infection following cesarean section, Obstet. Gynecol. 48:653-658, 1976.

The researchers examined puerperal morbidity in cesarean section patients divided into four groups: group I, those with no labor and no rupture of the membranes; group II, those with labor, but no rupture of the membranes; group III, those with ruptured membranes, but no internal fetal monitoring; and group IV, those with labor, ruptured membranes, and internal fetal monitoring. During the period of study, there were 4402 deliveries, of which 436 were by cesarean section. Of these 436 patients, 136 were excluded because of prior infection or prophylactic antibiotics, leaving 300 patients in the study. The results showed that patients without labor or ruptured membranes had the least infectious morbidity, those with labor but without ruptured membranes had a slightly greater morbidity than those who had ruptured membranes and labor. There was no difference in the patients who had ruptured membranes and labor in the infectious morbidity, regardless whether internal fetal monitoring was used. It was apparent in both groups III and IV that the highest incidence of morbidity was in those patients who had membranes ruptured longer than 12 hours. Standard morbidity was present in 51% of the group III patients and 44% of the group IV patients. Intrauterine infection was present in 43% of the unmonitored patients and 44% of the monitored patients. Antibiotics were used in 51% of the group III patients and 55% of the group IV patients. The incidence of bacteremia was 2.7% in the group III patients and 3.2% in the group IV patients.

COMMENT: The question of whether internal fetal monitoring contributes to postpartum endometritis and septicemia is an extremely important one. Considering its importance, that the literature presents conflicting reports is unfortunate. Wiechetek et al. (Puerperal morbidity and internal fetal monitoring, Am. J. Obstet. Gynecol. 119:230-233, 1974) can find no difference in postpartum morbidity among those patients who were monitored compared to those who were not. However, Larsen et al. (Intrauterine infection on an obstetric service, Obstet. Gynecol. 43:838-843, 1974) did find an increase in maternal morbidity following monitoring, and it is particularly interesting that their significant increase occurred when the duration of monitoring exceeded 8 hours. This did not seem to be borne out in the study by Gassner and Ledger. The study of Gibbs et al.—which does indeed attempt to get at the question of controls, albeit in a retrospective manner—does not seem to implicate internal monitoring in puerperal morbidity, but rather implicates the duration of rupture of the membranes. The duration of the ruptured membranes was not listed in the Gassner article; however, many of the monitored patients were monitored because they came into the hospital with ruptured membranes and were not in labor, which needed to be induced. Reason dictates that introducing a catheter through the vagina into the amniotic cavity would lead to some increase of infection. However, until a truly randomized control study is performed, the answer will not be completely known.

CHAPTER 16

Fetal and neonatal infection

■ Listwa, H. M., Dobek, A. S., Carpenter, J., and Gibbs, R. S.: The predictability of intra-uterine infection by analysis of amniotic fluid, Obstet. Gynecol. **48:**31-34, 1976.

The authors studied ninety-five patients who delivered vaginally at Walter Reed Army Medical Center in Washington, D.C. One hundred forty-three specimens of amniotic fluid were aspirated, and the uncentrifuged fluid was examined by Gram's stain and Wright's stain. Fifty-three samples from the first thirty patients were cultured for anaerobic and aerobic bacteria. Six patients fulfilled the criteria for infection. Positive evidence of infection included bacteria seen on Gram's stain during 2 minutes of searching or bacteria growing in the culture. Of the six, four were monitored for less than 8 hours and two were monitored for more than 8 hours. Thirty of the ninety-five patients had at least one amniotic fluid specimen with more than 1 polymorphonuclear neutrophil per high-powered field. Only three of the thirty became infected. Of the forty-nine patients who had amniotic fluid that was positive for bacteria on Gram's stain, only three showed intrauterine infection. Three of forty-six patients without bacteria on Gram's stain became infected. Microorganisms were grown in fifty of fifty-five specimens cultured from thirty-one patients; only two of these thirty-one patients became infected.

COMMENT: This study as well as another by Bobitt and Ledger (Quantitative analysis of amniotic fluid in the evaluation of obstetric infections, Obstet. Gynecol. [in press]) demonstrated the lack of predictability of white cells in the amniotic fluid as an indication of infection. This is unfortunate, since the early diagnosis of amnionitis may lead to the prevention of needless fetal death as well as serious maternal morbidity. It would appear that the only characteristic showing positive correlation with infection is the presence of bacteria either by culture or Gram's stain. The latter is more clinically useful because culture results are only returned well after some definitive action has been taken. Bacteria can be seen on an unspun specimen of amniotic fluid that has been Gram's stained.

The other methods of determining intrauterine infection, such as maternal febrile condition, tenderness of the uterus, and fetal tachycardia, are all important signs that should be frequently monitored in the patient who has premature rupture of the membranes.

■ Hanshaw, J. B., Scheiner, A. P., Moxley, A. W., Gaev, L., Abel, V., and Scheiner, B.: School failure and deafness after "silent" congenital cytomegalovirus infection, N. Engl. J. Med. **295:**468-470, 1976.

The investigators collected cord blood serum from all infants born at Strong Memorial Hospital, Rochester, New York, from 1967 through 1970. They were tested for antibodies to cytomegalovirus. Each cytomegalovirus IgM–positive infant was tested when between 3.5 and 7 years of age for developmental assessments. During that time period 9001 infants were born; 8644 of them were tested. Of these, fifty-three were positive. Five children could not be evaluated because the parents refused participation in the study, and two could not be located. Forty-four children were tested and an equal number of randomly chosen and matched controls were examined. The intelligence quotient of the children who were positive for cytomegalovirus was significantly lower than that of the controls. All seven children with an IQ of less than 79 were in the IgM-positive group. The majority, 68% of the positive group, came from families of low socioeconomic status. Only one of the cytomegalovirus IgM–positive children had neonatal symptoms suggestive of congenital infection. There was a significantly greater incidence of hearing loss in the cytomegalic-positive children compared to the controls.

COMMENT: This excellent article vividly points out a serious disease that may be responsible for some of the retarded children whose conditions were formerly attributed to hypoxia. There are undoubtedly other situations that we now classify as hypoxic brain damage that may be due to other causes.

■ Monif, G. R., Daicoff, G. I., and Flory, L. L.: Blood as a potential vehicle for the cytomegaloviruses, Am. J. Obstet. Gynecol. **126:**445-448, 1976.

The researchers are testing the hypothesis that cytomegalic inclusion disease may be transmitted to a pregnant woman from a blood transfusion. Other sources previously demonstrated for the mother include hand-to-mouth dissemination and infection through semen, and for the infant infected breast milk. The patient population consisted of three sources: pediatric patients undergoing cardiovascular surgery, women of childbearing age requiring transfusion, and older postmenopausal women on the gynecology service at the Shand's Teaching Hospital, Gainesville, Florida. Each patient's blood was treated before and after transfusion for presence of complement-fixing antibodies for cytomegalovirus, and the bloods given were tested. The study population consisted of 207 patients. They were given 897 units of blood. Complement-fixing antibody of 1 to 8 or greater was determined in 14.8% of these blood units. Prior to the transfusion, 140 individuals in the study had no antibodies. Fifty-four of these received a unit of blood with an antibody titer of 1 to 8 or greater. Of these, thirteen developed seroconversion. Of the eighty-six who received blood that did not contain antibodies, only three developed seroconversion.

■ Evans, T. J., McCollum, J. P. K., and Valdimarsson, H.: Congenital cytomegalovirus infection after maternal renal transplantation, Lancet **1:**1359-1360, 1975.

The authors report a 23-year-old primiparous patient who had a renal transplant. Four years later she became pregnant while taking 50 mg of azathioprine and 15 mg of prednisone. She delivered a seemingly healthy female infant at 35 weeks of gestation after spontaneous onset of labor. The child had purpuric hemorrhages over the face, trunk, and limbs, which faded during the first few days of life. She had mild jaundice on the third day that persisted until the fifteenth day. Probably intrauterine infection was diagnosed. Cytomegalovirus was cultured from the infant's throat and urine on the sixth day and also from the mother's cervix postpartum. The child did not develop chorioretinitis. There were no skull calcifications, and her development was normal at age 35 months.

COMMENT: Here is yet another situation in which cytomegalovirus may develop. Fortunately, this child faired significantly better than many of the others, as discussed in Monif et al. However, the report by Evans et al., as well as the one on acquired cytomegalovirus infection derived from blood transfusion, emphasizes the fact that this infection must be kept in mind.

■ Sarff, L. D., McCracken, G. H., Schiffer, M. S., Glode, M. P., Robbins, J. B., Orskov, I., and Orskov, F.: Epidemiology of *Escherichia coli* K1 in healthy and diseased newborns, Lancet **1:**1099-1104, 1975.

This study reports colonization rates of *Escherichia coli* containing the K1 capsular polysaccharide in term infants and their mothers and in premature infants and their mothers. A strain of *E. coli* has been shown to be responsible for three fourths of the neonatal *E. coli* meningitis cases. The K1 strains were found in 20% to 40% of the rectal cultures from healthy infants, children, and adult women. Of the infants born to mothers known to be carrying *E. coli* of this strain, 66% were also positive for the organism, whereas 11% of infants born to K1 negative mothers were colonized. In the full-term infants over 90% of those who were going to be colonized had, in fact, acquired the colonization with *E. coli* K1 strains by the third day of life. In contrast, in the seventy-one premature infants who became colonized, only 45% were colonized by the end of the first week of life. In the term infants, not only did they acquire the organism shortly after delivery, but also there was an 80% likelihood that the same sera type of *E. coli* K1 would be found in the infant as that recovered from the maternal rectal culture.

COMMENT: This study demonstrates that there is a basic difference in the pathogenicity between *E. coli* K1 and other organisms producing meningitis in early infancy. Although other pathogens such as meningococci, *H. influenzae* type B, and pneumococci share certain characteristics with *E. coli* K1, such as the presence of an encapsulated polysaccharide, the other organisms are not found as frequently among infants. The high carrier rate for *E. coli* K1 in newborn infants—and the fact that, when present, they are the predominant organism identified on the rectal cultures—distinguishes them from the other pathogens capable of producing purulent meningitis in early infancy. Thus, in addition to the characteristics of the organism itself, one must look for host-immune mechanisms to explain the relatively low infectivity rate among the large proportion of colonized newborn infants.

■ Ledger, W. J., Gee, C. L., Pollin, P. A., Lewis, W. P., Sutter, V. L., and Finegold, S. M.: A new approach to patients with suspected anaerobic postpartum pelvic infections. Transabdominal uterine aspiration for culture and metronidazole for treatment, Am. J. Obstet. Gynecol. **126:**1-6, 1976.

The author's population consisted of twenty-five febrile postpartum women. All had delivered vaginally. Twenty were willing to accept a new diagnostic procedure of aspiration of the endometrial cavity transabdominally with an 18-gauge spinal needle. In nineteen of these women less than 1 ml of bloody material was obtained after aspirating through a 10 ml syringe. This material was plated. Seven of these patients had positive bacterial growth. All twenty-five women had standard endometrial cultures obtained transcervically. Twenty-two of these patients had positive cultures. Both anaerobes and aerobes were identified; the most common anaerobe was *Bacteroides*. All the patients were treated with 250 mg orally of metronidazole every 6 hours for 10 days. Twenty of the patients responded to this therapy. Five others needed additional antibiotics for response.

COMMENT: Metronidazole seems to be extremely effective in the eradication of anaerobic organisms, particularly *Bacteroides*. Since the drug has relatively fewer side effects than either chloromycetin or clindamycin, metronidazole may prove to be a valuable drug in the treatment of postpartum infection.

The transabdominal aspiration technique, although probably giving a more accurate

yield of the bacterial content of the endometrial cavity, has the potential disadvantage of increased reluctance on the part of the patient to accept an invasive procedure and making certain that one is in the endometrial cavity at the time of aspiration.

■ Whalley, P. J., and Cunningham, F. G.: Short term versus continuous antimicrobial therapy for asymptomatic bacteriuria in pregnancy, Obstet. Gynecol. **49:**262-265, 1977.

The investigators identified asymptomatic bacteriuria in 300 women. The first 200 were randomly placed in one of two treatment groups. The first treatment group was given short-term therapy. The patients were treated for 14 days with sulfamethizole or nitrofurantoin. The second group was given continuous therapy. These patients were treated for the duration of their gestation with either sulfamethizole or nitrofurantoin. After one course of short-term therapy, 65% of the women were abacteriuric for the remainder of their pregnancy. In the continuous therapy group, 88% of the women had a sterile urine for the remainder of their pregnancy. Forty-seven, or 24%, of the women who were given short-term therapy initially became abacteriuric but relapsed within 2 weeks of completion of therapy. Two were not given further treatment, twenty-four remained abacteriuric following a second course of therapy, and five required a third course to eradicate bacteriuria. Sixteen women continued to relapse during their pregnancy. In three patients in the continuous therapy group bacteriuria persisted despite specific antimicrobial therapy. Of the eighteen patients in the short-term group with no response to initial therapy, one was not treated again, nine were cured with a second antimicrobial, one responded to treatment with a third, and seven continued to have persistent bacteriuria. Of the seven women in the continuous therapy group who did not respond, three became abacteriuric when a second drug was given and four demonstrated infection for the duration of gestation. The perinatal mortality rates and incidence of low birth rate infants were the same for both groups and did not differ significantly from the overall rate at the Parkland Memorial Hospital, Dallas, Texas.

COMMENT: Whether to use continuous or intermittent therapy in patients with asymptomatic bacteriuria has long been a controversial subject. This article would seem to indicate that intermittent therapy is reasonable; however, it does point out the importance of continuing to culture patients who have been treated with short-term therapy to make absoluely certain that their infection is eradicated and does not recur.

Asymptomatic bacteriuria does indeed lead to a higher incidence of pyelonephritis in pregnancy, and this is associated with a significant increase in perinatal mortality. Approximately 6% of all women had asymptomatic bacteriuria; thus it is important that cultures be performed on all pregnant patients at least once during their pregnancy and preferably at least once during each trimester.

■ Hemming, V. G., Overall, J. C., and Britt, M. R.: Nosocomial infections in a newborn intensive-care unit. Results of forty-one months of surveillance, N. Engl. J. Med. **294:** 1310-1316, 1976.

The authors studied 1161 infants admitted to the newborn intensive care unit at their hospital. Twenty percent were born in the hospital and 80% were transported from other hospitals. Among 904 infants discharged from the unit, 222 nosocomial infections were detected. The sites of infection were surface infection, 40.1%; pneumonia, 29.3%; bacteremia, 14%; surgical wound infection, 8.1%; urinary tract infection, 4.5%; and meningitis, 4%. The most commonly isolated agents were *Staphylococcus aureus,* 47.3%, and gram-negative enteric

TABLE 16-1

Nosocomial infections and mortality rates in the unit*

Datum	Number of infections	Number of infants	Deaths
No infection		766	104 (14%)
Total infections	222	138†	46 (33%)‡
Infection according to			
Body site			
Surface	89	86	13 (15%)
Pneumonia	65	58	15 (26%)
Bacteremia	31	28	11 (39%)
Surgical wound	18	16	4 (25%)
Urinary tract	10	9	5 (56%)
Meningitis	9	9	6 (67%)

*From Hemming, V. G., Overall, J. C., and Britt, M. R.: Nosocomial infections in a newborn intensive-care unit, reprinted by permission from The New England Journal of Medicine 294: 1310-1316, 1976.

†36 of the 138 infants had infection >1 body site; 14 had multiple infections at same body site.

‡21 of the 46 infants had infection at >1 body site; 1 infant had multiple infections at same site (three episodes of bacteremia).

bacilli, 45.1%. *Staphylococcus aureus* was the most common organism recovered from the skin and from patients with pneumonia. *E. coli* was frequently isolated from patients with bacteremia and those with urinary tract infections. *Klebsiella* was isolated in 7.7% of cases and *Pseudomonas* in 5.4%. Routine bathing of the infants with hexachlorophene was discontinued about midway through the study. Two staphylococcal skin abscesses were observed prior to discontinuing hexachlorophene bathing and twenty-six after. The infection rate was 4.2% in the first period of the study and 11.3% in the second period, a statistically significant difference. The infants with nosocomial infections had a significantly increased perinatal mortality. (See Table 16-1.)

COMMENT: This nosocomial infection rate is significantly higher than is reported in other areas of the same hospital by a factor of from three to twenty-four times. Obviously the babies in such a unit are significantly at risk for infection because of the very small size and the long hospitalization. The article points out vividly the marked difference that has occurred after discontinuing hexachlorophene bathing. In the absence of bathing the baby, the only logical answer is to make sure that all the personnel are meticulous in their hand care between infants. This seems to be the hardest job to accomplish in any nursery, particularly with the substitution of open radiant heaters for neonatal care instead of incubator care, a change that makes access to the baby much easier and thus increases the risk of a breach in hand-washing technique.

■ Lloyd, D. J., and Reid, T. M.: Group B streptococcal infection in the newborn: criteria for early detection and treatment, Acta Paediatr. Scand. 65:585-591, 1976.

These authors have examined the records of thirty-one newborn infants admitted to the special nursery of Aberdeen Maternity Hospital in Aberdeen, Scotland, from whom group B streptococci were isolated. The septicemia was associated significantly with a reduced birth weight (less than 2500 gm) and reduced gestational age (less than 37 weeks). There was also an association with asphyxia and a significant association with maternal pyrexia.

COMMENT: Since this is such a fulminant and fatal disease in the newborn, one must treat for disease in the newborn before or immediately after birth. A significant proportion of pregnant women have group B streptococci in their vagina, and the incidence of fetal injection is rather low; thus many newborns would be treated needlessly if all from positive mothers were treated. If only those infants whose mothers had no antibodies were treated, the magnitude of the needlessly treated newborns would be significantly smaller. The vaginal carriage rate for group B streptococci varied from 2.3% to 18%, and the authors point out in their article that during the period of the study the vaginal colonization rate in Aberdeen was 4.9%. The rate for an associated neonatal colonization was 1.9%. They have calculated the neonatal morbidity at 2.7/1000 and the neonatal mortality at 1/1000 births. This is comparable with other studies (Franciosi et al.: Group B streptococcal neonatal and infant infections, J. Pediatr. 82:707-718, 1973). In view of the fact that the vaginal colonization rate is so high in comparison to the relatively low neonatal morbidity and mortality rate, the question of treatment of all mothers with positive vaginal cultures arose. As the authors Lloyd and Reid point out, we are willing to screen for phenylketonuria, which has a much lower incidence (1/10,000), and so perhaps it would be logical to also do screening for this potentially lethal problem. Screening could take the form of vaginal cultures and antibody titers on all mothers in the last trimester of their pregnancy. If the vaginal culture is positive and the antibody titer is negative, the offspring of such mothers should receive therapy with penicillin, since the vast majority of these organisms are sensitive to penicillin. This would reduce the incidence of needlessly treated babies, yet protect those that are most at risk. If the baby is colonized, then one should begin prophylactic therapy with penicillin.

■ Baker, C. J., and Kasper, D. L.: Correlation of maternal antibody deficiency with susceptibility to neonatal group B streptococcal infection, N. Engl. J. Med. **294:**753-756, 1976.

Forty-one serum samples were tested; twenty-nine were from pregnant women at the Boston City Hospital who had type 3 strains of group B streptococcus isolated from the vaginal culture on one or more occasions during their pregnancy; seven from postpartum women at Jefferson Davis–Ben Taub Hospital in Houston, Texas, or Boston City Hospital whose infants contracted serious type 3 infections; and five out of the seven babies born to these women.

Antibody was considered to be present if the antigen-binding capacity of the serum sample was greater than 40%. Twenty-two of the twenty-nine women who had asymptomatic type 3 vaginal colonization had serum antibodies detected at a dilution of 1:2 or greater. Three neonates born to these women with antibodies showed antibody in their cord serum. None of the sera from the seven women delivering infected infants had antibodies, and the five babies' sera that were tested had no detectable antibodies.

■ Amstey, M. S., and Kobos, K.: An experimental model for disseminated herpesvirus infection of the neonate, Am. J. Obstet. Gynecol. **125:**40-44, 1976.

The author's model was CD-1 mice who were inoculated transvaginally during their pregnancy with herpes type 2 virus. Fifty-nine previously nonimmunized pregnant mice were inoculated vaginally. Of these, 40% died of overwhelming herpes infection, death occurring within 7 to 16 days. Virus was demonstrated in ten of the fifty-nine animals. Inoculation of twenty-six pregnant mice in the same way with culture medium free of virus produced no illnesses or death. Thirty-five nonpregnant mice were inoculated with the virus; one died, and the virus was not isolated from this animal, nor was there histologic evidence of infection.

Of the 309 newborn mice from mothers who were inoculated intravaginally with herpes type 2 virus, 45 died as a result of infection. Only three of 133 newborn mice died from unknown causes after having been delivered from mothers who were inoculated intravaginally with the virus-free culture medium. Two hundred mice were born to mothers who had been inoculated parenterally on the fifteenth day of gestation. Eight newborn mice died, and histologic evidence of virus was present in two animals. Of fifty adult mice that had been immunized subcutaneously with type 1 virus, nineteen survived and developed antibodies. Ten of these animals became pregnant and were inoculated with the virus-soaked tampons. These mice produced sixty-nine newborn, in which there were two deaths for unknown reasons. No virus was isolated from any of the neonates, all of whom were killed.

COMMENT (Amstey and Kobos): **This model would seem to shed light on the clinical fact that the majority of women with herpes in the vagina do not infect their newborns. A significant portion of the adult population (20%) has antibodies against herpesvirus. These antibodies, particularly the IgG, which may cross the placenta, could render the fetus protected during the labor and delivery process. If this is the case, it may be worthwhile to check mothers in the third trimester with a smear (Pap) for virus and to do antibody studies on those that are positive.**

■ Bolognese, R. J., Carson, S. L., Fuccillo, D. A., Traub, R., Moder, F., and Sever, J. L.: Herpesvirus hominis type II infections in asymptomatic pregnant women, Obstet. Gynecol. **48:**507-510, 1976.

This study consisted of 985 patients: 426 whites, 555 blacks, and 4 oriental. Venous blood was drawn in all three trimesters; cervical cultures were likewise taken in all three trimesters. The researchers also had amniotic fluids from 211 patients drawn for voluntary termination of pregnancy or obstetric indications. Sera from 352 patients revealed a predominance of type 2 antibodies. This followed the work of Rawls et al. (Measurement of antibodies to herpesvirus types 1 and 2 in human sera, **104:**599-606, 1969) which demonstrated that if the log of the antibody of titer of type 2 divided by the log of the antibody of titer of type 1 times 100 was 85 or greater, the patient had a type 2 infection. The bloods of 124 women did not contain both type 1 and type 2 antibodies from the sera, and 509 samples were identified as a type 2 over a type 1 index of 84 or less, indicating predominantly type 1 infection. The type 2 herpesvirus was isolated from cervical cultures done on 770 asymptomatic gravidas in first, second, and third trimester pregnancies. The incidence of antepartum infection type 2, virus in gravidas without herpetic lesions, was 0.065%. Of the patients who had a third trimester infection, two delivered before culture results were known, and one delivered by repeat cesarean section. None of the infants had disease. Four patients with a positive cervical culture had antibody available for determination. One demonstrated a type 2:1 index greater than 85, and the index was less than 85 in the remaining 3. Two hundred eleven amniotic fluid samples, obtained during the second and third trimesters by transabdominal amniocentesis, were cultured for herpesvirus infection and found negative.

COMMENT: Herpesvirus remains a significant and confusing problem in obstetrics. The disastrous consequences in an infected baby are well known to all. What is not known is the incidence of disease in women, and how often the patient who is asymptomatic delivers a baby who is infected with the virus. There is little doubt that the individual with active herpetic lesions in the vagina at term should be delivered and preferably by cesarean section. It has been pointed out (Nahmias et al.: Perinatal risk associated with maternal genital herpes simplex virus infection, Am. J. Obstet. Gynecol. 110:825-834, 1971) that if the membranes have been ruptured more than 4 hours, there is a significant risk that the child will develop herpesvirus infection even if cesarean section is done. Thus either the patient must be knowledgeable of the potential risk to the infant and come immediately to the hospital for cesarean section after rupture of the membranes or have an elective cesarean section at term.

- Speer, M. E., Taber, L. H., Yow, M. D., Rudolph, A. J., Urteaga, J., and Waller, S.: Fulminant neonatal sepsis and necrotizing enterocolitis associated with a "nonenteropathogenic" strain of Escherichia coli, J. Pediatr. 89:91-95, 1976.

This study documents an epidemic with a mucoid strain of *E. coli* in a newborn nursery. Study revealed a colonization rate of 14% with this nonendemic mucoid strain and an attack rate in colonized babies of almost 20%. In eight infants with proved infection, there was an 87.5% mortality and a high incidence of necrotizing enterocolitis. The sudden appearance of apnea, abdominal distention, and shock, followed by the other clinical signs of necrotizing enterocolitis, made this infection particularly striking. The investigators could not document the presence of heat-labile enterotoxin nor of intestinal invasiveness in this organism. In addition, the organism showed no evidence of K1 capsular antigen.

COMMENT: This study strongly suggested that particular organisms in the bowel flora may markedly increase the incidence of necrotizing enterocolitis and be unassociated with diarrhea. The fact that this occurred with an *E. coli* strain which was not producing enterotoxin and did not demonstrate particular invasiveness makes the finding more disturbing.

- Stoliar, O. A., Kaniecki-Green, E., Pelley, R. P., Klaus, M. H., and Carpenter, C. C. J.: Secretory IgA against enterotoxins in breast-milk, Lancet 1:1258-1261, 1976.

The investigators obtained breast milk 2 to 4 days postpartum from a group of twenty Guatemalan women and more milk 13 to 15 days postpartum from a separate group of twelve other Guatemalan nursing mothers. Milk was also obtained 15 to 30 days postpartum from a group of seven nursing mothers in Cleveland, Ohio. Colostrum completely inhibited cultures of *Vibrio cholerae* and *E. coli* enterotoxin. Breast milk also inhibited *E. coli* enterotoxin in relationship to the quantity of breast milk used. IgA was the predominant immunoglobulin found in highest concentration in the colostrum and in somewhat lower concentrations in the breast milk. IgM and IgG in breast milk and colostrum were extremely variable and did not correlate with the inhibition of enterotoxin. Some of the colostrum was fractionated into the globulins, and the IgA peak completely inhibited the cholera toxin.

COMMENT (Stoliar et al.): Pathology of the gastrointestinal system in the newborn infant, particularly the premature, has become a significant problem in recent years. The clinical observation has been made that the breast-fed infant is less likely to develop forms of enterocolitis than is the bottle-fed infant. This was believed to be on the basis of antibodies obtained through the colostrum and breast milk of the mother. This article would seem to place a solid, rational basis for that supposition, and again points out the importance of breast-feeding whenever that is possible.

■ Cederqvist, L. L., Francis, L. C., Zervoudakis, I. A., Becker, C. G., and Litwin, S. D.: Fetal immune response following prematurely ruptured membranes, Am. J. Obstet. Gynecol. **126:**321-327, 1976.

The authors have examined the sera, cord blood, and amniotic fluid from sixteen mothers with a history of premature rupture of the membranes. Their pregnancies were 33 to 41 weeks in duration. The fluids were examined for IgA, IgA_1, IgA_2, IgD, IgE, IgG, and IgM. Cord bloods in these patients compared with suitable controls showed a statistically significant increase in IgM, and a statistically significant decrease in IgD. There was a fivefold increase in the levels of IgA in the group with prematurely ruptured membranes compared to the controls. This was not a statistically significant difference due to the wide range of values found in the group with premature rupture of the membranes. The increased levels of IgA were found primarily in the IgA_1 group. There was no evidence that the duration of ruptured membranes or the duration of labor played any role in the degree of elevation of IgA and IgM.

COMMENT: It is interesting to note that no correlation was found between the duration of ruptured membranes or the duration of labor and the degree of elevation of IgA or IgM. One would expect just the opposite. On the other hand, since the fetus has to synthesize both IgA and IgM and the duration of rupture of the membranes is not given, it is quite possible that sufficient time had not elapsed between rupture of the membranes and delivery for synthesis. The fact that a patient with ruptured membranes for only 2 hours had the largest level of IgM may simply mean that there was some evidence of infection in that fetus prior to the onset of labor.

The fact that there was a fivefold increase in the level of IgA in the group with prematurely ruptured membranes could be interpreted to indicate that fetal infection is responsible for the premature rupture of the membranes.

■ Modlin, J. F., Herrmann, K., Brandling-Bennett, A. D., Eddins, D. L., and Hayden, G. F.: Risk of congenital abnormality after inadvertent rubella vaccination of pregnant women, N. Engl. J. Med. **294:**972-974, 1976.

The investigators have compiled information on 343 pregnancies complicated by inadvertent rubella vaccination. Of the 343 women, only 70 had hemagglutination inhibition serologic tests; before vaccination, all these seventy had titers of less than 1 to 10. There were 172 live-born infants, including thirty-eight from susceptible mothers. None of these infants had any evidence of congenital rubella infection or malformations attributable to rubella vaccine. Only passive antibodies were demonstrated in fifty-seven who had serologic testing. Fourteen spontaneous abortions and stillbirths did occur. (See Table 16-2.)

No virus was recovered from the products of conception in the two cases in which this was attempted. There were 145 therapeutic abortions and the products of conception were obtained in thirty-four cases. Twenty-eight of the women undergoing therapeutic abortion were susceptible to rubella. Rubella virus was isolated from gestational tissue in nine cases.

COMMENT: The article would seem to demonstrate that the risk of fetal malformation following inadvertent vaccination with rubella virus is slight indeed. However, the article

TABLE 16-2

Outcome of pregnancy for 343 women who received rubella-virus vaccine within two months before or during pregnancy*†

Rubella status before vaccination	Number of women	Outcome of pregnancy				Cases with virus isolated
		Therapeutic abortions	Spontaneous abortions or stillbirths	Live births	Outcome unknown	
Susceptible	70	28	3	38	1	6
Immune	14	1	0	13	0	0
Unknown	259	116	13	121	8	3
Totals	343	145	16	172	9	9

*From Modlin, J. F., Herrmann, K., Brandling-Bennett, A. D., Eddins, D. L., and Hayden, G. F.: Risk of congenital abnormality after inadvertent rubella vaccination of pregnant women, reprinted by permission from The New England Journal of Medicine **294:**972-974, 1976.
†129 cases followed by Center for Disease Control and 214 cases followed by other investigators.

does not give an exact incidence, as it cannot, for this possibility. It is estimated that there is certainly less than a 5% to 10% chance that the child will be damaged; however, even with this slight chance, we would feel that the patient still should have the option for therapeutic termination of the pregnancy if she so desires after understanding the relatively low chance for congenital malformation. Avoidance of vaccination during early pregnancy should be easier now with the beta subunit and receptor assays for human chorionic gonadotropin. This type of testing should be done in any individual considered for vaccination, and the patient should be told not to get pregnant for 2 months following the vaccination.

■ Schlievert, P., Johnson, W., and Galask, R. P.: Bacterial growth inhibition by amniotic fluid. V. Phosphate-to-zinc ratio as a predictor of bacterial growth–inhibitory activity, Am. J. Obstet. Gynecol. **125:**899-905, 1976.

The authors used human amniotic fluid at various stages of gestation. The fluid was obtained aseptically by transabdominal amniocentesis. Stages of gestation varied from 19 through 42 weeks. Fluid was subjected to ultrafiltration and the unfiltered fluid, ultrafiltrate, and retentate after ultrafiltration were checked for inhibitory activity against *E. coli*. Quantitative analyses of zinc and phosphate determinations were done. It was found that the zinc concentration in the amniotic fluid varied from 0.17 to 2.15 μg/ml, an average of 0.44 μg/ml. They demonstrated that the addition of 0.08 μg or more of zinc per milliliter of amniotic fluid added to noninhibitory control filtrates increased the antibacterial activity. The phosphate concentration in the same 22 amniotic fluids ranged between 14 and 200 μg/ml, with an average of 92 μg/ml. It was determined that the addition of phosphate decreased the inhibitory activity of amniotic fluid to *E. coli*. An ideal phosphate/zinc ratio was found to be 100 or less. In this instance bactericidal activity in the amniotic fluid was retained. Fluids with a phosphate/zinc ratio of 100:200 were bacteriostatic, and fluids with a phosphate/zinc ratio greater than 200 were noninhibitory. The minimum concentration of zinc in amniotic fluid that could be present and still have an inhibitory activity of the amniotic fluid was 0.08 μg/ml, but as stated previously, the phosphate/zinc ratio was also extremely important.

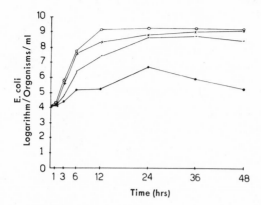

FIG. 16-1
Growth curves of *E. coli* in (●) amniotic fluid, (−) amniotic fluid plus brain-heart infusion
(BHI), (○) brain-heart infusion (control), and (×) Ringer solution (control). (From
Prevedourakis, C., Koumentakou, E., Zolotas, J., Zolotas, T., Xygakis, A., and Kotoulas, I.:
E. coli growth inhibition by amniotic fluid, Acta Obstet. Gynecol. Scand. **55**:245-248, 1976.)

■ Schlievert, P., Johnson, W., and Galask, R. P.: Bacterial growth inhibition by amniotic
fluid. VI. Evidence for a zinc-peptide antibacterial system, Am. J. Obstet. Gynecol. **125**:
906-910, 1976.

The investigators had previously demonstrated that zinc and phosphate were crucial in
the bacterial inhibition properties of amniotic fluid. Also, previous studies by Abelson and
Aldous (Ion antagonisms: interference of normal magnesium metabolism by nickel, cobalt,
cadmium, zinc, and magnesium, J. Bacteriol. **60**:401-413, 1950) found that the zinc concentration in a chemically defined medium needed to be 2 μg/ml for bacterial inhibition.
This was significantly higher than the 0.08 μg/ml found by the authors. In this study they
isolated what they believe is a protein (perhaps a polypeptide of a weight less than 10,000
daltons, possibly somewhere in the neighborhood of 5000 daltons) that is not a lysozyme but
is necessary for the bacterial inhibition of amniotic fluid at the reported levels of zinc and
phosphate.

■ Prevedourakis, C., Koumentakou, E., Zolotas, J., Zolotas, T., Xygakis, A., and Kotoulas, I.:
E. coli growth inhibition by amniotic fluid, Acta Obstet. Gynecol. Scand. **55**:245-248, 1976.

The authors are testing whether or not amniotic fluid will inhibit the growth of *E. coli*.
They have done so by collecting amniotic fluid samples from twenty-nine normal pregnancies
between the thirty-eighth and forty-first weeks of gestation. Samples were collected by amniocentesis either prior to vaginal delivery or at the time of cesarean section. *E. coli* organisms that had previously been cultured on nutrient agar were inoculated in 5 ml of brain-
heart infusion and incubated at 37° C for 18 hours. Aliquots of *E. coli* were added to
amniotic fluid, amniotic fluid enriched by brain-heart infusion, brain-heart infusion alone,
and Ringer's solution alone. Growth curves are available in Fig. 16-1 that demonstrate a
significantly slower growth of the *E. coli* in amniotic fluid and an inhibition of growth after
24 hours.

**COMMENT: It has been recognized for some time that amniotic fluid may be bacterio-
static. The work of Prevedourakis et al. would demonstrate that frequently the most common organisms found in this situation, *E. coli*, will grow in the amniotic fluid for 12 to**

24 hours, and then there seems to be a stasis of growth. The work of Galask and his colleagues in the articles by Schlievert et al. would seem to shed some light on the bacteriostatic property of the amniotic fluid. Their finding of a zinc/phosphate ratio that predicts the bacteriostatic property of the amniotic fluid is indeed significant. It is significant for the clinician in at least two ways: (1) If one could determine in individual cases with premature ruptured membranes that the amniotic fluid under consideration is bacteriostatic through its zinc/phosphate ratio, it may be significantly safer to let maturation of the fetus proceed in that situation, or conversely, if there are low bacteriostatic properties in the amniotic fluid, labor may need to be induced; (2) the second exciting part of this work is the potential ability to modify the bacteriostatic content of the amniotic fluid through a modification of the zinc/phosphate ratio either by diet or placing one or the other of these elements in the amniotic space.

- Shurin, P. A., Alpert, S., Rosner, B., Driscoll, S. G., Lee, Y. H., McCormack, W. H., Santamarina, B. A. G., and Kass E. H.: Chorioamnionitis and colonization of the newborn infant with genital mycoplasma, N. Engl. J. Med. 293:5-8, 1975.

The researchers studied 249 deliveries of live infants at Boston City Hospital. Vaginal cultures were obtained from forty mothers at the time of registration for prenatal care. During the 2 days after birth, duplicate vaginal swabs were obtained from 248 mothers. Placentas were obtained in 244 of the 249 cases. Placentas were analyzed for chorioamnionitis and graded on a scale from 0 to 3+. Cultures were obtained for *Mycoplasma hominis* and T mycoplasma. In the postpartum period, T mycoplasma was isolated from 62.1% and *Mycoplasma hominis* from 36.3% of the mothers. Cultures were also obtained for the same organisms from the infants born of these pregnancies. T mycoplasma was significantly associated with colonization of the newborn infant and the presence of placental chorioamnionitis, the T mycoplasma being isolated from the newborn infant in 37.5% of the cases with 2+ or 3+ inflammation of the placenta and only 19% of the cases with normal placentas.

COMMENT: Genital mycoplasma has been implicated in cases of spontaneous abortion (Driscoll et al.: Infections and first trimester losses: possible role of mycoplasmas, Fertil. Steril. 20:1017-1019, 1969), postpartum fever (McCormack et al.: Genital mycoplasmas in postpartum fever, J. Infect. Dis. 127:193-196, 1973), and chorioamnionitis (Caspi et al.: Amnionitis and T strain mycoplasmemia, Am. J. Obstet. Gynecol. 111:1102-1106, 1971). There has also been reported an increased fetal mortality rate in association with these organisms (Braun et al.: Birth weight and genital mycoplasmas in pregnancy, N. Engl. J. Med. 284:167-171, 1971). However, as has been pointed out in this article as well as others (McCormack et al.: Colonization with genital mycoplasmas in women, Am. J. Epidemiol. 97:240-245, 1973), these organisms are found very frequently in any population and in different locations in the body. Thus one needs to be extremely careful in choosing controls before making positive associations between various pathologic states and this organism; even if controls demonstrate a difference, it still may not imply a causal relationship.

- McCormack, W. M., Rosner, B., Lee, Y.-H., Rankin, J. S., and Lin, J.-S.: Isolation of genital mycoplasmas from blood obtained shortly after vaginal delivery, Lancet 1:596-599, 1975.

The authors obtained blood from 327 women within a few minutes after vaginal delivery. The blood was cultured for *Mycoplasma hominis* and T mycoplasma. Mycoplasma was isolated from the blood of 8%. Two of the ten women whose blood contained *Mycoplasma hominis* gave birth to stillborn infants. This is in contrast to only four stillborn infants among the 301 women whose blood did not contain mycoplasma.

■ Tafari, N., Ross, S., Naeye, R. L., Judge, D. M., and Marboe, C.: Mycoplasma T strains and perinatal death, Lancet **1**:108-109, 1976.

In this study the researchers have demonstrated the presence of mycoplasma T strain in the placenta and lungs of newborn infants who were stillborn or who died within 3 days of birth in Addis Ababa, Ethiopia. Samples were taken from the lungs of 290 such infants; forty-two (14.5%) had mycoplasma T strains grown from their lungs in the postmortem period. In twenty-four of the forty-two, T strains were the only organism. Sixteen of the twenty-four had organisms also located in the placenta. Late gestational examination of maternal urinary sediment did not reveal urinary tract infection in these mothers. Infants who had only T strain mycoplasma had congenital pneumonia and chorioamnionitis, with one exception. None of the mothers of these infants had ruptured their membranes prior to the onset of labor. Fourteen pregnancies (4.8%) had T strains grown from both placenta and lung; eleven of these had evidence of chorioamnionitis. T strains were grown from only 4 (2.7%) of successful pregnancies.

■ Monif, G. R., and Baer, H.: Polymicrobial bacteremia in obstetric patients, Obstet. Gynecol. **48**:167-169, 1976.

A series of septic patients was studied at the University of Florida at Gainesville from April, 1972, through April, 1975. There was septicemia in fifty-nine obstetric patients. In thirteen of these, more than one bacteria was concomitantly isolated from at least one set of blood culture bottles. Cultures had been done in thiol broth placed in two bottles, one of which was used for anaerobic and the other for aerobic cultures. The organisms most commonly isolated in these thirteen cases of polymicrobial bacteremia were *Hemophilus vaginalis* and the anaerobic streptococci and Bacterideaceae.

COMMENT (Monif and Baer)**: This article points out the importance of rigorous culture for anaerobic organisms in patients suspected of having sepsis. It also points out the fact that in roughly one fourth of the patients with septicemia both aerobes and anaerobes may be present. The most common anaerobic organisms demonstrated throughout obstetrics and gynecology septicemia is** *Bacteroides,* **which was again demonstrated in this article.**

■ Christensen, K. K., Christensen, P., Ingemarsson, I., Mardh, P., Nordenfelt, E., Ripa, T., Solum, T., and Svenningsen, N.: A study of complications in preterm deliveries after prolonged premature rupture of the membranes, Obstet. Gynecol. **48**:670-677, 1976.

The authors established a procedure in their hospital from October, 1974, through October, 1975, of treating all patients who had premature rupture of the membranes prior to the thirty-sixth week and a cervix that was dilated less than 4 cm with bed rest and terbutaline, a beta sympathomimetic agent. The patients were delivered after the beginning of the thirty-sixth week unless infection supervened. No antibiotics were given prior to delivery. There were twenty-six newborn patients delivered from twenty-four pregnant women. The mean length of pregnancy after premature rupture of the membranes was 10 days and 2 hours; five patients went longer than 2 weeks. The overall incidence of premature rupture of the membranes was 0.7%. Only one patient needed to be delivered because of infection, two others showed signs of endometritis postpartum, one had a *Bacteroides* septicemia, one baby died from probable neonatal infection, and two infants died of other causes.

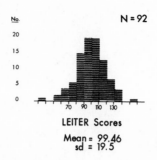

FIG. 16-2
Distribution of intelligence in rubella syndrome. (From Macfarlane, D. W., Boyd, R. D., Dodrill, C. B., and Tufts, E.: Intrauterine rubella, head size, and intellect, Pediatrics 55:797-801, 1975.)

COMMENT: These authors have tried to approach the problem of premature rupture of the membranes with pregnancy prolongation by using beta sympathomimetic agents; although their results were relatively good in that they had small numbers of infections, one must realize that they were dealing with a well-nourished Scandinavian population. Similar results might not be obtained in populations in the low socioeconomic group with which many health professionals in this country have to deal. The interesting clinical paradox that has frequently been observed between the higher socioeconomic group of patients and the low socioeconomic group in terms of their susceptibility to amnionitis following premature rupture of the membranes may indeed be explained on the basis of some of the fundamental studies done by Galask and co-workers, which were commented on earlier in this chapter in the two articles by Schlievert et al.

■ Macfarlane, D. W., Boyd, R. D., Dodrill, C. B., and Tufts, E.: Intrauterine rubella, head size, and intellect, Pediatrics 55:797-801, 1975.

This study reports on the relationship of IQ and head circumference to stature in ninety-two children who had had congenital rubella. The ninety-two children were obtained from a rubella clinic population of 111 children and included only those with vision sufficient to allow testing. Fig. 16-2 taken from their report shows that the mean IQ was 99.4 with a normal distribution. This is similar to the observation of Sheridan (Final report of a prospective study of children whose mothers had rubella in early pregnancy, Br. Med. J. 2:536-539, 1964), who also found an average IQ within the normal range in her study of 191 children who had prenatal rubella infection. Fig. 16-3 from the study by Macfarlane et al. presents the data that show the relationship between head circumference and stature relative to parental size.

COMMENT: This study demonstrates that the children with small head circumferences were also children who had experienced a reduction in their height. No correlation was found between IQ and head circumference. The authors emphasized the dangers in equating "microcephaly" with mental retardation. They stress the fact that children with congenital rubella are frequently delayed and educationally handicapped by their defects in hearing or vision; however, they warn against the assumption that these children are subnormal intellectually: to make such assumptions may lead to a self-fulfilling prophecy among the parents and health staff assisting the parents.

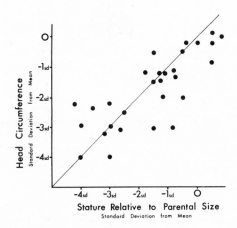

FIG. 16-3
Stature relative to parental size in rubella syndrome. (From Macfarlane, D. W., Boyd, R. D., Dodrill, C. B., and Tufts, E.: Intrauterine rubella, head size, and intellect, Pediatrics 55:797-801, 1975.)

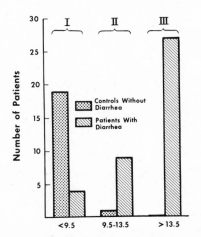

FIG. 16-4
Patient distribution according to the quantitative toxin production by each subject's most potent lactose-fermenting stool isolate. The mean Chinese hamster–ovary (CHO) cell response for all isolates from control patients without diarrhea was 5.26% (± 2.07% SD) of cells stimulated. Group *I* had only nontoxigenic isolates (< 2 SD above this mean); group *II*, isolates that gave intermediate responses (2 to 4 SD above this mean); and group *III*, highly toxigenic isolates (> 4 SD above this mean). (From Guerrant, R. L., Moore, R. A., Kirschenfeld, P. M., and Sande, M. A.: Role of toxigenic and invasive bacteria in acute diarrhea of childhood, reprinted by permission from The New England Journal of Medicine 293:567-573, 1975.)

■ Guerrant, R. L., Moore, R. A., Kirschenfeld, P. M., and Sande, M. A.: Role of toxigenic and invasive bacteria in acute diarrhea of childhood, N. Engl. J. Med. **293:**567-573, 1975.

This study examines the causes of diarrhea in infants and children from 9 days to 10 years of age admitted to one hospital in Brazil. Potential pathogens could be identified in thirty-one of forty consecutive children with diarrhea. Whereas among twenty control children without diarrhea no organisms were found producing heat-labial enterotoxin or tissue inva-siveness, *E. coli* or klebsiella producing heat-labile enterotoxin were found in twenty patients, and *E. coli* or salmonella with tissue-invasive properties was found in four of these forty pa-tients. Organisms that were both toxigenic and invasive were found in seven of the forty patients. Fig. 16-4 taken from their report demonstrates the results with one of the bioassays employed in a study showing the percentage of Chinese hamster ovary cells stimulated by specimens from patients with and without diarrhea.

COMMENT: It is clear from this study that *E. coli* with toxigenic or invasive properties was responsible for most of acute diarrheal disease in early infancy and childhood. It re-emphasizes the importance of diverting attention from classic typing of organisms toward the employment of more bioassays for the detection of specific compounds either produced by organisms with toxigenic properties or conferring increased invasiveness upon the or-ganism.

Index